WITHDRAWN

Mechanisms of Localized Bone Loss

(A special supplement to Calcified Tissue Abstracts)

The correct manner in which to refer to a paper from these proceedings is:

(Authors of Paper), (Title of Paper).
Proceedings, Mechanisms of Localized Bone Loss,
Eds. Horton, Tarpley, and Davis. Special
Supplement to Calcified Tissue Abstracts.
pp. 000, 1978.

Mechanisms of Localized Bone Loss

(A special supplement to Calcified Tissue Abstracts)

Proceedings of the first scientific
evaluation workshop on localized
bone loss.

November 14–15, 1977
Washington D.C.

Edited by
John E. Horton
Thomas M. Tarpley
William F. Davis

Co-sponsored by
Oral Biology & Medicine and General Medicine B
Study Sections
Division of Research Grants
National Institutes of Health

Information Retrieval Inc.
Washington D.C. and London

DONATION 12/78

International Standard Book Number   0-917000-03-X
Library of Congress Catalog Card Number   77-94859

Published as a Special Supplement to:
Calcified Tissue Abstracts
published quarterly by Information Retrieval Limited, London

Published by Information Retrieval Inc.
1911 Jefferson Davis Highway, Arlington, Va. 22202

Printed in the United States of America.

Preface

The concept for this conference emerged through discussions by the editors with a number of colleagues interested in the pathophysiology of localized disorders of bone. Recent progress in such diverse areas as immunology, microbiology, cell biology, anatomy, and transplantation, cancer and connective tissue studies had revealed new mechanisms in the expression and regulation of bone cell activities. These findings were highly relevant to bone loss associated with inflammatory, neoplastic, and reactive states, as exemplified in periodontal disease, rheumatoid arthritis, osteosarcoma, Paget's disease, and chronic osteomyelitis, as well as the localized osteoporosis of disuse. The need was therefore recognized to assemble current information from such diverse areas to focus on possible pathogenetic mechanisms operative in these bony lessions as distinct from those in generalized metabolic bone disease involving mineral homeostasis.

The Oral Biology and Medicine Study Section and the General Medicine B Study Section, Division of Research Grants, National Institutes of Health, were highly interested in this area and jointly agreed to co-sponsor a research conference on this subject. The purpose of the meeting would be to survey the recent progress and current status of this expanding area, provide information exchange amongst investigators in diverse areas, and improve review capabilities for interested members and groups. Proceedings of the meeting would be published and disseminated to the scientific community. In such fashion, areas of fruitful investigation could be defined for initiation and expansion and lead to approaches in therapeutic intervention for prevention and/or treatment regimens.

The conference program developed through consultations with a number of leading investigators throughout the nation. It soon became apparent that the fiscal mechanism available to support the program would impose restraints. Further, recent progress in some areas such as chronic osteomyelitis were limited, while others such as cellular transplantation and macrophage-osteoclast and macrophage-bone relationships were mushrooming. Thus the attempt was made to identify significant areas by focusing on functional as well as disease-related investigations in the expression of bone cell activities, thereby providing a balanced

program. Omissions of relevant and fruitful investigations therefore should not be viewed as an oversight, but rather due to con-
straining influences. Within this context, however, we believe
that the following published Proceedings attest to the success of
this initial attempt as well as the need to identify the distinct-
ness of this area of bone pathology. Undoubtedly, we shall propose to foster a succeeding conference as future progress develops.

The success of any endeavor is dependent upon the assistance
of numerous people. Notably these are the 1976-1977 members of
the Oral Biology and Medicine and the General Medicine B Study
Sections as well as Dr. Carl Douglass, Director, and Drs. S.
Stephen Schiaffino, Irving Simos and Mischa Friedman, Division
of Research Grants, without whose support this conference could
not have been possible. Additionally, gratitude is expressed to
Dr. David B. Scott, Director, National Institute of Dental
Research, whose support is deeply appreciated.

Secretarial assistance, while often not neglected, provides
the most necessary and respected tasks in preparation, coordin-
ation and typing of the program and published Proceedings. For
their outstanding and skilled accomplishments in such duties, we
are grateful to the Ms. Jeanette B. Crockett, Cathlyn Hill,
Patricia S. Hoff, Gretchen P. Jolles, Sue Meadows, Mary A. Smith,
Patricia F. Walker, and Virginia W. Wilson. Program illustrative
material was expertly accomplished by Mr. William F. Stancliff.

Finally, to our speakers, authors, and all participants, we
extend our thanks for their contributions to this meeting and
these Proceedings.

John E. Horton

Thomas M. Tarpley, Jr.

William F. Davis, Jr.

Planning Committee

John E. Horton,*
Program Chairman,
Departments of Microbiology and
    of Immunology,
USA Institute of Dental Research,
Walter Reed Army Medical Center,
Washington, D.C. 20012

*Present address:
Harvard School of Dental
    Medicine
Boston, MA 02115

Thomas M. Tarpley, Jr.
Executive Secretary,
Oral Biology and Medicine Study Section,
Division of Research Grants,
National Institutes of Health,
Bethesda, MD 20014

William F. Davis, Jr.,
Executive Secretary,
General Medicine B Study Section,
Division of Research Grants,
National Institutes of Health,
Bethesda, MD 20014

Speakers

Louis V. Avioli,
Division of Bone and Mineral
    Metabolism
Washington University School of
    Medicine,
The Jewish Hospital of St.Louis,
St.Louis, MO 63110

Jean J. Ballet,
Unité d'Immunohématologie,
Clinique Médicale Infantile,
Hôpital des Enfants-Malades,
75015 Paris, France

Carl D. Douglass,
Director,
Division of Research Grants,
National Institutes of Health,
Bethesda, MD 20014

Brian G.M. Durie,
Section of Hematology
    and Oncology,
University of Arizona Health
    Sciences Center,
Tucson, AZ 85724

Ernest Hausmann,
Department of Oral Biology,
State University of New York
    at Buffalo,
School of Dentistry,
Buffalo, NY 14226

Marijke. E. Holtrop,
Department of Orthopaedic
    Surgery,
Harvard Medical School,
The Children's Hospital Center,
Boston, MA 02108

John E. Horton,*
Departments of Microbiology and
    of Immunology,
USA Institute of Dental
    Research
Walter Reed Army Medical Center,
Washington, D.C. 20012

Jenifer O.M. Jowsey,
Orthopaedic Research,
Mayo Clinic,
Rochester, MN 55901

Hynda K. Kleinman,
Laboratory of Developmental
    Biology and Anomalies,
National Institute of Dental
    Research,
National Institutes of Health,
Bethesda, MD 20014

Stephan M. Krane,
Department of Medicine,
Harvard Medical School and the
    Medical Services (Arthritis
    Unit),
Massachusetts General Hospital,
Boston, MA 02114

Klaus E. Kuettner,
Departments of Biochemistry and
    of Orthopedics,
Rush Medical College and Rush
    College of Health Sciences,
Rush Presbyterian-St.Luke's
    Medical Center,
Chicago, IL 60612

J.L. Matthews,
A.Webb Roberts Center for Con-
    tinuing Education in the
    Health Sciences
Baylor University Medical Center,
Dallas, TX 75246

Gregory R. Mundy,
Division of Endocrinology and
    Metabolism,
Department of Medicine,
University of Connecticut Health
    Center,
Farmington, CT 06032

Mirdza E. Neiders,
Department of Oral Pathology,
State University of New York
    at Buffalo,
School of Dentistry,
Buffalo, NY 14214

Charles E. Olsen,
Laboratory of Microbiology and
    Immunology,
National Institute of Dental
    Research,
National Institutes of Health,
Bethesda, MD 20014

William A. Peck,
Department of Medicine,
The Jewish Hospital of
    St. Louis,
Washington University School
    of Medicine,
St. Louis, MO 63178

Lawrence G. Raisz,
Division of Endocrinology and
    Metabolism,
Department of Medicine,
University of Connecticut,
Farmington, CT 06032

Frederick R. Singer,
Section of Endocrinology,
Clinical Research Center,
University of Southern
    California School of
    Medicine,
Los Angeles, CA 90033

Paula Stern,
Department of Pharmacology,
Northwestern University
    Medical School,
Chicago, IL 60611

Roy V. Talmage,
Department of Surgery,
Orthopaedic Research Labora-
    tories,
School of Medicine,
University of North Carolina,
Chapel Hill, NC 27514

Armen H. Tashjian, Jr.,
Laboratory of Pharmacology,
Harvard School of Dental
    Medicine,
Department of Pharmacology,
Harvard Medical School,
Boston, MA 02114

Jean-Dominique Vassalli,
The Rockefeller University,
New York, NY 10021

Larry M. Wahl,
Laboratory of Microbiology
    and Immunology,
National Institute of Dental
    Research,
National Institutes of Health,
Bethesda, MD 20014

Donald G. Walker,
Department of Cell Biology
    and Anatomy,
The Johns Hopkins University
    School of Medicine,
Baltimore, MD 21205

Zena Werb,
Laboratory of Radiobiology,
University of California
    School of Medicine,
San Francisco, CA 94122

Glenda L. Wong,
Calcium Research Laboratory
Department of Biochemistry,
Veterans Administration Hospital,
Kansas City, MO 64128

Address of Welcome

It is a great pleasure to welcome participants of this scientific evaluation workshop on "Mechanisms of Localized Bone Loss" on behalf of the Division of Research Grants and the NIH as a whole. The sponsorship of the Oral Biology and Medicine and General Medicine B Study Sections and the hard work of the members of the Study Sections and John Horton, Tom Tarpley and Bill Davis represent important contributions, and we are most appreciative.

As you may know, the NIH under Dr. Fredrickson's leadership is undertaking a major effort to see to it that research results are applied for the practical health benefits of our citizens. He has recently announced the appointment of a new Associate Director for Clinical Trials and, also, the establishment of a new Office of Medical Application of Research. These moves are being made because of the clearly articulated demands by the Congress to see to it that improvements in health care flow from our research programs. Congress, of course, reflects the mood of the country in this interest in the application of research results. There is nothing wrong with this; in fact, it is a trend which is inevitable as our programs have grown and become more visible to the public.

Efforts such as this workshop and others which will be sponsored by our Study Sections will become ever more crucial as we use them to enhance research interests in particular areas, to identify gaps in our basic knowledge and even occasionally to decide that there are not promising opportunities for advances in particular research directions. If we are to maintain a balance between application of research and the pursuit of knowledge then such activities as this workshop will help keep our persepctive and our programs in balance because it is almost inevitable that without special attention and emphasis the demand for application will drain resources away from the pursuit of new knowledge.

Carl D. Douglass, Ph.D.

SESSION I

THE CELLS OF BONE—
THEIR MORPHOLOGY AND FUNCTION.

Proliferation and Specialization of Bone Cells Cultured in
Serum-Free Medium

William A. Peck and James K. Burks

The Department of Medicine, The Jewish Hospital of St. Louis,
Washington University School of Medicine, 216 S. Kingshighway,
St.Louis, MO 63110

Introduction

Highly specialized cells are responsible for bone formation
and resorption, and mediate ion fluxes between bone and blood.
Consequently, these activities define the mass and quality of
the skeleton, and aid in maintaining mineral and acid-base
homeostasis. The linneage of bone cells and the processes which
govern their acquisition of specialized characteristics are
poorly understood. A now classical formulation, derived from
histochemical and auto-radiographic studies, envisages osteoblasts and osteoclasts as arising from a common precursor cell
of mesenchymal origin (1-10). This mesenchymal cell, capable
of replication, first modulates into committed stem cells,
variously termed osteoprogenitor cells or preosteoblasts and
preosteoclasts, which in turn mature into nondividing differentiated foms.

A large body of experimental evidence now points to cells
of the monocyte-macrophage-histiocyte series of osteoclast
precursors (11-24). These precursors are thought to originate
in reticuloendothelial tissues, migrate to bone via the blood-
stream, and fuse in vitro to form the multinucleated bone
resorbing cells. Cells of thymic derivation may participate
as helper cells in the osteoclastic transformation of histio-
cytes. Whether skeletal mesenchymal cells can also differentiate
into osteoclasts has yet to be determined.

Use of isolated cell systems and application of sophisti-
cated cell culture techniques should enhance our knowledge of
mesenchymal cell proliferation and the formation of osteoblasts.
The most widely used method for cell isolation, in which rodent
calvaria are digested with crude collagenase, yields a mixed
population of cells that proliferate in primary culture and in
subculture, and respond to low concentrations of bone seeking
hormones (25-28). Recently reported modifications in this
method have improved cell viability and sensitivity to hormones
(29-31). Attempts to obtain populations which are enriched with
specific classes of cells (e.g. osteoblasts, osteoclasts) have
met with some success. The multiple sequential enzymatic
digestion technique of Wong and Cohn has been shown to liberate
separate cell populations which are highly enriched with

individual cell types (32,33). Luben, Wong and Cohn utilized a
variety of biological and biochemical criteria to characterize
the majority of the cells released initially as provisional
osteoclasts or osteoclast-like cells, and the more slowly
liberated cells as provisional osteoblasts or osteoblast-like
cells (34,35). The comparative responses of both cell populations to parathyroid hormone and to calcitonin lend support to
their provisional assignment. Furthermore, the osteoclast-like
cells appear to enhance the release of hydroxyproline, calcium
and phosphorus from devitalized bone in vitro (36). Although
the precise anatomical location of these various populations is
unknown, results of studies from our laboratory suggest that
osteoclast-like cells predominate in rodent periosteal tissues,
and osteoblast-like cells in subperiosteal bone (37).

Of considerable advantage in examining the many factors
which influence bone cell proliferation and specialization would
be an in vitro culture system that allows isolated cells to proliferate and differentiate in a chemically defined environment.
Hitherto, growth of enzymatically dispersed bone cells in vitro
has required the presence of serum in the incubation medium (25).
Uncertainties arising from the use of serum include not only
the presence of defined and as yet undefined growth-modifying
substances, but also non-uniformity from product to product,
the hazard of microbiological contamination (endotoxins,
bacteriophages, mycoplasma, and animal viruses have been detected in commercial sera), and potential shortages resulting from
future expansion in cell culture work. A wide variety of
established nonskeletal cell lines have been found to proliferate in defined medium, but these cells are not as suitable as
primary cultures for exploring specialized functions (38).
Indeed, there has been no convincing evidence that mammalian
cells proliferate in serum-free primary culture.

The present report describes the development of a system in
which cells proliferate and acquire specialized characteristics
during primary culture in a chemically defined incubation
medium. In addition, we provide evidence that cells so cultured
elaborate a factor (or factors) which enhances cell attachment
or growth (or both) in monolayer culture.

Methods

Bone cells were dispersed from the calvaria of rat fetuses
by incubation in crude collagenase as previously described (25).
Care was taken to remove adherent cartilage and periosteal
connective tissue before enzymatic digestion. Dispersed cells
were washed extensively in collagenase-free medium, and seeded
at an initial density of 10^6 cells per 35 mm Falcon plastic
petri dish. The culture medium was BGJ_b (39), as modified by
Fitton-Jackson (see - Grand Island Biologicals Company Catalo-
que), and altered so that its ionic composition resembled that of
the interstitial fluid of bone (40). The sodium and potassium
concentrations were 125 mM and 25 mM respectively, the final
pH was 7.50 to 7.55, and the mean tonicity 350 mOsm. The medium
was supplemented with Pentex albumin, 10 mg/ml, ascorbic acid,

and glutamine. Cells were cultured in a humidified atmosphere of 2% CO_2 and 98% air. The incubation medium was totally replaced within the first 24 hours of culture, and every 2-3 days thereafter. DNA synthesis and proliferation were determined periodically in three ways; incorporation of ^3H thymidine (41), hemocytometer counts of the number of cells released from the culture dishes during brief exposure to trypsin, and DNA content per cell layer by the indole method of Hubbard et al. (42). Total alkaline phosphatase activity was measured in the incubation medium by the method of Koyama and Ono (43), and cellular alkaline phosphatase content by the histochemical method of Ackerman (44). Electron microscopic localization of cellular alkaline phosphatase was carried out in collaboration with Dr. Steven Doty (National Institute of Dental Research, National Institutes of Health, Bethesda, Maryland).

RESULTS AND DISCUSSIONS

The plating efficiency of the inoculum was 35%; 75% of the unattached cells, removed at the time of the first medium replacement, excluded Trypan blue, suggesting that many viable cells failed to attach. Sequential study of the cultures revealed unequivocal evidence for proliferation during the first nine days. Cell number and DNA content per culture nearly tripled between days 1 and 9 (Table I). Microscopic examination of the cell layers confirmed proliferation, and revealed the presence of frequent mitoses. Tritiated thymidine incorporation reached a maximum on day 7, then gradually declined (Table I). Bone cells did not proliferate, and underwent gradual attrition over a 12-day period when cultured at one-half the initial population density used in the previous experiments. Cells dispersed from rat skin and from periosteal tissues by collagenase digestion did not survive in the serum-free medium at high or at low population densities.

The dependence of proliferation on population density suggested that the cultured cells were "conditioning" the incubation medium, by contributing a factor or factors that promoted growth. To test this possibility, we inoculated bone cells in serum-free medium harvested from 10- and 12-day-old bone cell cultures. Medium which had bathed cells for the first 24 hours of culture was not used in order to exclude degradation products of unattached cells. Incubation in "conditioned" medium appeared to enhance cell attachment and markedly increased the rate of cell proliferation. Five-day-old cultures contained nearly 50% more cells when grown in the presence than in the absence of "conditioned" medium (Table II). Microscopic examination of the cultures, however, indicated a substantial increase in plating efficiency when the cells were seeded in conditioned medium. In order to discriminate between enhanced attachment and increased growth, we studied the effect of conditioned medium on the proliferation of cells which had been cultured for 12 days in unconditioned medium. In this experiment, the conditioned medium was dialyzed exhaustively and lyophilized before use. Addition of the lyophilized powder at a final concentration of 10 µg/ml increased cell number to a modest degree, and markedly increased

TABLE I

PROLIFERATION AND APPARENT SPECIALIZATION OF CELLS CULTURED

IN SERUM-FREE MEDIUM

Day in Culture	Cell Number	DNA (µg/culture)	DNA (pg/cell)	^{3}H Thymidine Incorporation (DPM/culture)	Alkaline Phosphatase (µmole/hr/mg/DNA)
1	339,000 ± 11,000	3.5 ± 0.2	10.3	26,987* ± 3512	164
5	564,000 ± 37,000	6.6 ± 0.5	11.7	42,160 ± 2232	325
9	779,000 ± 44,000	9.0 ± 0.6	11.6	29,952 ± 386	503
12	848,000 ± 25,000	8.8 ± 0.5	10.4	17,237 ± 1281	859

*performed on day 2 of culture

Data are pooled from studies with 6 separate isolations and sets of cultures, and are presented as means, or as means and standard errors where indicated. A mean of 985,000 cells was seeded per culture dish - the figures obtained on day 1 reflect plating efficiency.

TABLE II

EFFECT OF CONDITIONED MEDIUM ON BONE CELL ATTACHMENT AND GROWTH

	Day in Culture	Cell Number	^{3}H Thymidine Incorporation DPM/culture
Experiment I			
Control medium	5	653,000 ± 27,000	-
Conditioned medium	5	887,000 ± 110,000	-
Experiment II			
Control medium	14	700,000 860,000	10,813 13,317
Conditioned medium dialysate	14	900,000 1,040,000	32,665 32,535

In experiment I, cells were exposed to either 100% non-conditioned or 50% conditioned - 50% non-conditioned medium for the entire 5 day culture period. Means and standard errors of 3 separate cultures are given. In experiment II, treated cells received 10 µg/ml of lyophilized conditioned medium dialysate on day 12 and were studied with controls on day 14. All cultures were exposed to ^{3}H thymidine for 1 hour before termination.

Figure 1. Electron photomicrograph of 12 day culture (original magnification x 10,000). Alkaline phosphatase reaction carried out for 10 minutes at room temperature at pH of 9.4 using the method of Mayahara as modified by Kurashashi and Yoshiki, Arch. Oral. Biol. 17, 155-176 (1972). The reaction product is most intense on the cell membrane, particularly at cell-cell junctions. Reaction product is also present on the nuclear envelope. Fine glycogen particles are seen throughout the cytoplasm.

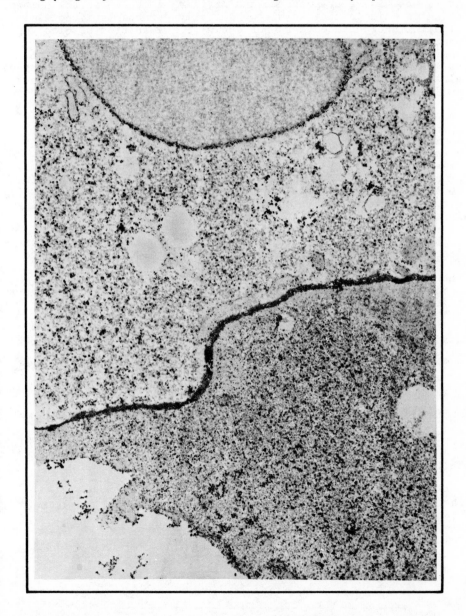

^{3}H thymidine incorporation (Table II). These results indicate that conditioned medium fosters cell attachment and also contains a macromolecular growth promoting factor (or factors).

Proliferation of cells in primary culture was accompanied by a progressive increase in alkaline phosphatase activity in the incubation medium (Table I). The greatest increment appeared after proliferation had ceased, between days 9 and 12 in culture. There was also a progressive and striking increase in the number of cells which contained histochemically detectable cytoplasmic alkaline phosphatase (data not shown). Examination of electron photomicrographs revealed that cellular alkaline phosphatase was largely confined to plasma membranes (Figure 1). Because osteoblasts are known to contain copious plasma membrane-located alkaline phosphatase, we have provisionally characterized these cells as osteoblasts.

Since bone cell populations enriched with osteoblasts respond preferentially to parathyroid hormone with marked increases in cyclic AMP, we explored the effects of parathyroid hormone on the cyclic AMP content of cells cultured in serum-free medium. Brief exposure to parathyroid hormone (100 ng/ml) caused a ten-fold increase in cyclic AMP (data not shown). In contrast, these cells failed to respond to salmon calcitonin with a cyclic AMP rise (data not shown), also a typical finding in osteoblast-enriched cell populations (34,35,37).

The types of cells which proliferate and apparently specialize in the present system remain to be defined. That they are in fact cells which are unique to bone is suggested by the absence of proliferation in cultures of skin fibroblasts and periosteal cells. It is tempting, therefore, to speculate that mesenchymal or osteoprogenitor (preosteoblasts) cells attach preferentially, multiply and mature over the 12 day culture period. In that case, the system should be most useful in examining the regulation of these processes. Further study will be necessary to exclude the possibility that apparent osteoblastic differentiation represents only a recovery of cells from damage suffered during isolation and preparation

Acknowledgement

We thank Ms. Janet Weil and Ms. Gale Kohler for their technical assistance.

This project was supported by research grant AMO9865 from the National Institute of Arthritis, Metabolism and Digestive Diseases, National Institutes of Health

REFERENCES

1. Pritchard, J.J. 1952. Cytological and histochemical study of bone and cartilage formation in rat. J.Anat., 86, 259-277.

2. Pritchard, J.J. 1956. The Osteoblast. In: Bourne, G.H., ed. The Biochemistry and Physiology of Bone, New York, Academic Press, 1956, 179-212.

3. Kember, N.F. 1960. Cell division in endochondral ossification. A study of cell proliferation in rat bones by the method of tritiated thymidine autoradiography. J. Bone and Joint Surg. 43B, 824-839.

4. Young, R.J. 1962. Cell proliferation and specialization during endochondral osteogenesis in young rats. J. Cell Biol., 14, 357-370.

5. Young, R.W. 1962. Regional differences in cell generation time in growing rat tibiae. Exp. Cell Res. 26, 562-567.

6. Owen, M. 1963. Cell population kinetics of an osteogenic tissue. J.Cell Biol., 19, 19-32.

7. Owen, M. and MacPherson, D. 1963. Cell population kinetics of an osteogenic tissue. J. Cell Biol, 19, 33-44.

8. Scott, B.L. 1967. Thymidine-^{3}H electron microscope radioautography of osteogenic cells in the fetal rat. J. Cell Biol. 35, 115-126.

9. Vaughan, J.M. 1970. The Physiology of Bone, Clarendon Press, Oxford.

10. Owen, M. 1971. Cellular dynamics of bone. In: Bourne, G.H., ed., The Biochemistry and Physiology of Bone, Academic Press, New York, 1971, 271-298.

11. Frost, H.M. 1965. A synchronous group of mammalian cells whose in vivo behavior can be studied. Henry Ford Hosp. Med. Bull. 13, 161-172.

12. Fischman, D.A. and Hay, E.D. 1962. Origin of osteoclasts from mononuclear leucocytes in regenerating newt limbs. Anat. Rec. 143, 329-337.

13. Jee, W.S.S. and Nolan, P.D. 1963. Origin of osteoclasts from the fusion of phagocytes. Nature, 200, 225-226.

14. Kahn, A.J. and Simmons, D.J. 1975. Investigation of cell lineage in bone using a chimaera of chick and quail embryonic tissue. Nature, 258, 325-327.

15. Walker, D.G. 1972. Congenital osteopetrosis in mice cured

by parabiotic union with normal siblings. Endocrinology, 91, 916-920.

16. Walker, D.G. 1973. Osteopetrosis cured by temporary para-biosis. Science, 180, 875.

17. Marks, S.C. Jr. 1973. Pathogenesis of osteopetrosis in the ia rat: reduced bone resorption due to reduced osteoclast function. Am. J. Anat., 138, 165-189.

18. Gothlin, C. and Ericcson, J.L. 1973. On the histogenesis of the cells in fracture callus. Electron microscopic auto-radiographic observations in parabiotic rats and studies on labeled monocytes. Virchow's Archiv (B) Zellpathol. 12, 318-329.

19. Toyama, K., Moutier, R. and Lamendin, H. 1974. Résorption osseuse après parabiose chez les rats "op" (ostéopécrose). C. R. Acad. Sci. (D) (Paris), 278, 115-117.

20. Hall, B.K. 1975. The origin and fate of osteoclasts. Anat. Rec. 183, 1-11.

21. Walker, D.G. 1975. Bone resorption restored in osteopetro-tic mice by transplants of normal bone marrow and spleen cells. Science, 190, 784-785.

22. Walker, D.G. 1975. Spleen cells transmit osteopetrosis in mice. Science., 190, 785-787.

23. Walker, D.G. 1975. Control of bone resorption by hemato-poietic tissue. The induction and reversal of congenital osteopetrosis in mice through the use of bone marrow and splenic transplants. J. Exp. Med. 142, 651-663.

24. Walker, D.G. 1973. Experimental osteopetrosis. Clin. Orthop. 97, 158-174.

25. Peck, W.A., Birge, S.J. Jr., Fedak, S.A. 1964. Bone cells: biochemical and biological studies after enzymatic isolation. Science., 146, 1476-1477.

26. Peck, W.A., Messinger, K., Brandt, J. and Carpenter, J. 1969. Impaired accumulation of ribonucleic acid precursors and depletion of ribonucleic acid in glucocorticoid-treated bone cells. J. Biol. Chem. 244, 4174-4184.

27. Peck, W.A., Messinger, K. and Carpenter, J. 1971. Regula-tion of pyrimidine ribonucleoside incorporation in isolated bone cells. Stimulation by insulin and by 2,3-dihydroxy-1, 4 dithiobutane (dithiothreitol), J. Biol. Chem., 246, 4439-4446.

28. Peck, W.A., Carpenter, J., Messinger, K. and DeBra, D. 1973. Cyclic 3'5' adenosine monophophate in isolated bone cells:

Response to low concentrations of parathyroid hormone. Endocrinology 92, 692-697.

29. Rodan, S.B. and Rodan, G.A. 1974. The effect of parathyroid hormone and thyrocalcitonin on the accumulation of cyclic adenosine 3'5'-monophospahte in freshly isolated bone cells. J. Biol. Chem., 249, 3068-3974.

30. Dziak, R. and Brand, J.S. 1974. Calcium transport in isolated bone cells. I. Bone cell isolation procedures. J. Cell Physiol., 84, 75-83.

31. Dziak, R. and Brand, J.S. 1974. Calcium transport in isolated bone cells. II. Calcium transport studies, 84, 85-96.

32. Wong, G.L. and Cohn, D.V. 1974. Separation of parathyroid hormone and calcitonin-sensitive cells from non-responsive bone cells. Nature, 252, 713-715.

33. Wong, G.L. and Cohn, D.V. 1975. Target cells in bone for parathormone and calcitonin are different: Enrichment for each cell type by sequential digestion of mouse calvaria and selective adhesion to polymeric surfaces. Proc. Natl. Acad. Sci. USA, 72, 3167-3171.

34. Luben, R.A. and Cohn, D.V. 1976. Effects of parathormone and calcitonin on citrate and hyaluronate metabolism in cultured bone. Endocrinology, 98, 413-419.

35. Luben, R.A., Wong, G.L. and Cohn, D.V. 1976. Biochemical characterization with parathormone and calcitonin of isolated bone cells: provisional identification of osteoclasts and osteoblasts. Endocrinol. 99, 526-534.

36. Wong, G.L., Luben, R.A. and Cohn, D.V. 1977. 1,25-Dihydroxycholecalciferol and parathormone: Effects on isolated osteoclast-like and osteoblast-like cells. Science, 197, 663-665.

37. Peck, W.A., J.K. Burks, J. Wilkins, S.B. Rodan and G.A. Rodan. 1977. Evidence for preferential effects of parathyroid hormone, calcitonin and adenosine on bone and periosteum. Endocrinology, 100(5), 1357-1364.

38. Higuchi, K. 1976. Cultivation of mammalian cell lines in serum-free chemically defined medium. Methods in Cell Biol. XIV, ed. David M. Prescott, Academic Press, New York, 12, 131-143.

39. Biggers, J.D., Gwatkin, R.B.L. and Heyner, S. 1961. Growth of embryonic avian and mammalina tibiae on a relatively simple chemically defined medium. Exp. Cell Res. 26, 41-58.

40. Neuman, W.F., and Ramp, W.K   1971.   Cellular mechanisms for calcium transfer and homeostasis, G. Nichols, Jr. and R.H. Wasserman, Eds. Academic Press, New York, 197-206.

41. Hubbard, R.W., Matthew, W.T. and Dubowik, D.A. 1970. Factors influencing the determination of DNA with indole. Anal. Biochem. 38, 190-201. Hubbard, R.W. Matthew, W.T., Moulton, D.W. 1972. Factors influencing the determination of DNA with indole II. Recovery of hydrolyzed DNA from protein precipitates. Anal. Biochem. 46, 461-472.

42. Thymidine, (Methyl-^{3}H) 20 Ci/mMole, New England Nuclear.

43. Ackermann, G.A. 1962. Substituted naphthol as phosphate derivatives for the localization of leukocyte alkaline phosphatase activity., Lab Invest. 11, 563-567.

44. Parathyroid Hormone, residues 1-34, Beckman.

The Response of Osteoclasts to Prostaglandin and Osteoclast
Activating Factor as Measured by Ultrastructural Morphometry.

Marijke E. Holtrop, Lawrence G. Raisz and Gregory J. King.

Department of Orthopaedic Surgery, Harvard Medical School,
The Children's Hospital Medical Center, Boston, Massachusetts,
and
Department of Medicine, University of Connecticut Medical School,
Farmington, Connecticut.

Osteoclasts are cells specialized for the breakdown of bone
matrix. Electron microscopic and microcinematographic studies
have shown convincingly that osteoclasts are involved in bone
resorption and that the ruffled border is the active site of
resorption (1). The ruffled border lies adjacent to the bone
surface and consists of many infoldings of the cell membrane resulting in finger-like projections of cytoplasm and providing
an extensive surface area well suited for intensive exchange
between the cell and the extracellular space (Fig. 1). The
clear zone is an area of the cytoplasm encircling the ruffled
border along the cell membrane at the bone surface and
of an amorphous fine granular material with bundles of actin-
like filaments perpendicular to the bone surface (Fig. 1). It
is likely that this area forms a mechanism of attachment for
the cell to the bone surface (2). The bone underlying the
ruffled border is frayed, but under the clear zone it is smooth.
The cytoplasm of the osteoclast contains an abundance of mitochondria and little rough endoplasmic reticulum, making it easy
to recognize profiles of the osteoclasts in electron microscopic
sections. Vesicles and vacuoles of variable number and size can
be found and are often associated with the ruffled border.

The breakdown of bone matrix in an organism can be the result of a number of different processes. A generalized process
of bone resorption is seen in the remodelling during growth and
the replacement of bone tissue during adult life. In both
these processes osteoclasts are involved in the resorption of
bone matrix. Calcium homeostasis is regulated by parathyroid
hormone (PTH). It has been questioned what cells are involved
in the release of calcium from the bone. Recently we have
demonstrated that PTH activates osteoclasts both in vitro and
in vivo within a short period of time, followed later by an
increase of their number* (3).

---

*King, G.J., M.E. Holtrop and L.G. Raisz: The relation of ultra-
structural changes in osteoclasts to resorption in bone cultures
stimulated with parathyroid hormone. Submitted.

FIGURE LEGEND

Figure 1   Electron micrograph of a part of an osteoclast with
            ruffled border (rb) and clear zone (cz), outlined as
            they would be traced for measurement. x 13,250.

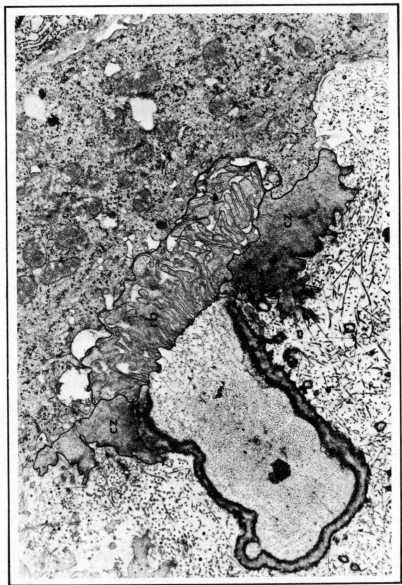

Top of Figure.

Localized bone loss is seen in certain bone diseases. The cell responsible for the loss of bone matrix is in many cases not well defined. Prostaglandin (PGE) synthesis has been linked with inflammation (4,5,6) and with tumors associated with hyper-calcemia (7,8); osteoclast activating factor (OAF) has been assoc-iated with gingivitis (9) and myeloma (10). These agents stimulate bone resorption in vitro (11,12), presumably by osteo-clast activity. Repeated PGE_1 injections onto the calvarium of rats caused extensive bone loss, but multinucleated cells were infrequent (13).

In this study we have compared the effects of PGE_2 and OAF with the effects of PTH on osteoclasts in cultured bones. We have tested the changes in ultrastructural morphology as a mea-sure of cell activity, changes in the number of osteoclasts as a measure of cell differentiation, and compared these parameters with the resorptive activity of the tissue determined by the release of calcium from the bones into the culture medium.

METHODS

Long bones from 19-day-old fetal rats were pre-labelled with ^{45}Ca by injection of the mother one day previously. These bones were then cultured in control medium or in medium with PGE_2 10^{-6} M, OAF, or PTH 10^{-8} M for various time intervals. At the end of the culture period the calcium released from the bones into the medium was determined and the bones were prepar-ed for electron microscopy. Details of the culture technique and the preparation for electron microscopy have been described previously (14,15).

Morphometry:

Osteoclasts are sparsely distributed in bone and as a re-sult the common methods of morphometry cannot be applied. We have developed a method of obtaining quantitative information on the size of cells and cell organelles in osteoclasts. We based our method on the principle that larger cells will yield larger average area of cell profiles in sections, provided that the cell profiles are sampled randomly. We accomplished this by selecting at random one section per bone and photographing all osteoclast profiles in that one section. In this way no osteoclast was represented by more than one cell profile. The negatives of the electron micrographs of these profiles were projected onto a digitizing table interfaced with a computer. By means of a sensor the areas of interest were traced and expressed in μ^2. The areas that we measured in cell profiles were cell area, ruffled border area, and clear zone area. The cell area is bounded by a membrane and therefore is easy to recognize. The ruffled border area was defined as the area of the osteoclast adjacent to the bone characterized by highly convoluted membranes not including vacuoles and vesicles. The clear zone area was defined as the area adjacent to the bone and the ruffled border filled with amorphous or filamentous material excluding the usual cellular organelles. An example how these areas were traced is given in Figure 1. From each experimental or control group four bones were selected at random and from these at least 25 osteoclast profiles were photographed on 35 mm film. After measuring the area, the means and standard errors for the areas in each population were calculated and differences between populations were tested using the Student's t-test. More details about this technique and its interpretation have been published elsewhere (16).

The numbers of osteoclasts were estimated in 6 pieces of bone that were selected at random from each cultural group. One random section of 1μ thickness, stained with toluidine blue, was examined with the light microscope at a standard magnification and the number of osteoclasts in this one section was counted. These numbers were accepted as a representative sample of the population of osteoclasts in that area of bone.

RESULTS

The results of the measurements of osteoclasts in control bones and treated bones from 2 to 4 different experiments are pooled. These are represented in Table 1.

All agents tested caused approximately a two-fold increase in the size of the osteoclast after 12 to 24 hours of culture, and this increase was maintained up to 48 hours. The total nuclear area per cell profile increased at the same rate, resulting in a constant nucleus-cell ratio. In one experiment (Table 2) the area of individual nuclear profiles was enlarged significantly in the OAF treated osteoclasts and enlarged but not significantly in the PGE_2 treated cells after 12 hours of treatment, but not after 24 hours. The number of nuclear profiles per cell increased after 12 hours and 24 hours significantly for the PGE_2 treated cells.

The ruffled border areas had increased approximately five-fold in the osteoclasts in PGE_2- and OAF treated bones after 12 hours and remained large. Clear zones were significantly larger in the OAF-treated osteoclasts after 3 hours and had enlarged approximately three-fold in PGE_2 and OAF osteoclasts after 12 hours. In the osteoclasts treated with PTH, the increases in ruffled border and clear zone were seen earlier, at 3 hours, but were of the same magnitude as in the osteoclasts treated with PGE_2 or OAF.

The numbers of osteoclasts per bone section were variable between different experiments and could therefore not be pooled. Generally, in the PGE_2- or OAF-treated bones no increases in numbers occurred compared to their corresponding controls. Only in one experiment the number of osteoclasts had increased slightly, but not significantly, after treatment with PGE_2 for 24 hours. In the PTH-treated bones, however, the number of osteoclasts increased two-fold ($p < 0.05$) between 6 and 24 hours. Calcium release from the bones into the medium was usually significantly increased 12 to 24 hours after exposure to PGE_2 or OAF, and 12 hours after exposure to PTH.

Table 1: The areas (μ^2) of cell, ruffled border and clear zone in profiles of osteoclasts of fetal rat bones cultured with and without PGE_2, OAF or PTH for 3, 12, 24 or 48 hours

	hr	n	cell	ruffled border	clear zone
Co	3	109	318.9 ± 54.5	2.5 ± 1.1	6.2 ± 1.0
PGE_2		42	349.6 ± 53.0	6.5 ± 2.9	8.7 ± 1.9
OAF		35	335.5 ± 74.8	2.7 ± 0.8	10.4 ± 1.8*
PTH		87	317.0 ± 33.6	5.9 ± 0.6*	10.1 ± 1.2*
Co	12	107	292.3 ± 27.9	2.2 ± 0.8	4.8 ± 0.7
PGE_2		56	591.7 ± 87.0***	11.9 ± 2.2***	15.1 ± 2.5***
OAF		50	598.2 ± 89.4***	10.2 ± 2.0***	17.0 ± 2.8***
PTH		86	384.1 ± 36.1	11.2 ± 1.8***	10.1 ± 1.2***
Co	24	84	254.1 ± 23.8	3.5 ± 0.9	5.9 ± 0.9
PGE_2		35	488.1 ± 64.8***	24.1 ± 6.0***	19.3 ± 3.1***
OAF		25	476.7 ± 69.9***	9.7 ± 3.0*	18.9 ± 3.9***
PTH		62	425.6 ± 51.8***	21.3 ± 3.3***	17.5 ± 2.5***
Co	48	50	284.6 ± 33.1	5.0 ± 1.4	7.9 ± 1.6
PGE_2		29	612.9 ± 79.3***	13.0 ± 4.7	27.3 ± 6.0***
OAF		25	715.7 ± 106.0***	59.8 ± 22.7*	50.7 ± 22.0
PTH		24	511.9 ± 81.4*	53.8 ± 11.8***	19.0 ± 3.5**

n = number of osteoclast profiles

*Significantly different from corresponding controls $p < 0.05$

**$p < 0.01$

***$p < 0.005$

Table 2: The number of nuclear profiles per cell profile, the area (μ^2) of nuclear profiles and the total area of nuclear profiles per cell profile of osteoclasts in fetal rat bones cultured with and without PGE_2 or OAF for 12 or 24 hours.

	hrs	n profiles	n nuclei/cell	area/nucleus	total nuclear area
Co	12	68	1.17 ± 0.18	23.2 ± 1.5	27.6 ± 4.4
PGE_2		66	2.86 ± 0.74*	28.0 ± 2.2	65.0 ±17.5*
OAF		46	1.84 ± 0.35	31.7 ± 2.3***	56.9 ±11.4***
Co	24	51	0.98 ± 0.13	23.2 ± 1.9	24.0 ± 3.6
PGE_2		61	1.85 ± 0.33*	26.9 ± 2.0	51.8 ± 8.9***
OAF		42	1.83 ± 0.54	23.5 ± 2.4	45.4 ±11.2

n profiles: total number of nuclear profiles

n nuclei/cell: number of nuclear profiles per cell profile, mean ± S.E.

area/nucleus: area of nuclear profile in μ^2, mean ± S.E.

total nuclear area: total area of nuclear profiles per cell profile, mean ± S.E.

*significantly different from corresponding control p < 0.05

***p < 0.005

DISCUSSION

Osteoclasts in cultured bones responded in a qualitatively similar way to PGE_2, OAF and PTH by increasing the size of cells, ruffled borders and clear zones. The changes in the ruffled borders occurred at a slower rate in the PGE_2- or OAF-treated osteoclasts than in the PTH-treated cells. Calcium release from the bones into the medium was usually also slower than with PTH. The number of osteoclasts did not increase in bones exposed to PGE_2 or OAF, whereas a two-fold increase was seen in bones treated with PTH. These new cells entering the population were probably small and, as a result, decreased the average size of the cells. This could explain the differences in cell size between PTH-treated osteoclasts and osteoclasts treated with the other agents at 12 to 48 hours.

Cell area and total nuclear area per cell profile increased at the same rate for all agents tested. The individual nuclei became sometimes larger in the PGE_2- and OAF-treated cells. The number of nuclear profiles per cell profile also increased, although not always significantly. The latter figures are not a reliable representation of the number of nuclei per cell, since larger nuclei will have a greater chance to be included in any one section through a cell. Nevertheless, it seems that the increase in total nuclear area per cell is the result of enlargement of individual nuclei in addition to an increase in number. Since osteoclast nuclei have never been seen to divide, the increase in number is probably the result of fusion of osteoclasts with pre-existing preosteoclasts.

These results suggest that PGE_2 and OAF stimulate the activity of existing osteoclasts by an increase in cell and re-sorbing apparatus, but not the proliferation and subsequent differentiation of progenitor cells. Osteoclast activity is stimulated at the same rate, but later than with PTH.

ACKNOWLEDGEMENT

This work was supported by Grant AM 17834 from the National Institutes of Health.

REFERENCES

1. Holtrop, M.E. and G.J. King, 1977. The ultrastructure of the osteoclast and its functional implications. Clin. Orthop. Rel. Res., 123, 177-96.

2. King, G.J. and M.E. Holtrop, 1975. Actin-like filaments in bone cells of cultured mouse calvaria, as demonstrated by binding to heavy meromyosin. J. Cell. Biol., 66, 445-51.

3. Holtrop, M.E., G.J. King and L.G. Raisz, in press. Factors influencing osteoclast activity as measured by ultrastructural morphometry. In: Proc. 6th Parathyroid Conference 1977.

4. Goodson, J.M., F. Dewhirst and A. Brunetti, 1974. Prostaglandin E_2 levels and human periodontal disease. Prostaglandins, 6, 81-85.

5. Gomes, B.C., E. Hausmann, N. Weinfeld and C. DeLuca, 1976.
    Prostaglandins: bone resorption stimulating factors re-
    leased from monkey gingiva. Calcif. Tiss. Res., 19, 285-93.

6. Robinson, D.R., A.H. Tashjian, Jr. and L. Levine, 1975.
    Prostaglandin-stimulated bone resorption by rheumatoid
    synovia. J. Clin. Invest., 56, 1181-88.

7. Voelkel, E.F., A.H. Tashjian, R. Franklin, E. Wasserman and
    L. Levine, 1975. Hypercalcemia and tumor-prostaglandins:
    the VX_2 carcinoma model in the rabbit. Metabolism, 24,
    973-86.

8. Seyberth, H.W., G.V. Segre, J.L. Morgan, B.J. Sweetman,
    J.T. Potts and J.A. Oates, 1975. Prostaglandins as
    mediators of hypercalcemia associated with certain types
    of cancer. New Engl. J. Med., 293, 1278-83.

9. Horton, J.E., L.G. Raisz, H.A. Simmons, J.J. Oppenheim and
    S.E. Mergenhagen, 1972. Bone resorbing activity in super-
    natant fluid from cultured human peripheral blood leukocytes.
    Science, 177, 793-95.

10. Mundy, G.R., L.G. Raisz, R.A. Cooper, G.P. Schechter and
    S.E. Salmon, 1974. Evidence for the secretion of an osteo-
    clast stimulating factor in myeloma. New Engl. J. Med.,
    291, 1041-46.

11. Klein, D.C. and L.G. Raisz, 1970. Prostaglandins: stimula-
    tion of bone resorption in tissue culture. Endocrinology,
    86, 1436-40.

12. Raisz, L.G., R.A. Luben, G.R. Mundy, J.W. Dietrich,
    J.E. Horton and C.L. Trummel, 1975. Effect of osteoclast
    activating factor from human leukocytes on bone metabolism.
    J. Clin. Invest., 56, 408-13.

13. Goodson, J.M., K. McClatchy and C. Revell, 1974. Prostag-
    landin-induced resorption of the adult rat calvarium. J.
    Dent. Res., 53, 670-77.

14. Raisz, L.C. and I. Niemann, 1969. Effect of phosphate,
    calcium and magnesium on bone resorption and hormonal
    responses in tissue culture. Endocrinology, 85, 446-52.

15. Holtrop, M.E., L.G. Raisz and H.A. Simmons, 1974. The
    effects of parathyroid hormone, colchicine and calcitonin on
    the ultrastructure and the activity of osteoclasts in organ
    culture. J. Cell Biol., 60, 346-55.

16. Holtrop, M.E., in press. Quantitation of the ultrastructure
    of the osteoclast for the evaulation of cell function. In:
    Proc. Second Int. Workshop on Bone Histomorphometry 1976.
    Ed. P.J. Meunier.

An Appraisal of Bone Cellular Function in Senescence.

Louis V. Avioli

Schoenberg Professor of Medicine; Director, Division of Bone and Mineral Metabolism, Washington University School of Medicine, The Jewish Hospital of St. Louis, St. Louis, MO 63110

There is unanimity of opinion that skeletal mass decreases with age, a phenomena which appears independent of major differences in activity, diet and expectations of aging. It has been suggested that this age-related loss of bone is quite independent of other aspects of senescence; and simply reflects the product of age-dependent changes in renal, neural, vascular gastrointestinal and hormonal activities (1). Since bone growth, modeling and remodeling in the pre-pubescent years, and the re-modeling which continues following ultimate skeletal maturation and epiphyseal closure results from a cybernetic interplay be-tween osteoblastic controlled bone formation and osteoclastic-osteocytic modulated bone resorption, senescent osteopenia must invariably result from a discordant interplay between the cell-ular component.

The aging of human bone has been associated with: (1) an imbalance between osteoblasts and osteoclasts at the expense of osteoblastic function; (2) reduced metabolic rates of osteo-blasts and osteoclasts; (3) alterations in remodeling resulting in an accumulation of incompletely resorbed osteons as inters-titial lamallae resulting in a "pseudomosaic" bone pattern; (4) an enlargement of the marrow space, cortical thinning and enlargement of Haversian canals; (5) a slight decrease in the "soluble" collagen and a proportional increase in its biological half-life; (6) an increase in the more mature "insoluble" colla-gen fraction with an accumulation of more highly "cross-linked" forms: (7) reduced glycosoaminoglycan synthesis (and metabolism) and an overall reduction in bone protein synthesis; and (8) a decrease in the hexosamine-uronic acid and hexosamine-hydroxy-proline ratios (2). The cause-effect relationship between these isolated observations is still conjectural, although it has been assumed that the "uncoupling" of osteoclastic-osteoblastic activity with osteoclastosis predominating, plays a pivotal role in modulating the bone loss which attends the aging process.

Studies which detail the effect of age on the metabolic activity of cells obtained from human bone are relatively rare. In 1965, Flanagan and Nichols, in studies of bone samples ob-tained from thirteen human subjects ranging in age from the newborn to 67 years, reported that the cellularity of bone de-creased with age (3). Since in this study cortical bone contained one-quarter as many cells as did mixed bone samples

21

(cortical and trabecular), the authors concluded that the relative amounts of cortical or trabecular bone included in any one biopsy sample will condition its overall cellularity. Despite the wide age range of the subjects biopsied in the study, the O_2 utilization rates were fairly constant at 0.47 ± 0.09 μmoles O_2/mg DNA/hr (3). Similarly, the rates of bone aerobic lactate production were also fairly constant in this mixed population at 0.79 ± 0.12 mmoles/mg DNA/hr, although a tendency for lactate production to decrease with age was observed in the rat (3). The authors concluded that the most important factor controlling the overall metabolic rate of bone cells in humans is the number, rather than the relative metabolic activity of the cellular component. These preliminary studies should be interpreted with caution since the "cellular fraction" was never clearly defined and simply represented alkali extracted material.

Recently, Schulz and Delling have shown that osteoblastic activity is reduced with advancing years (4), a process which is accompanied by an antagonistic increase in the inactive osteoid surface without osteoblasts. The rise in the inactive osteoid surface of trabecular bone becomes most significant in the sixth decade. This age-related decrease in osteoblastic activity when coupled with age-related increments in osteoclastic activity (5) could readily account for a steady and progressive loss of bone with age.

"Osteocyte differential counts" also vary with age (6). The percentage of small osteocytes, enlarged osteocytes and empty lacunae constitute the osteocyte differential count. The small osteocytes usually represent more than 50% of the count in Haversian systems and in the cancellous bone trabeculae; this value increases gradually until the 40th year and then diminishes, a pattern which is to be contrasted with that of the large osteocytes, which actually increase in number after 40 years of age (6). Whereas the small osteocyte is considered to play an active part in the transport of substances in bone, the large osteocyte functions primarily to resorb bone, i.e. "osteocytic osteolysis" (7). Since activation of osteocytes is a sensitive indicator of parathyroid function, the age-related increments in these cells may actually represent a biological response to mild but progressive increments in parathyroid hormone (8).

Regardless of the documented decrements in osteoblastic bone forming cellular components, and progressive increments in bone resorbing osteoclasts and osteocytes in aging individuals, the nature of the cellular response to hormones must still be considered. Although parathyroid hormone, vitamin D (via its biologically active 25-hydroxycholecalciferol and 1,25-dihydroxycholecalciferol metabolites) and calcitonin have been considered the guardians of skeletal development, remodeling and mineral homeostasis, estrogens, testosterone, somatomedin(s), thyroid hormone, insulin and cortisol are also essential in this regard.

There is evidence that changes in ovarian function do

affect the skeletal mass; with loss of ovarian estrogens the estrogen-dependent endosteal bone mass is reduced. This response in the early post-menopausal years cannot, however, account for the progressive bone loss seen in the elderly (70-90 yr) female who is losing skeletal mass originally formed 50-60 years previously. The manner in which estrogens alter bone cellular function is still unknown. Although bone "receptors" for calcitonin, parathyroid hormone and 1,25-dihydroxy-cholecalciferol have been identified, such is not the case for estrogens. It has been proposed however, that the rapid loss of skeletal mass seen in some post-menopausal women (with estrogen levels comparable to age-related less fracture prone females) results from a defect in estrogen binding to cellular receptors in bone (9). An analagous defect in estrogen binding to bone cells has also been proposed to account for the skeletal loss in older men with normal gonadal functions.

Changes in endocrine functions with age include an increase in circulating parathyroid hormone, and a decrease in triiodo-thyronine, estrogens, testosterone, calcitonin, somatomedin(s) and 1,25-dihydroxycholecalciferol (8,10). Thyroxine, cortisol, insulin and glucagon remain relatively constant. Bone cell metabolism may be altered in diabetics with documented premature loss of skeletal mass (11) since insulin stimulates the uptake of amino acids in bone (12) and exerts a stimulatory effect on collagen synthesis in bone organ cultures (13). The decreased bone mass in diabetics may also represent premature senescence of the osteoblast, a theory compatible with the observations of Goldstein et al (14). These investigators demonstrated a decreased proliferative capacity of the diabetic fibroblast in tissue culture and suggested an early senescence of all cells as basic to the diabetic problem.

Thus, relative degrees of estrogen, calcitonin and insulin insufficiency, coupled with age-related progressive increments in circulating parathyroid hormone levels may well account for the histological findings of decreased osteoblastic and increased osteoclastic-osteocytic activity and the resultant loss of skeletal tissue. Until more definitive techniques are developed for the isolation and cell culture of osteoblasts, osteocytes and osteoclasts obtained from human bone (15), and the life cycle of bone forming and bone resorbing cells defined (16), we must be satisfied with an analysis of age-related bone-cellular changes in animal models such as the growing rat and miniature pig (3). Data thus derived must still be interpreted with caution until the hormonal milieu which characterizes the aging human is also reproduced.

References

1. Garn, S.M. 1975. Bone-loss and aging. The Physiology and Pathology of Human Aging, Goldman, R., and Rockstein, M. (editors), Academic Press, New York, pgs. 39-57.

2. Schmidt, U.J., Kalbe, I., and Sielaff, F. 1975. Bone aging. Cell Impairment in Aging and Development, Cristofalo, V.J. and Holeckova, E. (editors), Plenum Press, New York, pgs. 371-374.

3. Flanagan, B. and Nichols, G., Jr. 1965. Metabolic studies of human bone in vitro. I. Normal Bone. J. Clin. Invest. 44, 1788-1794.

4. Schulz, A., and Delling, G. 1976. Age-related changes of new bone formation--determination of histomorphometric parameters of the iliac crest trabecular bone. Proceedings of the First Workshop on Bone Morphometry, Univ. of Ottawa, 28-31 March, 1973, Univ. of Ottawa Press, pgs. 189-190.

5. Schulz, A. and Delling, G. 1976. Age-related changes of bone resorption parameters in iliac crest trabecular bone. Proceedings of the First Workshop on Bone Morphometry, Univ. of Ottawa, 28-31 March, 1973, Univ. of Ottawa Press, pgs. 161-162.

6. Baud, C.A. 1975. Histophysiology of the osteocyte: an introduction to the morphometry of peri-osteocytic lacunae. Proceedings of the First Workshop on Bone Morphometry, Univ. of Ottawa, 28-31 March, 1973, Univ. of Ottawa Press, pgs. 267-272.

7. Belanger, L.F., Robichon, J., Migicovsky, B.B., Copp, D.H., and Vincent, J. 1963. Resorption without osteoclasts (osteolysis). In Mechanisms of Hard Tissue Destruction. Sognnaes, R.F., (editor), Sognnaes, Washington, American Association for the Advancement of Science, pgs. 531-556.

8. Berlyne, G.M., Ben-Ari, J., Kushelevsky, A., Idelman, A., Galinsky, D., Hirsch, M., Shainkin, R., Yagil, R. and Zlotnik, M. 1975. The aetiology of senile osteoporosis: secondary hyperparathyroidism due to renal failure. Quart. J. Med. 44, 505-521.

9. Bartizal, F.J., Coulam, C.B., Gaffey, T.A., Tyan, R.J. and Riggs, B.L. 1975. Impaired binding of estradiol to vaginal mucosal cells in post-menopausal osteoporosis. Calc. Tiss. Proceedings on XIth European Symposium, Pors Nielsen, S., and Hjorting-Hauen, E. (editors), pgs. 412-416.

10. Davis, P.J. 1977. Endocrines and aging. Hosp. Prac. September, 1977, pgs. 113-128.

11. Levin, M.E., Boisseau, V.C., and Avioli, L.V.   1976.
Effects of diabetes mellitus on bone mass in juvenile and
adult-onset diabetes.   N. Engl. J. Med. 294, 241-245.

12. Hahn T.J., Downing, S.J., and Phang, J.M.   1971.   Insulin
effect on amino acid transport in bone: dependence on protein synthesis and Na$^+$. Am. J. Physiol. 220, 1717-1723.

13. Wettenhall, R.E.H., Schwartz, P.L., Bornstein, J.   1969.
Actions of insulin and growth hormone on collagen and chron-
droitin sulfate synthesis in bone organ cultures.   Diabetes
18, 280-184.

14. Goldstein, S., Littlefield, J.W., Soeldner, J.S.   1969.
Diabetes mellitus and aging: diminished plating efficiency
of cultured human fibroblasts. Proc. Nat. Acad. Sci. 64,
155-160.

15. Luben, R.A., Wong, G.L. and Cohn, D.V.   1976.   Biochemical
characterization with parathormone and calcitonin of isolated bone cells: provisional identification of osteoclasts and
osteoblasts.   Endocrinology 99, 526-534.

16. Yaeger, V.L., Chiemchanya, S. and Chaiseri, P.   1975.
Changes in size of lacunae during the life of osteocytes in
osteons of compact bone.   J. Gerontol. 30, 9-14.

Discussion for Session I; The Cells of Bone - Their Morphology and Function.

The manner of reproducing the discussion periods comprised recording of each discussion on magnetic tape and preparation by the editors of written proceedings therefrom.

DR. TASHJIAN: In your experiments, Dr. Peck, with conditioned medium from bone cells showing a stimulation of adherence and possibly a proliferation, do you have any evidence that it is a specific effect of conditioned medium from bone cells; or does conditioned medium from any kind of cell reproduce that effect?

DR. PECK: We have no specific evidence at present. We are examining the possibility that this could be a non-specific stimulator of growth in other cultured cells.

Unfortunately, it is difficult to test this material in the absence of serum because the other cells that we are using for test objects require serum for growth. Nevertheless, we are adding it to the serum.

DR. TASHJIAN: Can you grow cells up to density and then condition them?

DR. PECK: Yes.

DR. TASHJIAN: Dr. Holtrop, could you distinguish cells stimulated with OAF, parathyroid hormone and prostaglandin E-2 on the basis of shape by electron microscopy?

DR. HOLTROP: No.

DR. STERN: I have a question for Dr. Holtrop. You mentioned that with parathyroid hormone, you seemed to get more recruitment. I wonder whether this is related to fibroblastic proliferation. In other words, can any cell in the area be recruited to form an osteoclast by the resorbing stimuli, or is it a specific type of cell?

Further, do prostaglandins and OAF cause the kind of fibroblastic proliferation that you see with parathyroid hormone?

DR. HOLTROP: In this culture system, we do not see that many fibroblasts even though they are there. However, if there are any changes with each stimulant I was not aware of it without measuring and counting.

DR. STERN: Then you think that parathyroid hormone is a specific stimulus for proliferation of an osteoclast, rather than the fact that with parathyroid hormone there are more cells around?

DR. HOLTROP: Yes. There are cells that I consider progenitor cells, because they have a lot of mitochondria but not as many as an osteoclast. I feel these are progenitor cells which are activated, differentiate and get into the population of osteoclasts.

DR. PUZAS: I have a question and a comment for Dr. Peck. You said that when you seed a million cells, 30 percent adhere, which is 300,000 cells. However, when you seed half a million cells, or 500,000 cells, the culture fails, presumably due to lack of attachment. The difference is only approximately 150,000 cells. Isn't that a fine difference for the success or failure of a culture?

DR. PECK: That is a fine difference, and it was just the difference that we selected in the first series of experiments. We have subsequently examined a variety of initial cell densities and five times 10^5 cells is really the borderline between success of the culture and non-success. It probably relates to how much growth factor the cells are releasing into the medium.

DR. PUZAS: Secondly, using a technique for determining DNA specifically on the rat bone cells that we have developed, we find that the DNA content is probably closer on the order of six picograms per cell. Perhaps your figure of 10 to 11 may be due to active DNA synthesis that is going on during proliferation.

DR. WURTHIER: Dr. Peck, your factor is non-dialyzable. I feel that you thought it was protein; but is it possible that it might be RNA, messenger RNA, or something like that?

DR. PECK: We are obviously testing that possibility. Those of you who are fans of growth factors will know that this is a very rapidly-growing area. As reviewed elegantly in the Annual Review of Biochemistry last year, there are probably 40 or 50 such growth factors that have been described. To my knowledge, they are all proteinaceous or glycoproteinaceous in nature. Although we have to prove it, I think it is quite likely that this is either a protein, or more likely a glycoprotein.

However, we can't exclude the possibility that other factors have left the dialysis sac which may also be active in our system.

DR. WURTHIER: Have you started to characterize this?

DR. PECK: Yes, but I am a little reluctant to give you the results of data that haven't been corroborated.

DR. PARFITT: I have a question addressed to Dr. Holtrop, and it has to do with a possible ambiguity in her use of a term, "area". When one does morphometric studies of this kind, one can measure a length or perimeter in the section, and from that, one can extrapolate from two dimensions to three dimensions and estimate the surface area of the structure in three dimensions.

Alternatively, one can measure the area in the section, and from that, extrapolate to the three dimensions as a volume. So the term "area" can be what you measure in the section, which is a two-dimensional structure giving information about three dimensions, or it can be something that one extrapolates from the one-dimensional measure or perimeter.

I would like to ask exactly what, in which sense, the term "area" was used in her measurements.

DR. HOLTROP: The "area" used was the area in the two-dimensional section. If the average area in two-dimensional sections is larger in one population than in another, then we know that the volume is larger as well. There is a conversion possible between the average area and average volume that I didn't get into, which also assumes that the shape of the object remains the same; I have not worked with this conversion.

If the average area is larger, the average volume is larger, too. We underestimate, really, what the enlargement is, because area is enlarged by the square and volumes enlarge by the cube. If you do the conversion to volumes, then the enlargement of the ruffled border volume is just incredible.

The reason that I did not do the conversion is that one can convert from average area to average volume but lose the standard error; statistics would be then invalid on those new figures.

DR. COHN: My question is also for Dr. Holtrop. The "clear zones", ruffled borders, and areas with the different agents that you tested could change at somewhat different rates. I wonder if you could tell us how these changes correlated with the release of calcium into the medium by these different agents.

DR. HOLTROP: The release of calcium with parathyroid hormone is between six and 12 hours, and the release of calcium with PGE and OAF is between 12 and 24 hours. So in the release of calcium we also see a difference in rate, in time.

DR. COHN: Did you find one morphological feature to change preferentially? Which of those changes do you think correlated best with the release of calcium, and did you find any particular morphological change that cut across the different inducing agents which you tested that also might indicate which of these might play a role in the release of calcium, presumably by these osteoclasts?

DR. HOLTROP: The change that correlates best with the calcium release is the change in ruffled border and clear zone, which go at the same time. Usually the cell change is a little later.

DR. MINKIN: A question for Dr. Holtrop. In the material that you examined, did you see or look for any cells that one might call macrophages, as opposed to osteoclasts? Were they present in these bones, and did they change in response to the various treatments to which you subjected them?

DR. HOLTROP: In these cultures, the marrow cells don't do so well; so, no; I can't say anything about that. We are very aware now in our in vivo studies to look at the macrophages; but I cannot say anything about it in the culture system.

DR. MINKIN: They don't survive in the culture system?

DR. HOLTROP: No. Or they regress; I don't know what happens to them.

DR. TALMAGE: I would like to review a couple of points with Dr. Avioli. The first is in regard to his slide where he showed calcitonin content in elderly people was going down. Now, in most rats, which of course are not people, the aged rat has a fairly high content of calcitonin.

It just happens that very recently I had cause to have my calcitonin content examined and found my calcitonin content extremely high; and I am obviously a very normal individual! I bring up the point that possibly calcitonin in elderly humans also is higher than in the middle-aged; not as high as the young, but it probably goes back up again, in the elderly.

Also, I wondered about your definition of the osteoclasts in your slides when you said there were whole areas of osteoid which were not covered by osteoblasts. Now, I don't know what you meant; were they covered by any cells at all?

We in our group, Dr. Grubb and Dr. VanderWiel have been studying aged people as well as young people, and our conclusion is that there is no osteoid in any age of human being that isn't covered with some type of cell. I wonder if you would like to comment on that.

DR. AVIOLI: Your point is well taken. Time did not allow me to say that the data published in terms of calcitonin and age have been directed primarily to the aging female. Measured estrogen levels have been shown to be relatively lower as a female ages; further, the response to calcium loading in the aging female is blunted. Those are data. What, or how, they relate to the aging male is another story, because obviously, one of the biggest problems we have today in so-called bone disease is not the male. It is the female. Now, maybe there is a calcitonin story there.

Your second question or comment is an interesting one, and perhaps someone like Dr. Jowsey could answer that, or Dr.

Teitelbaum. We see a lot of patients who do have relatively inactive bone.

DR. TEITELBAUM: Dr. Talmage is right. All bone, not only bone that is covered by visible osteoid, but all bone that isn't being resorbed by osteoclasts is covered by either osteoblasts or so-called bone lining cells. We don't know what those cells are, those flat, fusiform cells that cover the surface.

But so far as the number of osteoblasts is concerned, in the aging bone, I am not sure those data are correct, vis-a-vis the percentage of surface that we see covered by osteoid. We have been looking at bone biopsies of aging women and trying to categorize them into biopsies that are actively turning over and those which fulfill the classical concept of suppressed bone turnover. Most of our patients appear to have an increase in bone turnover; when we see an increased number of osteoclasts, we also see an increased number of osteoblasts; when we do double-tetracycline labeling on these patients, bone formation is not suppressed, but increased.

Now there is sub-population of individuals, in our series it was about 30 percent, in which there is an actual suppression of bone turnover. One sees very few osteoclasts and very few osteoblasts.

DR. AVIOLI: One final comment I would make to that, and maybe Dr. Jowsey could respond, is the data I showed came from Europe. I am convinced that it depends on the endemic population. They may be a lot more vitamin D deficient than here, and what we are really seeing in these individuals is a very early form of D-deficient rickets with senescence, and that is why they see fewer cells lining osteoid than we do.

DR. JOWSEY: It is very important to realize that some of the differences may be based on whether one has a D-replete or a D-deficient population. If you look at bone from Europe and Canada, one finds an increase in osteoid, inactive osteoid, with age; but not in a D-replete population in the United States of America. So there is bound to be a difference, which is a real difference, because of population differences.

DR. TURNER: This question is directed to Dr. Peck. How do you distinguish your isolated cells from fibroblasts? You mentioned the fact that the fibroblasts did not survive very well; your flattened cells look very much like fibroblasts.

DR. PECK: We can't determine whether or not there are fibroblasts in our cell system. Obviously, the population of cells is heterogeneous. What we can say is that deliberate culturing of fibroblasts isolated by this same technique and cultured under similar conditions does not yield evidence of pro-liferation, or indeed survival, in the absence of serum in primary culture.

This suggests that either the fibroblast-like cells that do

survive that are derived from bone are special kinds of fibro-blasts, bone fibroblasts, as opposed to skin or periosteal fibroblasts; or that they just appear to be fibroblasts by this very crude morphological assay and aren't at all, but are more mesenchymal cells that have the capacity to differentiate.

DR. TURNER: Did they synthesize and secrete collagen?

DR. PECK: We haven't tested that. I can tell you that on the multiple electron photomicrographs that we have seen, in cultures that are in the absence of serum and in the absence of any added hormones, there is no evidence of banded structure that looks like collagen.

DR. TURNER: Do you seen any evidence of differentiated behavior?

DR. PECK: Only with respect to alkaline phosphatase activity. In data that I didn't show, with respect to response to bone-seeking hormones, the cultures respond to parathyroid hormone at very low concentrations, as little as half a nanogram per milliliter, with a profound increase in cyclic AMP. They fail to respond to calcitonin. These cells resemble the deeper cells, or the later-release cells, of Wong, Cohn, and Lubin, and also the cells that we have described to be derived from bone that is periosteum-free. Presumably, osteoblast-like cells are those that respond preferentially to parathyroid hormone in terms of cyclic AMP production.

Those are the only criteria for differentiation that we have applied at this point. We have done some preliminary studies with the synthesis of gamma carboxyl glutamic acid-containing protein, but the data are really too preliminary to quote.

DR. RAISZ: I have two slides by E. Canalis which show that there is a dissociation in our system between collagen synthesis and thymidine incorporation.

This slide is of fibroblast growth factor. At 100 nanograms per mil, which is about at the top of the dose response curve in other cell systems, it reduces percent collagen synthesis without any effect on non-collagen protein.

The next slide shows that in these particular 24-hour studies, there is a substantial increase in both thymidine and uridine incorporation into the whole bone explant.

In other words, what we find, and this shows up morphologi-cally, is that fibroblastic proliferation can be stimulated by fibroblast growth factor and seems to be at the expense of osteoblasts. This is a phenomenon which we believe we are seeing in a lot of cells. I think there is, from all the work that has been done by others, some kind of cycle in which proliferation is followed by differentiation. This was brought out in Dr. Peck's introduction.

The question I would now ask of Dr. Peck concerns the character of cells which are stimulated to replicate. Do they look as though they are differentiating back, or do they look the same as the cells which are replicating less rapidly in your system?

DR. PECK: The only valid test of that would be the 14-day-old cultures; that is, the cells that have been used to test putative bone cell growth factor after attachment has already occurred. Under those conditions, after two days of exposure, there was no increase in alkaline phosphatase activity.

But as you saw from the data indicating tripling of thymidine incorporation, these cells are, at the time we assayed them, still in a proliferative phase, or DNA synthetic phase. It would be too soon to determine whether specialization would follow.

We are also testing fibroblast growth factor in our system. It will be of interest to compare that with whatever it is in our dialysate.

DR. MUNDY: I would just like to press Dr. Peck a little bit more on an answer to an earlier question. I wonder if the products of your cells, like the growth factor or the liberated protein, would be altered by hormones which you might expect could affect osteoblast function, like parathyroid hormone?

DR. PECK: It is an intriguing question. I have no data. We have done experiments with parathyroid hormone, with glucocorticoids, and with calcitonin, but the data aren't available.

DR. PARFITT: Just two quick comments on the previous remarks by Dr. Avioli and Dr. Teitelbaum. If you look at elderly people, very elderly people, who have had hip fractures, you find, just as in Europe, that a significant number of them have very low plasma 25-OH-D-3 levels and increased osteoid surface; so it would be a mistake to imply that this does not occur in the United States.

Secondly, the fact that in some old people there is increase in the number of osteoblasts, and the total rate of bone formation, is correct; but this is consistent with there also being a defect in the function of each individual osteoblast.

Our data suggest that all old people have defective osteoblast function, irrespective of whether bone turnover is high, normal, or low.

DR. AVIOLI: I cannot deny or argue against data which have been accumulated. I can only suggest that it may be a mistake to take one determinant, like a 25-hydroxyl level, and compare it, correlated with the amount of osteoid content in bone, and assume that there is a relationship, because we could talk for a year about the relationship between circulating 25-hydroxy-D levels and what is seen in bone in many diseases. Just because the 25-hydroxy level is low, I am not willing to buy, immediately, that these individuals have a form of D-lack rickets.

I think there may be much more going on in those old bones. Some of these people have elevated PTH's. Are we to buy the fact that PTH increases collagen synthesis, and maybe it is a combination of too much PTH or too little 25? I think it is a nice correlate; but we have seen so many people who have fluoride osteomalacia on bone biopsies whose 25-hydroxy levels are normal; and we have seen individuals whose levels look like they are low normal whose bone biopsies, in terms of dynamics, are relatively normal.

I look at these numbers with a jaundiced eye. Given a number in blood, and given a bone sample in terms of histometric analysis, we should be very cautious before we go from that number to what is going on in bone, unless you know about all the hormones: insulin, PTH, estrogens, etc.

DR. WURTHIER: Dr. Peck, back to the synthesis of alkaline phosphatase in your cultured cells. I am wondering if this may not be a reflection of something which one sees in, say callous formation in which one recapitulates what one sees in embryogenesis. Maybe you are looking at something which is almost like a hypertrophic chondrocyte. In this sense there would be a tremendous influx of alkaline phosphatase synthesis. Do you have any data that might support that type of "pathway", so to speak, in your cultured cells?

DR. PECK: I can't speak directly to that. I can tell you that the cells that are initially cultured are not chondroblasts, because we obviously take great care in preparing the bones before we isolate the cells. But I can't exclude the possibility that this is a phase of chondroblastic transformation in cells that may ultimately become bone, bone cells, or osteoblast-like cells.

One of the reasons for embarking on the culture system was the hope that we could replicate a sequence of differentiation. We have no right to predetermine what that sequence of differentiation will be. Ultimately, it would be nice to see that these cells would emerge as osteoblasts which were capable of forming bone.

DR. TEITELBAUM: I would like to respond to Dr. Avioli's comments about bone loss with age, and to Dr. Parfitt. This may be a cliché, but we all know that there is a coupling phenomenon which exists between osteoblasts and osteoclasts. In the remodeling skeleton, as one increases, the other increases; and as one decreases, the other decreases.

On the other hand, rate does not necessarily follow the number of cells. In other words, one can have an increased number of osteoblasts and a decrease in the rate of bone formation, if, as Dr. Parfitt says, the rate of bone formation of the individual osteoclast, decreases with age.

So Dr. Parfitt's statement is very much in keeping with what Dr. Avioli pointed out, as regards the decrease in bone formation with age.

SESSION II

THE MATRIX OF BONE — ITS DISSOLUTION
AND DEMINERALIZATION

Regulation of the Synthesis of Bone Matrix in Organ Culture

Lawrence G. Raisz, Barbara E. Kream, and Ernesto M. Canalis

Division of Endocrinology and Metabolism, Department of Medicine, University of Connecticut Health Center, Farmington, CT 06032 and

Endocrine Unit, St. Francis Hospital and Medical Center, Hartford, CT 06015

Although studies concerned with the pathogenesis of bone loss have emphasized mechanisms by which bone resorption is increased, it is likely that such mechanisms can only produce substantial bone loss when bone formation is also impaired. Bone resorption and bone formation are closely coupled in the adult skeleton. This coupling is largely anatomic and is the basis for the concept of the bone remodeling unit (1). It is expressed in Haversian remodeling which is initiated by vascular invasion and the formation of an osteoclast cutting cone which produces a large canal. This is subsequently filled by concentric lamellae of new bone formed by osteoblasts just behind the resorption site. Similar phenomena occur on the bone surface. Bone is removed by osteoclasts and the resulting Howship's lacunae are replaced by variable amounts of new bone, thus altering the shape of cortical or trabecular bone. Bone loss requires that this coupled process be uncoupled either in time or space. Bone loss could occur with little increase in the resorption rate if bone formation were arrested. This may be the case in the osteopenia of glucocorticoid excess. On the other hand there are disorders in which bone resorption is clearly accelerated and bone loss does not occur. In primary hyperparathyroidism and in hyperthyroidism there is a marked increase in bone resorption but this is accompanied by an equal increase in bone formation in many patients. Small doses of parathyroid hormone may actually increase bone mass. Localized bone loss could occur if the increases in resorption and increases in formation were at different sites.

The regulation of bone formation must involve local as well as systemic factors. First there is the anatomic coupling by which osteoclastic bone resorption is regularly followed by osteoblastic bone formation. Additional local factors enable the skeleton to adjust to changing mechanical and gravitational stress. There appears to be a resorptive response to pressure and a formative response to tension. A striking example is the ability of orthodontic forces to move teeth in the alveolar bone. The mechanisms by which mechanical and gravitational stress alter bone remodeling are not known. Piezo-electric effects are implicated and it is of interest that collagen rather than bone mineral may be the source of currents generated in response to stress in the skeleton (2). Recently Rodan et al

(3) demonstrated that electrical fields could influence thymidine incorporation into DNA in isolated cartilage cells and suggested that this was due to alterations in ion transport. It is also possible that mechanical stress may produce humoral mediators which modulate bone cell activity. Certainly humoral factors are important in the regulation of overall skeletal growth. Clinical data and animal experiments indicate that normal growth depends on the concerted action of the calcium regulating hormones, parathyroid hormone (PTH), the active metabolites of vitamin D, and calcitonin, and more general regulators such as the thyroid hormones, glucocorticoids, insulin, and growth hormone. The last probably acts through somatomedins (4).

Bone formation is most likely to be regulated by influencing the rate of synthesis of bone matrix by osteoblasts and osteocytes, since matrix formation precedes and directs bone mineralization. It is possible that hormones could influence bone mineralization and have indirect effects on matrix synthesis. When mineralization is impaired in vitamin D deficiency, matrix formation continues for a certain period but then slows. The existence of a cell syncytium connecting osteoblasts and osteocytes could provide a feedback mechanism for control of matrix synthesis. When a portion of the newly synthesized osteoid has become mineralized this might signal the surface osteoblasts to synthesize additional matrix. This would not explain the initiation or cessation of osteoblastic activity. When active osteoblasts stop making matrix the remaining osteoid becomes fully mineralized to the bone surface.

If osteoblastic matrix synthesis is the major regulated system in bone formation then it seems likely that this regulation will be at the level of collagen synthesis, since this protein constitutes 90 percent of mature bone matrix. The possibility that regulation occurs by control of noncollagen components of the matrix cannot be ruled out, and is attractive since noncollagen components may determine bone mineralization.

We selected to study the regulation of bone collagen synthesis in organ culture as the first point at which to attack some of the following questions: 1) Do agents which produce pathologic increases in bone resorption have any direct influence on bone formation? If so, is this to enhance coupling, that is, increase bone formation or to produce uncoupling, that is, decrease bone formation? 2) Are there systemic hormones which stimulate osteoblastic collagen synthesis and oppose localized or generalized bone loss? 3) Are there intrinsic regulators in bone or periosteal tissues which might be important in physiologic and pathologic changes in bone formation?

For these studies we have used organ cultures of half calvaria from 21-day old fetal rats incubated in chemically defined medium supplemented with bovine serum albumin or 5 percent serum. Collagen synthesis is measured by labeling the tissue with proline after various periods of treatment and determining the incorporation of proline into collagen using purified bacterial collagenase. Using this method it is also possible to

detect effects of various agents on the synthesis of noncollagen
protein. In addition we have measured the labeled hyrdoxyproline
formed, the release of collagen into the medium, and the incorporation of labeled uridine into RNA and labeled thymidine into
DNA to assess the mechanisms by which changes in collagen synthesis occur.

Stimulators of bone resorption

A number of agents have been shown to stimulate bone resorption directly in organ culture. These include calcium regulating
hormones, PTH (5) and the active metabolites of vitamin D (6),
and thyroid hormones (7), which are not considered calcium regulators but are certainly important in bone turnover (8). Other
agents such as prostaglandins (9) and osteoclast activating
factor (OAF) (10) are certainly of pathologic importance but
may also be important as local physiologic mediators of resorption. Exogenous substances such as bacterial products may also
stimulate bone resorption (11).

We studied the effects of all of these agents on bone collagen synthesis with the exception of bacterial products (12). The
results indicate that, _in vitro_, agents which stimulate bone resorption appear to be uncouplers; that is, they inhibit bone
formation. However, there are substantial differences in dose
response, time course, and structure-activity relations among
these agents which may be of great importance in determining
their ability to produce pathologic bone loss.

Confirming many previous studies, both _in vivo_ and _in vitro_,
we have found that high concentrations of PTH inhibit bone collagen synthesis (13). This inhibition is progressive with time
and occurs at the same concentrations which stimulate bone resorption _in vitro_. A major difference between the effects of
bone resorption and bone formation is that prolonged bone resorption can be induced by brief exposure to PTH, while inhibition
of bone formation requires the continuous presence of the hormone
and does not persist when it is removed. These _in vitro_ observations were obtained at high concentrations of PTH and it is
possible that lower concentrations stimulate bone collagen synthesis resulting in the so-called anabolic effect of PTH (14).
A possible explanation for the anabolic effect _in vivo_ is that
it depends on the intermittent release of PTH. A pulse of PTH
may produce a prolonged resorptive effect but only transient
inhibition of osteoblasts. Since PTH causes proliferation of
fibroblastic potential precursor cells it is possible that between these pulses osteoblastic activity rebounds to exceed control values. Recently it has been suggested that PTH might impair collagen synthesis by inhibiting hydroxylation rather than
affecting the rate of translation of collagen (15). However, in
our cultures the collagen in PTH inhibited cultures show no decrease in hydroxyproline content (12).

Since vitamin D is considered to be a growth hormone for
the skeleton we wondered whether any of its active metabolites
might be couplers, that is whether they stimulated bone

resorption and formation since such an effect would favor orderly skeletal growth. However, we found that 1,25-dihydroxyvitamin D_3 and 1,24,25-trihydroxyvitamin D_3 which are potent stimulators of bone resorption also inhibited collagen synthesis at low concentrations (10^{-11} to 10^{-9}M) (16). 25-Hydroxyvitamin D and 24R,25 dihydroxyvitamin D did not alter bone collagen synthesis at concentrations (10^{-5}M) which stimulate bone resorption. Further studies are needed to determine whether these or other metabolites could enhance bone formation under different conditions. Nevertheless these results support the possibility that 1,25-dihydroxyvitamin D is not the form of vitamin D which stimulates physiologic bone growth.

Thyroid hormones have been shown to stimulate bone resorption at relatively low concentrations but only after prolonged exposure (7). Halme et al (17) found that high concentrations of triiodothyronine inhibited collagen synthesis in cartilagenous long bone rudiments. We have seen only minimal inhibition of collagen synthesis in calvaria with high concentrations of thyroid hormones (Canalis, Mundy, and Raisz, unpublished observation).

Preparations containing potent OAF activity have been shown to inhibit bone collagen synthesis in both rat (18) and mouse (19) calvaria. Since OAF has not yet been completely purified, this inhibition may not be due to the same material that stimulates bone resorption. One interesting aspect of the inhibitory effects of OAF and PTH on bone collagen synthesis is that they can be demonstrated in microphthalmic mutant mice which are highly resistant to the stimulatory effects of these agents on bone resorption (19). Assuming that microphthalmic mice have a genetic defect in osteoclast precursors (20), the unaltered response of osteoblasts supports the concept that these cells are derived from different precursors.

A number of different prostaglandins can stimulate bone resorption, although prostaglandins of the E series appear to be by far the most potent (21). Inhibition of bone collagen synthesis was seen with prostaglandins of the E series but only at concentrations considerably higher than those which stimulate bone resorption (22). Moreover prostaglandins of the F series which are approximately 10 percent as potent as the E compounds in stimulating bone resorption showed no inhibitory effect on collagen synthesis at concentrations as high as 10^{-4}M. These results suggest that the structure-activity as well as the dose-response relations for prostaglandins are different for bone resorbing and bone forming cells. Evidence for a possible role of prostaglandins as endogenous local regulators is presented below.

Systemic Bone Growth Factors

Thus far we have identified two agents which clearly stimulate bone collagen synthesis in organ culture, insulin (23) and somatomedin (24). Because the effects of these two compounds are not additive and because insulin is effective at low physiologic concentrations (10^{-9}M) we have postulated that both agents are acting on the same receptor, possibly an insulin receptor, and that somatomedin is acting as nonsuppressable insulin-like activity. There are probably additional factors in normal serum which stimulate osteoblasts. We observed greater synthesis with normal serum than with serum from hypophysectomized rats or hypopituitary patients which did not appear to be attributable to either insulin or somatomedin (24). We have obtained negative results with a number of other peptides which have been considered to be possible stimulators of bone growth including calcitonin, glucagon and growth hormone itself (13, 23, 24).

Endogenous Local Factors

Changes in the local synthesis and secretion of various prostaglandins could provide a humoral mechanism to mediate local changes in bone remodeling. We have previously shown that bone can produce prostaglandins in organ cultures (25). Recent studies have indicated that endogenous prostaglandin production may modulate collagen synthesis as well as resorption (B.E. Kream, S.C. Gworek, and L.G. Raisz, unpublished observations). Bones cultured in the presence of small amounts of complement sufficient serum show decreased collagen synthesis compared to cultures in the same serum with an inhibitor of prostaglandin cyclo-oxygenase added to the medium. Moreover cultured calvaria can release substantial amounts of PGE_2 into the medium as measured by immunoassay (A.L. Sandberg, unpublished observations). Addition of the precursor, arachidonic acid, to the medium can enhance PGE_2 production in such systems and result in further inhibition of collagen synthesis.

Conclusion

Pathologic bone loss probably requires not only an enhancement of resorption but some inhibition of the natural processes of repair. A number of agents have been identified which influence bone collagen synthesis including potential local factors which might be responsible for local impairment of bone formation in pathologic conditions. The study of this problem has just begun and more factors will undoubtedly be identified. However, identification of such potential factors is only the first step. Proof that a particular agent is responsible for bone loss requires demonstration that the agent is localized to the site of pathologic change. Such a demonstration has not yet been achieved for any putative mediator of localized bone loss.

Acknowledgement

This work was supported by Research Grant AM 018063 from the National Institutes of Arthritis, Metabolism, and Digestive Diseases. Dr. Kream is supported by USPHS postdoctoral Fellowship AM-05055.

REFERENCES

1. Rasmussen, H. and Bordier, P. 1974. The physiological and cellular basis of metabolic bone disease, Williams and Wilkins, Baltimore.

2. Marino, A.A., Becker, R.O., and Soderholm, S.C. 1971. Origin of the piezo-electric effect in bone. Calcified Tissue Research 8:177.

3. Rodan, G.A., Bourret, L.A. and Norton, L.A. 1978. Science, in press.

4. Raisz, L.G. and Bingham, P.J. 1972. Effects of hormone on bone development. Ann. Rev. of Pharmacology, 12:337.

5. Gaillard,P.J. 1957. Parathyroid gland in bone in vitro. Schwcitz. Med. Wochenschr, 14:447.

6. Raisz, L.G., Trummel, C.A., Holick, M.F., and DeLuca, H.F. 1972. 1,25-dihydroxy cholecalciferol: A potent stimulator of bone resorption in tissue culture. Science, 175:4023.

7. Mundy, G.R., Schapiro, J.L., Bandelin, J.G., Canalis, E.M., Raisz, L.G. 1976. Direct stimulation of bone resorption by thyroid hormone. J. Clin. Invest, 58:529.

8. Krane, S.M., Brownell, G.L., Stanbury, J.B. and Corrigan, H. 1976. The effects of thyroid disease on calcium metabolism in man. J. Clin. Invest., 35:874.

9. Klein, D.C. and Raisz, L.G. 1970. Prostaglandins: Stimulation of bone resorption in tissue culture. Endocrinology, 86:1436.

10. Horton, J.E., Raisz, L.G., Simmon, H.A., Oppenheim, J.J., and Mergenhagen, S.E. 1972. Bone resorbing activity in supernatant fluid from cultured human peripheral blood leukocytes. Science, 168:862.

11. Hausmann, E., Raisz, L.G. and Miller, W.A. 1970. Endotoxin: Stimulation of bone resorption in tissue culture. Science, 168:862.

12. Raisz, L.G., Canalis, E.M., Dietrich, J.W., Kream, B.E., Gworek, S.C., 1978. Hormonal regulation of bone formation. Recent Progress in Hormone Research, in press.

13. Dietrich, J.W., Canalis, E.M., Maina, D.M., Raisz, L.G. 1976. Hormonal control of bone collagen synthesis in vitro: Effects of parathyroid hormone and calcitonin. Endocrinology, 98:943.

14. Parsons, J.A., 1976. Biochemistry and Physiology of Bone, G.H. Bourne, editor, Academic Press, New York, Volume 4, in press.

15. Cohn, D.V., Wong, G.L., and Luben, R.A. 1977. Proceedings of the 6th Parathyroid Conference, in press.

16. Raisz, L.G., Maina, D.M., Gworek, S.C., Dietrich, J.W., and Canalis, E.M. 1978. Hormonal control of bone collagen synthesis in vitro: Inhibitory effects of 1,25-hydroxylated vitamin D metabolites. Endocrinology, in press.

17. Halme, J., Uitto, J., Kivirikko, K.I., and Saxen, L. 1972. Effect of triiodothyronine on the metabolism of collagen in culture embyronic bone. Endocrinology, 90:1476.

18. Raisz, L.G., Luben, R.A., Mundy, G.R., Horton, J.E., and Trummel, C.A. 1975. Effect of osteoclast activating factor from human leukocytes on bone metabolism. J. Clin. Invest., 56:408.

19. Raisz, L.G., Simmons, H.A., Gworek, S.C. and Eilon, G. 1977. Studies on congenital osteoporosis in microphthalmic mice using organ culture. Impairment of bone resorption in response to the physiologic stimulators. J. Exp. Med., 145:857.

20. Walker, D.G. 1975. Spleen cells transmit osteopetrosis in mice. Science, 190:785.

21. Dietrich, J.W., Goodson, J.M., and Raisz, L.G. 1975. Stimulation of bone resorption by various prostaglandins in organ culture. Prostaglandins, 10:231.

22. Raisz, L.G. and Koolemans-Beynen, A. 1974. Inhibition of bone collagen synthesis by prostaglandin E_2 in organ culture. Prostaglandins 8:377.

23. Canalis, E.M., Dietrich, J.W., Maina, D.M. and Raisz, L.G. 1977. Hormonal control of bone collagen synthesis in vitro: Effects of insulin and glucagon. Endocrinology, 100:668.

24. Canalis, E.M., Hintz, R.L., Dietrich, J.W., Maina, D.M. and Raisz, L.G. 1977. Effect of somatomedin and growth hormone on bone collagen synthesis in vitro. Metabolism, 26:1079.

25. Raisz, L.G., Sandberg, A., Goodson, J.M., Simmons, H.A. and Mergenhagen, S.E. 1974. Complement dependent stimulation of bone resorption mediated by prostaglandins. Science, 185:789.

The Effect of Parathormone on the Synthesis of Collagenous Matrix by Isolated Bone Cells.

Glenda L. Wong and David V. Cohn.

Calcium Research Laboratory, Veterans Administration Hospital, Kansas City, Missouri 64128; University of Missouri-Kansas City School of Dentistry, Kansas City, Missouri 64108; and University of Kansas School of Medicine, Kansas City, Kansas 66103.

We previously described a proteolytic digestive technique that permits one to obtain from mouse calvaria two types of cells that are metabolically and morphologically different (1-4). The cells that are released early in the digestive procedure, designated CT cells, express osteoclast-like functions such as the stimulation by parathyroid hormone of their hyaluronate synthesis, acid phosphatase activity and their ability to solubilize mineral and matrix from dead bone (Table I). Those cells obtained later in the digestion procedure, designated PT cells, demonstrate osteoblast-like characteristics such as the inhibition by parathormone of their alkaline phosphatase activity, citrate decarboxylation and collagen yield (Table I). Calcitonin antagonized the action of parathormone in the CT cells but did not affect PT cell metabolism. Since the biosynthesis of collagen is fundamental to bone matrix formation and represents a major activity of osteoblasts, we have attempted to more closely define this function in the separated CT and PT cells and to evaluate the effect of parathormone on this metabolism. This report presents these data.

Methods

CT and PT bone cells were prepared by sequential digestion with collagenase-trypsin of calvaria from 2-3 day old mice (Charles River Laboratories, Wilmington, Mass.) as previously described (2,3). In some experiments an additional 20 min digestion period was included yielding in all 6 populations of cells. Generally, populations 2 and 3 exhibited the characteristics of CT populations (3), and 4, 5 and 6 those of PT populations (3). The isolated cells of each population were then cultured in Minimum Essential Medium containing 10% fetal calf serum for 6 days. They were subdivided in fresh Minimum Essential Medium containing 0.57 mM-asorbic acid and 10% fetal calf serum when indicated. Other experimental details are provided in the figure and table legends and text.

(^{3}H)proline (25 Ci/mMole) and (^{14}C)proline (0.3 Ci/mMole) were purchased from New England Nuclear Corp., Boston, Mass. Minimum Essential Medium, fetal calf serum, crude collagenase and trypsin were obtained from GIBCO, Grand Island, N.Y.

TABLE I

CHARACTERIZATION OF BONE CELLS WITH PARATHORMONE

	DIRECTION of CHANGE	
	CT CELLS	PT CELLS
cAMP	↑	↑
Hyaluronate Synthesis Acid Phosphatase Dissolution of Matrix	↑	0
Alkaline Phosphatase Citrate Decarboxylation Collagen Yield	0	↓

Purified collagenase was obtained from Sigma Chemical Company, St. Louis, Missouri. It was further purified, when required, by gel filtration as described by Peterkofsky (5).

Results

Six day old CT and PT cells were subdivided as described in Methods and grown in culture containing (^{3}H)proline for 48 hours after which the collagenase-digestible protein of the cell layer and medium was determined. There was little difference between the amounts of non-collagenous protein produced by the CT and PT cells (Table II). In the PT cells, however, almost 18% of the protein synthesized was collagenase-digestible compared to only 3% in the CT cells. Thus, in keeping with the previously established osteoblastic nature of the PT cells, collagen production represented a major synthetic activity.

Consistent with the chemical data on collagen formation, in electron micrographs of pellets of PT cells one could routinely observe extracellular collagen fibrils (Fig. 1). These were less commonly noted in CT cell pellets.

In preliminary studies we have analyzed the type of collagen produced by the PT cells. Fig. 2 shows the results of polyacrylamide gel electrophoresis of denatured, pepsin-digested collagen produced by these cells. Based on the ratio of radioactivity into α1- and α2-chains of close to 2, it appears that the bulk of collagen was Type 1.

We next examined the effects of parathormone on collagen formation in PT cells. When the PT cells were grown in standard growth medium containing 10% fetal calf serum, parathormone neither affected the total yield of collagen nor its distribution between the medium and cell layer (Fig. 3). An unexpected effect of parathormone, however, was that the collagen associated with the cell layer was substantially more extractable in phosphate buffered saline (approximately 0.15M salt).

The lack of effect of parathormone on yield of collagen was not in accord with the reported action of parathormone in decreasing collagen synthesis in cultures of intact bone (6,7). Since in some such experiments serum had been omitted (7), we tested the action of parathormone on collagen yield and extractability when serum was omitted from the incubation medium. Table III shows that under this condition the amount of collagen was substantially less in the hormone-treated cells than in the controls in agreement with the data of Dietrich et al in intact bone (7). Table III also shows that the fraction of cell-layer collagen that was extractable was greater in the hormone-treated cells and in this regard the action of parathormone was similar whether or not serum was present. These results suggested that serum in part either masked the action of parathormone on collagen metabolism or caused the hormone to act differently.

TABLE II

Collagen synthesis by isolated bone cells

Replicate samples of 1 x 10^5 cells (populations 2 and 3 for CT cells and 4, 5 and 6 for PT cells) were cultured for 48 hours in Minimum Essential Medium containing 10% fetal calf serum, [^{14}C]proline (0.2 µCi/ml), and 0.57 mM ascorbic acid. At the end of the culture period, the collagen in both the medium and cell layer was measured as the radioactivity rendered non-acid precipitable after collagenase digestion and the non-collagenous protein (NCP) as that fraction which resisted collagenase. Results are expressed as dpm/10^5 cells seeded.

Bone Cell Type [a]	Collagen (dpm)	NCP (dpm)	Collagen % of Total [b]
CT	6.0 ± 1.2	38.6 ± 3.5	2.7
PT	57.8 ± 4.7	48.8 ± 9.1	17.9

[a] Average of CT populations 2 and 3 and PT populations 4-6.
[b] Calculated by assuming the proline content of collagen is 5.48 times greater than non-collagenous protein.

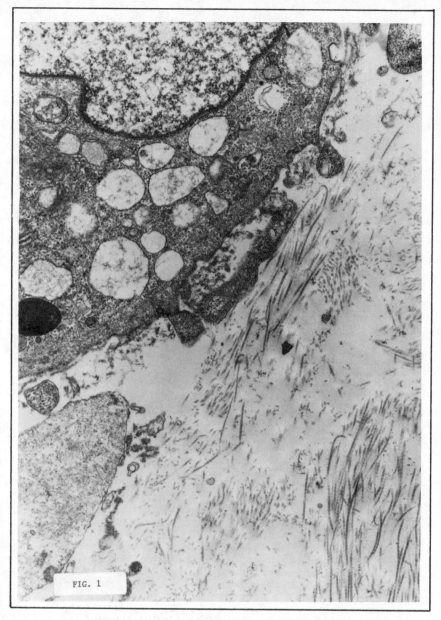

Fig. 1. Electron micrograph of collagen fibrils associated with PT cells. After 6 days in primary culture PT cells were harvested by scraping with a rubber policeman, pelleted by centrifugation and fixed in 2% glutaraldehyde, followed by exposure to osmium tetroxide. (x27,00) (Photograph courtesy of Dr. S. Teitelbaum, Washington University School of Medicine, St. Louis)

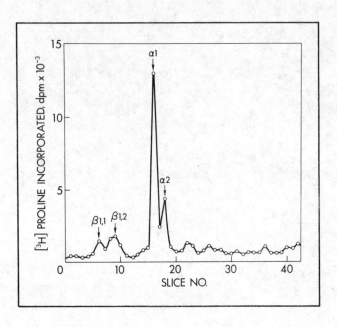

FIG 2. SDS-gel electrophoresis of collagen
produced by isolated PT bone cells. 6 day
old cultures of PT cells were grown in (^{3}H)
proline (50 μCi/ml) for 24 hours in Minimum
Essential Medium containing 0.57 mM ascorbic
acid. The medium was removed from the cells,
made 1M with acetic acid and digested overnight with pepsin at 4C. After lyophilization,
the material was suspended in and dialyzed
against 1% sodium dodecylsulfate, 0.05M urea
in 0.01M phosphate, pH 7.2. Samples for gel
electrophoresis were then made 5% with merca-
ptoethanol and heated at 60°C for 1 hour
before being applied to 7% acrylamide-0.14%,
N,N'-diallyltartardiamide (DATD) gels containing 0.1% sodium dodecylsulfate and 0.5M urea
as described by Clark (11). The radioactivity
in the α1 and α2 peaks were 14,870 dpm and
5,960 dpm respectively.

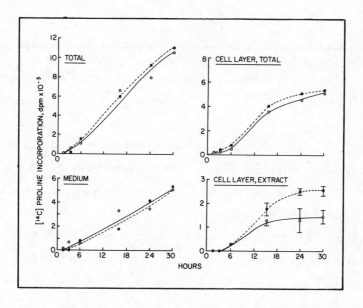

FIG. 3. Effects of parathormone on collagen
metabolism in PT cells. 1 x 10⁵ cells were
grown in Minimum Essential Medium containing
10% fetal calf serum, 0.57 mM ascorbic acid
and (^{14}C) proline (0.5 µCi/ml) with (o---o)
or without (o---o) 2 x 10⁸M parathormone.
After 30 hours the medium was removed. The
cell layer was frozen and extracted 3 times
with 5 ml of phosphate buffered saline.
These washes were pooled to give the cell
layer extract fraction. Collagen in the
medium, cell layer extract, and cell layer
residue was assayed as acid-precipitable
collagenase-digestible radioactivity in 2
mM Tris, pH 7.2, containing 20 µg/ml N-
ethylmaleimide, and 2 units/ml of purified
bacterial collagenase (Sigma). The cell
layer total is the sum of the extract and
residue fractions. Each point is the average
of 6 cultures.

TABLE III

Effects of parathormone on collagen yield in the absence or presence of serum

PT cells were subdivided into multiwell dishes (1 x 10^5 cells per well) and cultured overnight in Minimum Essential Medium containing 10% fetal calf serum and 0.57 mM ascorbic acid. The experiment was initiated by the addition of fresh medium containing 0.57 mM ascorbic acid, $[^{14}C]$-proline (1,0 μCi/ml) and, where indicated, either or both 10% fetal calf serum and 2 x 10^{-8}M parathormone. Incubation was continued for 30 hours. Collagen in the medium, cell layer extract and residue was assayed as described in Fig. 3.

Collagen Fraction	− Serum (dpm x 10^3)		+ Serum (dpm x 10^3)	
	Control	Parathormone	Control	Parathormone
Total	7.2 ± 0.9	3.5 ± 0.4	10 ± 1.6	11.0 ± 0.7
Medium	3.2 ± 0.3	1.7 ± 0.2	5.0 ± 0.5	5.4 ± 0.6
Cell Layer	4.0 ± 0.8	2.2 ± 0.3	5.0 ± 1.5	5.6 ± 0.3
% Extractable	20 ± 6	36 ± 7	28 ± 7	50 ± 4

In order to determine if the effect of parathormone on decreasing the yield of collagen in the absence of serum was due
to a decrease in rate of synthesis or an increase in the rate of
degradation, or both, we performed pulse and chase experiments in
the PT cells. Table IV indicates that parathormone did not
affect the rate of collagen synthesis at any period up to 25
hours after exposure to the hormone. Identical results were
obtained when the experiments were performed in the presence of
serum. In the chase experiments, on the other hand, while parathormone did not affect the loss of previously synthesized
radioactive collagen in cultures containing serum, it stimulated
its degradation in those cultures in which serum was absent (Fig.
4).

Discussion

The present results show that the PT cells manufacture a
substantial amount of collagen compared to the CT cells. This
finding reinforces our assumption that the PT cells are osteoblasts or osteoblast-related (3) and thus may represent valid
in vitro models for studying those aspects of bone metabolism
that are under osteoblastic control.

Our data also provide some new insight into the action of
parathormone on collagen metabolism in the PT cells. The data
reveal that parathormone caused a substantial increase in degradation of collagen when serum was omitted from the incubation
medium. This action of the hormone might be due to a direct
effect on the PT cells themselves or on osteoclast-like CT cells
that might be present as a contaminant in somewhat heterogeneous
PT populations. In either case the accelerated degradation of
collagen most likely was catalyzed by collagenase-like activity.
It has been reported that $\alpha 2$ macroglobulins present in serum can
inhibit the action of collagenase (8). Such an inhibition could
account for the failure to observe an increased degradation of
collagen in parathormone-treated cells when serum was present.
If enhanced collagenase activity were still expressed under these
latter conditions, (albeit much inhibited), this might have
modified the compactness of the cell layer matrix and could
account for its greater extractability. On the other hand, the
increased extractability could be due to undefined changes including a diminution in cross-linking of extracellular collagen
strands (9) or a change in other factors responsible for the
aggregation of collagen and other macromolecules in the culture
dish.

Based on these and our previous results (3,4), it is
attractive to speculate that the parathormone-induced acceleration of collagen degradation in the PT cells plays a role in the
overall breakdown of matrix during parathormone-induced bone
resorption. If the effect of the hormone is on the PT cells
themselves, we may postulate that brief exposure to parathormone
leads to resorption of both mineral and matrix by the osteoclasts
and increases the solubility and possibly the rate of destruction
of newly formed collagen by the osteoblasts. This may then be
followed by inhibition of precursor cell differentiation into

TABLE IV

Lack of effect of parathormone on rate of collagen synthesis

Replicate cultures of PT bone cells were permitted to attach overnight in Minimum Essential Medium containing 10% fetal calf serum and 0.57 mM ascorbic acid. Fresh medium containing no serum, 0.57 mM ascorbic acid and, where indicated, parathormone (2×10^{-8}M) was added at 0 hours. At various times thereafter, [^{14}C]proline was added to a final concentration of 1.0 μCi/ml for 90 min, and the collagen synthesized during that pulse was assayed as collagenase digestible radioactivity.

Culture Period	[^{14}C]Proline Incorporated (Dpa)	
hrs	Control	+ Parathormone
3	3,200 ± 500	3,000 ± 800
7	2,900 ± 600	3,250 ± 250
18	4,400 ± 500	5,000 ± 200
25	3,700 ± 150	3,900 ± 400

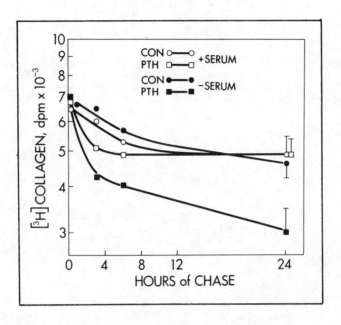

FIG. 4. Effects of parathormone on the degradation of radioactive collagen by PT cells cultured
in the presence or absence of serum. Cultures
of 1 x 10⁵ PT cells were precultured for 24
hours in Minimum Essential Medium containing 0.57
mM ascorbic acid, 10% fetal calf serum, and where
indicated, 2 x 10⁻⁸M parathormone. The medium
was removed and replaced with either Minimum
Essential Medium alone or with 2 x 10⁻⁸M parathormone
and with or without 10% fetal calf serum, all
containing (³H) proline (50 µCi/ml). Culture
was resumed for 70 minutes (pulse) at which
time radioactive medium was removed. The cells
were rinsed thrice with Minimum Essential
Medium containing 1 mM proline and then culture
was resumed for up to 24 hours of chase in
the same medium for the pulse except for the absence
of radioactive proline. Note that the ordinate
is a logarithmic scale.

osteoblasts (10), resulting in a marked decrease in collagen synthesis, as shown when bones are cultured for two weeks in parathyroid hormone (6).

REFERENCES

1. Wong, G. and D.V. Cohn 1974. Separation of parathyroid hormone and calcitonin-sensitive cells from non-responsive bone cells. Nature, 252, 713-715.

2. Wong, G.L. and D.V. Cohn 1975. Target cells in bone for parathormone and calcitonin are different: Enrichment for each cell type by sequential digestion of mouse calvaria and selective adhesion to polymeric surfaces. Proc. Natl. Acad. Sci. U.S.A., 72, 3167-3171.

3. Luben, R.A. and D.V. Cohn 1976. Effects of parathormone and calcitonin on citrate and hyaluronate metabolism in cultured bone. Endocrinology, 98, 413-419.

4. Luben, R.A., G.L. Wong and D.V. Cohn 1977. Parathormone-stimulated resorption of devitalized bone by cultured osteoblast-type bone cells. Nature, 265, 629-630.

5. Peterkofsky, B. and R. Diegelmann 1971. Use of a mixture of proteinase-free collagenases for the specific assay of radio-active collagen in the presence of other proteins. Biochemistry, 10, 988-994.

6. Goldhaber, P., B.D. Stern, M.J. Glimcher and J. Chao 1968. The effects of parathyroid extract and thyrocalcitonin on bone remodeling in tissue culture. In Parathyroid Hormone and Thyrocalcitonin (Calcitonin), R.V. Talmage and L.F. Belanger, eds. Excerpta Medica Foundation, Amsterdam, pp. 182-195.

7. Dietrich, J.W., E.M. Canalis, D.M. Maina and L.G. Raisz 1976. Hormonal control of bone collagen synthesis in vitro: Effects of parathyroid hormone and calcitonin. Endocrino-logy, 98, 943-949.

8. Reynolds, J.D. and Z. Werb 1975. The relation of phagocyto-sis to the secretion of non-lysosomal enzymes by connective tissue cells. In Extracellular Matrix Influences on Gene Expression, H.C. Slavkin and R.C. Greulich, editors. Academic Press, New York, pp. 225-230.

9. Levene, C.I., S. Shoshan and C.J. Bates 1972. The effect of ascorbic acid on the cross-linking of collagen during its synthesis by cultured 3T6 fibroblasts. Biochem, Biophys. Acta, 257, 384-388.

10. Gaillard, P.J. 1965. Observations on the effect of para-thyroid products on explanted mouse limb-bone rudiments. In Parathyroid Glands, P.J. Gaillard, R.V. Talmage and A.M. Budy, editors. Univ. Chicago Press, pp. 145-169.

11. Clark, C.C. 1976. Separation of collagen components by acrylamide gel electrophoresis. In The Methodology of Connective Tissue Research, D.A. Hall, editor. Joynson-Bruvvers Ltd, Oxford, pp. 205-226.

Attachment of Bone Cells to Collagen.

Hynda K. Kleinman, J. Clifford Murray, Ermona B. McGoodwin, George R. Martin and Itzhak Binderman.

Laboratory of Developmental Biology and Anomalies, National Institute of Dental Research, Bethesda, MD 20014

Summary

Prior studies have shown that attachment to collagen of cells from such established lines as 3T3, SV3T3 and CHO is mediated by a glycoprotein, c-CAP (cell attachment protein) which is made by cells and which is also present in serum. Primary cultures of periosteum cells were also found to require serum for attachment to collagen. CSP, a cell surface glycoprotein presumed to be the precursor of the serum glycoprotein also promoted attachment. Osteosarcoma cells adhered poorly to collagen even in the presence of serum. Only these adherent cells (35% of the total) were found to be tumorigenic. A central role for c-CAP in the differentiation, growth and resorption of bone is suggested.

Introduction

In addition to its structural role, collagen has other effects on cells with which it interacts. For example, (i) a greater cellular outgrowth occurs from tissues cultured on collagen substrates than on artificial substrates such as glass or plastic (1). (ii) Cells become senescent less rapidly when cultured on collagen (2). Collagen also affects (iii) the morphology of cells in culture (3) and (iv) increases the rate and extent of attachment (4). Hauschka and Konigsberg (5) found that (v) myoblast cells require a collagen substrate in vitro to differentiate into multinucleated muscle fibers. Certain CNBr peptides of type I collagen, $\alpha 1(I)$-CB7, and to a lesser extent, $\alpha 1(I)$-CB8, are active in promoting myogenesis (6) suggesting that the effect is specific. Ketley et al. (7) carried out related studies testing the ability of various collagen types (I-IV) to stimulate myogenesis. They found equal myogenic inducing activity with all collagen types, but non-collagenous proteins were inactive. (vi) Collagen fibers will also induce the aggregation of platelets (8).

Recently Klebe (4) reported that cells do not bind directly to collagen but that a high molecular weight serum derived glycoprotein, c-CAP (collagen cell attachment protein), binds the cells to collagen. There are three requirements for the attachment of cells to collagen. c-CAP first binds to collagen substrate. In the presence of Ca^{++} or Mg^{++} the cells then bind to the c-CAP-collagen complex. Metabolic energy is required to maintain a long term attachment to the c-CAP-collagen complex. These events are summarized in figure 1.

Serum-derived c-CAP is a high molecular weight glycoprotein with subunits linked by disulfide bonds. Pearlstein (9) suggested tht c-CAP is identical to cell surface protein, CSP (10), the major protein on the fibroblast cell surface. This protein or family of proteins is also known as LETS (11), fibronectin (12) etc. Chemically and antigenically these proteins resemble cold insoluble globulin (13,14). A variety of investigators have studied this glycoprotein and many of its properties are known. It is constantly shed into the culture medium (12). Although it is sensitive to trypsin (10), it is resynthesized one hour after enzyme treatment (10). After viral transformation this glycoprotein is almost totally absent from the cell surface (hence the name LETS, large external transformation sensitive protein) (11) but its absence may not be due to a reduced rate of synthesis (15). When LETS is added exogenously to transformed cells in vitro the cells spread and resemble more closely their non-transformed counterparts (16). However, the growth rate and tumorigenicity are unaffected (17).

We were interested in determining whether c-CAP binds to a specific site on the collagen molecule. Since the binding of c-CAP to collagen-coated dishes was inhibited by prior incubation of the serum with collagen or collagen peptides, it was possible to assay for the binding site. Such studies on type I collagen revealed that the $\alpha 1(I)$ chain was more active in binding c-CAP than the $\alpha 2$ chain (18). Cyanogen bromide digestion of the $\alpha 1(I)$ chain resulted in some loss of activity but two peptides, $\alpha 1(I)$-CB7, $\alpha 1(I)$-CB8, were found to contain activity; $\alpha 1(I)$-CB7 contained 80% of the activity while $\alpha 1(I)$-CB8 contained the remainder. Both peptides are similar in molecular weight ($\sim$24,000) and lack carbohydrate. Type II collagen was also found to be active. A peptide homologous to $\alpha 1(I)$-CB7, $\alpha 1(II)$-CB10, was found to contain the c-CAP binding site. Subsequently, employing proteolytic digestion of $\alpha 1(I)$-CB7, we isolated a fragment comprising residues 758-791 which is active in binding c-CAP (Kleinman et al., unpublished observations). Cleavage of the bond between residues 779-780 by chymotrypsin destroyed the activity. In addition, digestion of native collagen with animal collagenase destroyed activity, suggesting the importance of the bond at residues 775-776. These results are schematically summarized in figure 2. A portion of this region of the collagen chain (residues 774-785) is unique for a helical segment since both proline and hydroxyproline are lacking. This might lead to a less stable helix (19), thus allowing a specific sequence of amino acids to react with c-CAP.

Little is known about the specificity of attachment of different kinds of cells to the various types of collagen. Since different collagens show a tissue specific location, it

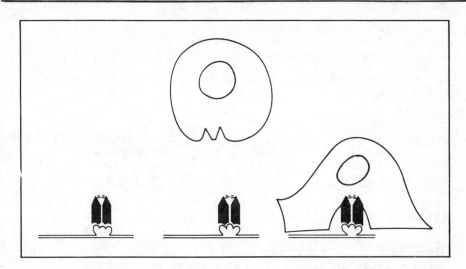

Figure 1.   Schematic model of major events in cell attachment.
First, c-CAP which contains disulfide bonds binds to
a specific site on the collagen chain.   Next a
freshly trypsinized cell lacking the attachment protein from its cell surface contacts the c-CAP-
collagen complex.   Finally, the cell flattens in
the presence of ATP and divalent cations.

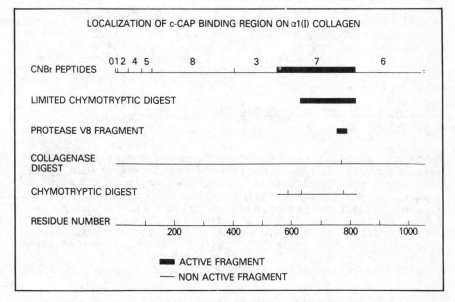

Figure 2.   Localization of c-CAP binding region along the
α1(I) chain of type I collagen.   Active fragments: ▬
and petide bond cleavage sites: ┴ .

is possible that some cells might produce a c-CAP specific for
the type of collagen which they synthesize. In this study we
have examined the attachment of periosteum cells and osteosarcoma cells to various types of collagen. Marked differences
were noted between the attachment properties of periosteal
cells and osteosarcoma cells.

Materials and Methods

Preparation of collagen. Type I collagen was prepared from the
skins of lathyritic rats (20), type II collagen from a rat
chondrosarcoma (21), type III collagen from a pepsin digest
of fetal calf skin (22), and type IV collagen from a murine
tumor producing a basement membrane-like matrix (23). Reduced
and methylated Ascaris lumbricoides cuticle collagen was a
gift of Ms. Catherine Sullivan (24).

Preparation of collagen-coated petri dishes. Collagen was dissolved in 0.5 N acetic acid (1 mg/ml) and stored at 20° until
needed. Stock solutions of the collagen were diluted with
water, 10 µg was applied to a 35 mm bacteriological plate and
alowed to dry.

Cell attachment assay. The attachment of cells was measured as
previously described (4). One ml of Eagles minimal essential
medium (MEM) containing 200 µg of bovine serum albumin and
varying amounts of bovine serum were added to the petri dish
and incubated for one hour at 37° in the presence of 95% air
and 5% CO_2. The cells (usually 10^5) suspended in MEM were
subsequently added to the plate in Eagles MEM and incubated for
an additional 1.5 hours to permit attachment. After incubation,
the unattached cells were decanted and the surface of the dish
was washed three times with 0.02 m phosphate buffered saline
(PBS), pH 7.2. The attached cells were then removed enzymatically (0.1% trypsin, 0.1% EDTA in PBS) and counted in a Coulter
counter (ZBI).

Preparation of periosteum and osteosarcoma cells. Rat periosteum cells were obtained from calvaria of embryonic rats
(16-20 days of gestation). Calvaria comprising the frontal,
parietal and occupital bones were removed washed in PBS and
separated by scraping into periosteum and bone proper. The
periosteum was minced with scissors and disaggregated by incubation for 0.5 hours at 37° with a solution of 0.2% collagenase, as previously described (25). The cells were harvested
by centrifugation, resuspended in culture medium and plated at
2.5×10^5 cells per 35 mm Falcon tissue culture dish. Cultures
were maintained in a humid atmosphere of 95% air, 5% CO_2.
Some cells were grown in BGJ_G medium (26) supplemented with
10% fetal calf serum. The medium was replaced every 3-4 days.
Usually the cells became confluent during the first week in
culture.

The osteosarcoma, type R-355Y/52A, originally raised at
Panicolaou Cancer Institute was given to us by Dr. G.A. Rodan
of the University of Connecticut. The tumor, which is grown

in ACI rats, was removed, digested with collagenase and cultured as described above.

A study was made to determine whether there was a difference between osteosarcoma cells which adhered to collagen and those that did not adhere with respect to their ability to produce tumors in rats. Cultures of osteosarcoma cells were trypsinized and allowed to attach on petri plates coated with type I collagen in the presence of 1% serum. After 1.5 hours the unattached cells were removed, collected by centrifugation and resuspended in MEM at a concentration of 10^6 cells/ml. The attached cells were removed with a rubber policeman and treated similarily. Cell viability as measured by trypan blue exclusion was found to be 75% for the unattached cells and 95% for the attached. One ml of the cell suspension (which is ten fold excess more cells than is required to yield tumors) was injected subcutaneously into either side of ACI rats in a manner similar to that by which this tumor is maintained.

Results

The binding of periosteum cells to collagen substrates was examined under a variety of serum conditions. As illustrated in figure 3, the attachment of these cells to collagen was markedly stimulated by pretreatment of the collagen-coated dishes with MEM containing serum. Most cells (85%) attached after pretreatment with 10% serum, the highest concentration tested. In the absence of a collagen substrate, increasing serum concentrations caused some stimulation of cell attachment to the plastic surface. However, under those conditions the cells did not flatten. No clear difference was observed in the extent of binding of the cells to any of the four collagen types, and complete attachment was seen on each.
Purified CSP (a gift of Dr. K. Yamada, NCI) was tested for its ability to promote cell attachment. As illustrated in figure 4, in the absence of serum 5-15 µg of CSP was capable of promoting cell attachment to the same extent as 5% serum (see ⊘ in figure 4). Under these conditions the cells also failed to show any clear preference among types I-IV collagen substrates. Ascaris collagen, in contrast, supported less attachment than untreated plastic.

The attachment properties of the periosteum cells and cultured osteosarcoma cells were compared. Both cell types were found to adhere at a similar rate with maximal attachment reached within one hour (not shown). However, as illustrated in figure 5, the attachment of the osteosarcoma cells was not stimulated by serum. In addition, in the absence of serum the osteosarcoma cells appeared slightly less adherent than the periosteum cells. No specificity for any collagen type was found. Neither type of cell appeared to bind well to ascaris collagen.

The osteosarcoma cells which adhered to collagen were tested for the strength of adhesion as judged by the rate at

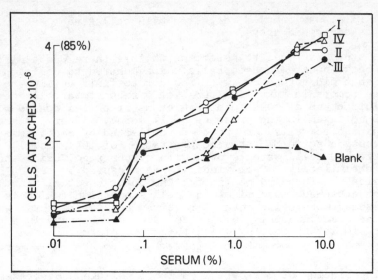

Figure 3. Attachment of periosteum cells to collagen types I, II, III, and IV in the presence of increasing concentrations of serum. Control bacteriological plates contained no collagen.

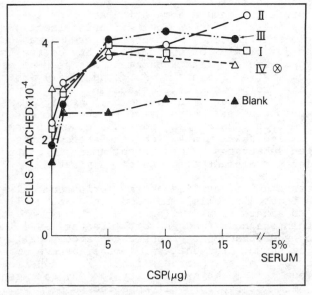

Figure 4. Attachment of periosteum cells to types I, II, III and IV collagens in the presence of increasing amounts of CSP. Control bacteriological plates contained no collagen. For comparison, cell attachment on type I collagen in the presence of 5% serum was also assayed (⊗).

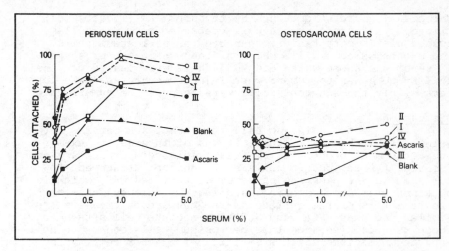

Figure 5. Attachment of periosteum and osteosarcoma cells to types I, II, III and IV collagens, ascaris collagen and uncoated plates in the presence of increasing serum concentrations.

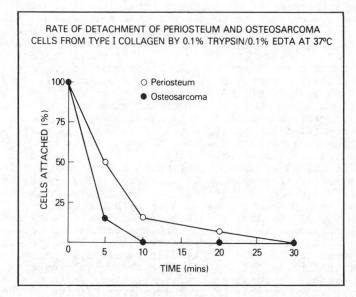

Figure 6. Rate of detachment from type I collagen of periosteum and osteosarcoma cells with trypsin-EDTA. After 1.5 hours in the presence of 1% serum, the cells were washed three times with phosphate buffered saline, pH 7.2, and incubated with 0.1% trypsin, 0.1% EDTA. At the times shown the released cells were counted electronically.

which they could be detached by trypsin. As illustrated in figure 6, the osteosarcoma cells detached from the collagen coated plates more rapidly than did the periosteum cells. Those osteosarcoma cells which did adhere in the presence of 1% serum and those which did not adhere were tested for their ability to generate tumors when injected subcutaneously into rats. Only the adherent cells were found to be tumorigenic.

Discussion

Since most studies on cell attachment are carried out using established cell lines, it was of interest to examine the attachment properties of freshly dissociated primary cells. Cultured rat periosteum cells show enhanced attachment to collagen in the presence of serum or purified CSP, which is obtained from chick embryo fibroblasts. This suggests that the receptors on the surface of the rat and chick cells are similar and that c-CAP and SCP both mediate cell attachment. These results also show that periosteum cells adhere to collagen via mechanisms which are similar for other cell types. In these studies the cells showed no preference among the various types of collagen. These cells did not bind well to ascaris collagen, a collagen similar in composition to other collagens. Previously, ascaris collagen was found to be inactive as a substrate for the attachment of a variety of other cell types and to be inactive in promoting myogenesis.

The attachment of osteosarcoma cells was also examined to determine how transformation alters this phenomenon. Cultured tumor cells are known to have reduced levels of the LETS protein (27), increased levels of proteolytic enzymes (28) and a reduced serum requirement for growth. It was therefore expected that tumor cells might behave differently in the attachment assay. A small proportion of the osteosarcoma cells did adhere irrespective of the presence or absence of serum but there was no enhancement of attachment with serum as is seen with the periosteum cells as well as with hepatocytes and skin fibroblasts (Kleinman et al., unpublished observations). It is interesting to note that only the adherent cells produced tumors in rats. Since the binding of the osteosarcoma cells was not inhibited by serum, they may not have been binding to the c-CAP-collagen complex. If there were binding to the collagent via c-CAP on their cell surface, serum might have decreased cell attachment as is seen with chondrocytes (Kleinman et al., unpublished observations). Since osteosarcoma cells synthesize more collagen than the periosteum cells (Binderman et al, unpublished observations), it is possible that trypsin treatment did not fully remove all the collagen or c-CAP or that these cells synthesize these proteins at a rapid rate. Therefore, a small proportion of these cells may "recover" more quickly and establish themselves irrespective of the substrate composition, a characteristic consistent with their tumorigenicity. In this respect, osteosarcoma cells showed enhanced attachment with serum on uncoated bacteriological plates to a similar level to that observed on a collagen substrate.

The failure of a large number of osteosarcoma cells to attach is not due to a decrease in cell viability since 95% of the osteosarcoma cells are viable as determined by trypan blue exclusion. Studies are in progress to determine the type of collagen synthesized by these cells, their cell surface proteins and cell associated proteases.

The above data suggest c-CAP may play a vital role in bone formation and destruction. Specific c-CAPs produced by cells may determine the manner in which collagen matrices are colonized by various cell types. c-CAP could therefore determine the course of differentiation of cell population. Finally, since c-CAP and collagenase recognize the same site on collagen, these two substances may be involved in the regulation of collagen degradation.

References

1. Ehrmann, R.L. and Gey, G.C. 1956. The growth of cells on a transparent gel of reconstituted rat tail collagen. J. Nat. Cancer Inst., 16, 1375-1390.

2. Gey, G.C., Svotelis, M., Foard, M. and Bang, F.B. 1974. Long term growth of chicken fibroblasts on a collagen substrate. Exptl. Cell Res., 84, 63-71.

3. Weiss, P. 1961. Guiding principles in cell locomotion and cell aggregation. Exptl. Cell Res., 25 (suppl. 8), 260-281.

4. Klebe, R.J. 1974. Isolation of collagen-dependent cell attachment factor. Nature, 250, 248-251.

5. Hauschka, S.D. and Konigsberg, I.R. 1966. The influence of collagen on the development of muscle clones. Proc. Nat. Acad. Sci., USA, 55, 119-126.

6. Hauschka, S.D. and White, N.K. 1972. In: Research Concepts in Muscle Development and the Muscle Spindle, eds. Banker, B., Preyoylyski, R., and Van der Meulen, J., and Victor, M., pp. 53-71. Excerpta Medica, Amsterdam.

7. Ketley, J.N., Orkin, R.W. and Martin, G.R. 1976. Collagen in developing chick muscle in vivo and in vitro. Exptl. Cell Res., 99, 261-268.

8. Zucker, M.B. 1972. In: Hematology, eds., Williams, W.J., Beutler, E., Erslow, A.J. and Rundle, R.W., p. 1014, McGraw Hill, New York.

9. Pearlstein, E. 1976. Plasma membrane glycoprotein which mediates adhesion of fibroblasts to collagen. Nature, 262, 497-500.

10. Yamada, K.M. and Weston, J.A. 1974. Isolation of a major cell surface glycoprotein from fibroblasts. Proc. Nat. Acad. Sci., USA, 71, 3492-3496.

11. Hynes, R.C. 1973. Alteration of cell-surface proteins by viral transformation and proteolysis. Proc. Nat. Acad. Sci., USA, 70, 3170-3174.

12. Rouslahti, E., Vaheri, A., Kuusela, P. and Linder, E. 1973. Fibroblast surface antigen: a new serum protein. Biochim, Biophys. Acta, 322, 352-358.

13. Mossesson, M.W., Chen, L.B. and Huseby, R.M. 1975. The cold-insoluble globulin in human plasma: studies of its essential features. Biochim, Biophys. Acta, 386, 509-524.

14. Rouslahti, E. and Vaheri, A. 1975. Interaction of

soluble fibroblast surface antigen with fibrinogen and fibrin. Identity with cold insoluble globulin of human plasma. J. Exptl. Med., 141, 497-501.

15. Vaheri, A., Rouslahti, E., Westermark, B. and Pontén, J. 1976. A common cell type specific surface antigen in cultured glial cells and fibroblasts: loss in malignant cells. J. Exptl. Med., 143, 64-72.

16. Ali, I.U., Mautner, V., Lanza, R. and Hynes, R.C. 1977. Restoration of normal morphology, adhesion and cytoskeleton sensitive surface protein. Cell, 11, 115-126.

17. Willingham, M.C., Yamada, K.M., Yamada, S.S., Pousségur, J. and Pastan, I. 1977. Microfilament bundles and cell shape are related to adhesiveness to substratum and are dissociable from growth control in cultured fibroblasts. Cell, 10, 375-380.

18. Kleinman, H.K., McGoodwin, E.B. and Klebe, R.J. 1976. Localization of the cell attachment region in types I and II collagens. Biochem. Biophys. Res. Commun., 72, 426-432.

19. Ramachandran, G.N. and Ramakrishan, C. 1976. In: Biochemistry of Collagen, eds., Ramachandran, G.N. and Reddi, A.H., pp. 45-81, Plenum Press, New York.

20. Bornstein, P. and Piez, K.A. 1966. The nature of the intramolecular cross-links on collagen. The separation and characterization of peptides from the cross-link region of rat skin collagen. Biochemistry, 5, 3460-3473.

21. Smith, B.D., Martin, G.R., Miller, E.J., Dorfman, A. and Swarm, R. 1975. Nature of the collagen synthesized by a transplanted chondrosarcoma. Archiv. Biochem. Biophys. 166, 181-186.

22. Epstein, E. 1974 $[\alpha 1(III)]_3$ Human skin collagen. Release by pepsin digestion and preponderance in fetal life. J. Biol. Chem., 249, 3225-3231.

23. Orkin, R.W., Gehron, P., McGoodwin, E.B., Martin, G.R., Valentine, T. and Swarm, R. 1977. A murine tumor producing a matrix of basement membrane. J. Exptl. Med., 145, 204-219.

24. Evans, H.J., Sullivan, C.E. and Piez, K.A. 1976. The resolution of Ascaris cuticle collagen into three chains. Biochemistry, 15, 1435-1439.

25. Peck, W.A., Birge, S.J. and Fedak, S.A. 1964. Bone cells: biochemical and biological studies after enzymatic isolation. Science, 146, 1476-1473.

26. Binderman, I., Duksin, D., Hasell, A., Katzir (Katchalski), E., Sachs, L. 1974. Formation of bone tissue in culture

from isolated bone cells. J. Cell Biol., 61, 427-439.

27. Chen, L.B., Gallimore, P.H. and McDougall, J.K. 1976.
    Correlation between tumor induction and the large external
    transformation sensitive protein on the cell surface.
    Proc. Nat. Acad. Sci., USA, 73, 3570-3574.

28. Unkeless, J.C., Tobin., A., Ossowski, L., Quigley, J.A.,
    Rifkin, D. and Reich, E. 1973. An enzymatic function
    associated with transformation of fibroblasts by oncognic
    viruses. J. Exptl. Med., 137, 85-115.

The Demand for Bone Calcium in Maintenance of Plasma Calcium
Concentrations

Roy V. Talmage, Stephen A. Grubb, Carole J. Vander Wiel, Samuel
H. Doppelt, and Hiromichi Norimatsu

Department of Surgery, Orthopaedic Research Laboratories,
School of Medicine, University of North Carolina,
Chapel Hill, North Carolina 27514

An eighty-five year old woman was rushed from an outlying
clinic to the State Hospital. She was reported to have plasma
calcium concentrations in the range of 18 mg/100 ml. Before
the House Staff could lower her plasma calcium, she underwent
cardiac arrest. Autopsy identified a parathyroid adenoma. A
cyst in the gland had recently hemmorhaged and there was evidence that similar episodes had occurred in the past. However,
her bone structure was excellent for a woman her age, and
showed none of the typical signs of osteitis fibrosa cystica.
Resorption centers and osteoclast numbers appeared normal.

The thesis we would like to discuss in this report is as
follows: 1) with adequate exogenous calcium supplies plasma
calcium concentrations are controlled by balancing the rates of
calcium efflux and influx between blood and bone fluid; 2)
the primary first source of calcium used by parathyroid hormone
(PTH) in maintaining plasma calcium is obtained from bone
fluid and the surfaces of bone; and 3) only when these supplies
are exhausted will PTH call on bone resorptive processes for
the needed calcium.

The concept that bone surfaces supply calcium for body
fluids is certainly not new. In 1933, Hastings and Huggins
(1) reported that if blood, decalcified with lead phosphate,
was returned to its donor (dogs), the temporary drop in circulating plasma calcium levels due to the infusion of low
calcium blood was quickly corrected. In control dogs, the
plasma level for this cation returned rapidly to normal
(+10 mg/100 ml). If the dogs had been previously thyroparathyroidectomized (TPTX), the plasma calcium returned to its
previous level (in the range of 6 to 7 mg/100 ml). These
studies were confirmed in rats by Copp et al.(2) using versene
(EDTA) infusion and by our group (3) using the peritoneal
lavage technique. In 1955, McLean and Urist (4) reported
their postulate correlating a negative feedback control for
parathyroid hormone secretion with a "basic" equilibrating
process between calcium in blood and in bone. Although they
later suggested (5) that this basic process involved some
cellular activity in bone, they concluded that the difference
in the basic and normal plasma calcium levels was due to parathyroid hormone action on osteoclastic bone resorption. This

concept soon became dogma; a dogma which we vigorously supported for many years. Our present view differs from this
McLean and Urist model by suggesting that under normal physiological conditions, in the presence of adequate dietary calcium,
parathyroid hormone action is merely to increase the activity
of the basic process. This process consists of controlling the
rates of calicum efflux and influx between blood and bone fluid.

We reported experiments years ago in which we took great
pains to try to explain our results by the osteoclastic bone
resorption model. In our earliest studies, using continuous
peritoneal lavage, (3) we reported that in 200 gm parathyroidectomized rats, it was possible to remove calcium from
bone at the rates up to 13 mg/k/hr. without stimulating osteoclastic proliferation. In the presence of the parathyroid
glands, this rate, from the first peritoneal lavage period
before increased osteoclastic activity could be identified,
was increased to and maintained at a maximum rate of 16 mg/k/hr.

Working with Elliott, (6) we compared the effect of citrate administration to that of PTH. The rats were administered
^{45}Ca either 1 day or 10 days prior to the citrate or PTH. The
effects of citrate on plasma ^{45}Ca changes in both the "1 day"
and "10 day" radioisotope pretreated conditions were identical
to those produced by PTH. Since at that time we were advocat-
ing that PTH procured its calcium by resorbing so-called "deep"
bone, we therefore reported in amazement that somehow citrate
must be able to reach these same specific areas of bone. How
much more rational the explanation would have been if we had
concluded that the similarity in results was due to the fact
that both citrate and parathyroid hormone procured their calcium from the surfaces of bone. It took the aging process to
heed the words of the late American humorist and philosopher,
Josh Billings, "I have lived in this world just long enough to
look carefully the second time into things I was most certain
of the first time".

Two studies reported by our group in 1965 refocused our
thoughts and led to the formulation of our current concepts.
The first study was by Cooper et al. (7) in which it was reported that control of plasma calcium concentrations appeared to
reside primarily in compact bone which has a low density of
osteoclasts, rather than in trabecular bone where most osteoclasts are found. In the second report by Doty et al. (8)
parathyroid function was studied in rats injected 1-5 days previously with plutonium. As previously reported by Arnold and
Jee, (9) osteoclasts are damaged by plutonium and bone remodelling is inhibited. Osteoblasts are not damaged. In our rats,
the ability of PTH to maintain plasma calcium levels was not
affected, though the plutonium not only prevented the increase
in osteoclast numbers, but actually decreased the concentration
of these cells. Those remaining were heavily burdened with
plutonium.

Our major problem when adhering to the McLean-Urist model
was in the interpretation of plasma ^{45}Ca data. We assumed

that if the radioactivity had been in the animal for days, and if an administered agent raised plasma ^{45}Ca levels, it meant that calcium was being derived from preformed "deep" bone. Rowland (10) clearly demonstrated that a large portion of injected ^{45}Ca (over 50%) was distributed throughout compact bone. Would not interpretations of plasma ^{45}Ca data be simplified if it were assumed that regardless of the time of injection of ^{45}Ca, it was the radioactivity on the surfaces of compact bone that produced the rapid changes in plasma ^{45}Ca activity? The diagram in Fig. 1 demonstrates this concept. This is a diagrammatic drawing of compact bone with lining cells and layers of osteocytes, each further removed from the primary extracellular fluid (ECF). The relative activity on the surfaces of bone are represented by the vertical bars on either side. The darker the bar the greater the ^{45}Ca concentration. The bar on the left represents this distribution a few hours after ^{45}Ca injection into fasted rats. The bar on the right represents the relative ^{45}Ca surface distribution a week or more later in rats maintained under normal feeding conditions. The difference in the two situations is due more to the result of entrance of unlabelled (cold) calcium into the system after the ^{45}Ca was administered, than due to the actual movement of ^{45}Ca deeper into bone. A very simple principle can be used as a basis for interpretation of rapid plasma ^{45}Ca changes regardless of when the radioactivity was administered. The ^{45}Ca specific activity (CPM ^{45}Ca/mg calcium) after injection remains higher in plasma than that on the surface of bone until unlabelled calcium enters plasma from exogenous sources. When unlabelled calcium enters the system, ^{45}Ca specific activity (^{45}Ca S.A.) in plasma will always be reduced and will eventually be lower than that on the surface of bone. This is illustrated in an experiment shown in Fig. 2. (11) In this experiment, a single dose of PTH was injected into TPTX rats which had been either fed or fasted overnight. ^{45}Ca was injected in one group of rats >6 days before PTH; in a second group it was injected only 18 hours before the hormone. In the fasted "18 hour" ^{45}Ca group, plasma ^{45}Ca S.A. falls rapidly after PTH because under this situation there is a marked difference between the pre-existing ^{45}Ca S.A. in plasma and the ^{45}Ca S.A. in bone fluid at the surface of bone (ECF >bone fluid). If the rats were fed, plasma ^{45}Ca S.A. was reduced and only slightly above that in bone fluid and the adjacent bone surfaces. Hence, PTH raised plasma calcium with only a minor drop in plasma ^{45}Ca S.A. (relative to controls). The opposite situation exists in the ">6 day" ^{45}Ca situation, where the differences in the specific activities in plasma and on the surface of bone are less in the fasted state and greater in the fed state. Therefore, in the fed state PTH will produce the greater change in ^{45}Ca S.A.

The above discussion is given as an explanation of what changes should occur if parathyroid hormone were acting at the surfaces of bone. This explanation might also be valid if PTH was using only preformed "deep" bone. An experiment demonstrating the involvement of surface calcium is illustrated

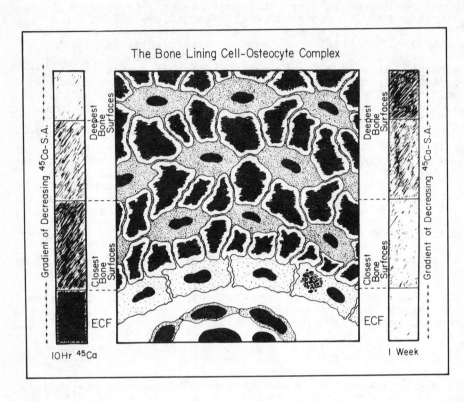

Figure 1. The distribution of ^{45}Ca in extracellular fluid and on the surfaces of bone. The osteocyte-lining cell complex (illustrated diagrammatically) is given in the center. The vertical bars on either side represent the relative amount of ^{45}Ca present in fluid and on the surfaces of bone at each location. The darker the shading, the greater the concentration of ^{45}Ca. The bar on the left represents the condition 10 hours after ^{45}Ca injection in fasted rats; on the right six or more days later in rats fed regularly.

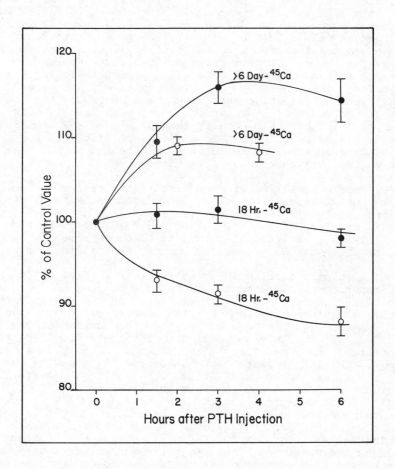

Figure 2. Plasma ^{45}Ca specific activity (^{45}Ca CPM/mg calcium) changes in fed and fasted rats following a single dose of parathyroid hormone. ● = fed rats. O = fasted rats. >6 day ^{45}Ca = ^{45}Ca given more than 6 days before injection of PTH. 18 hour ^{45}Ca = ^{45}Ca injected 18 hours before PTH injection. All values are normalized first to initial values and then to appropriate controls. (Taken from Ref. 11.)

in Fig. 3. (11) In this figure, plasma ^{45}Ca changes in CPM/ml following a single injection of PTH are summarized. PTH was injected 1 hour, 10 hours, or 18 hours, after injection of ^{45}Ca into TPTX rats. In each case, the immediate result was to increase the plasma ^{45}Ca content relative to controls being run concurrently. In the "1 hour" ^{45}Ca group, this was reflected as a net decrease in the rate of ^{45}Ca disappearance from plasma; in the "18 hour" ^{45}Ca group, there was an actual increase in the content of ^{45}Ca/ml of plasma following PTH injection. The important point is that if all data are illustrated as percent change from their controls, they fall on a single curve as shown in the lower right panel. Our interpretation of these data is that PTH in this acute situation is taking calcium from a single compartment; this compartment must be on the surface of bone and be the same as that which received calcium from blood.

In our next series of ^{45}Ca tracer studies, we would like to present experiments which we feel demonstrate that both PTH and calcitonin (CT) affect (in opposite directions) the rate of calcium efflux from bone fluid to blood. Therefore, they influence the rate of return to blood of some of that calcium which has most recently entered bone fluid from blood.

The primary calcitonin study is given in Fig. 4. (12). In this experiment, calcitonin infusion was started 10 hours after ^{45}Ca injection into fasted normal rats. At the start of the calcitonin infusion, plasma calcium levels fell rapidly and then remained constant at the lower concentration for the remainder of the infusion period. (These are not illustrated). In contrast there was a biphasic effect of CT on plasma ^{45}Ca levels. These fall faster than in control rats during the time when plasma calcium concentrations were falling. However, after the plasma calcium levels stabilize, plasma ^{45}Ca values in CT infused rats fell slower than controls. It was shown that this was not due to an effect of endogenous PTH in another experiment by infusion of CT into TPTX rats (Fig.5) (12). The initial fall in plasma ^{45}Ca levels during CT infusion could be the result of either an increased movement of ^{45}Ca from plasma or a decreased return of the isotope back to plasma. To demonstrate that this fall was not an increased movement of calcium from plasma, the radioactivity was injected one hour after CT infusion had begun (Fig. 6). (12) When this was done, continued CT infusion reduced the rate of loss of ^{45}Ca from plasma. This sequence of data is interpreted as showing that CT produces a decrease in the amount of ^{45}Ca returned to plasma during the period when plasma calcium is falling. Once the rates of calcium efflux and influx are equilibrated at lower levels, the rate of ^{45}Ca loss from plasma is reduced.

Parathyroid hormone infusion produces the opposite effect as can be seen in Fig. 7. (13) The time table for the development of the biphasic effect is considerably longer for PTH than for CT. The data clearly indicate that the rate of loss of ^{45}Ca from plasma is decreased (upper left panel) during the

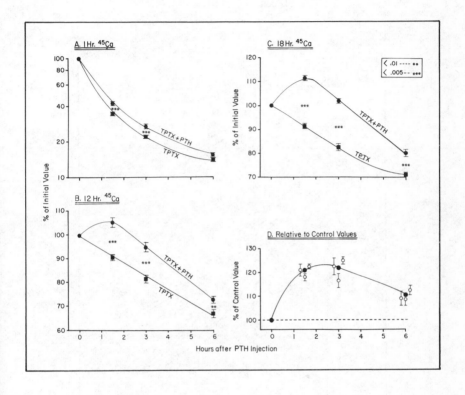

Figure 3. Observed plasma ^{45}Ca changes following PTH injection into fed thyroparathyroidectomized rats. A through C: ●
= PTH injected into TPTX rats; ▓ = TPTX control rats. All
values expressed as percent of initial value. Graph D: ●
= Average of values from A through C, corrected to the control
animals value. O = Averages of individual groups (A,B,C)
+ S.E. corrected to controls which are superimposed left to
right at each point: 1 hour ^{45}Ca; 12 hour ^{45}Ca; 18 hour ^{45}Ca.
(Taken from Ref. 11.)

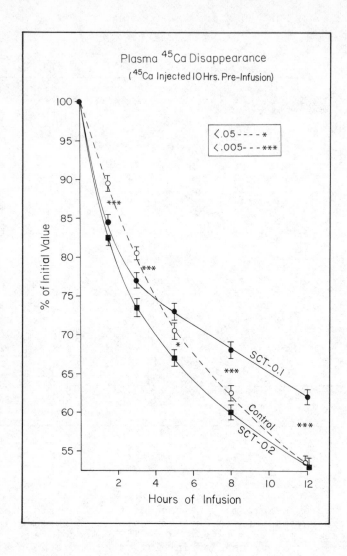

Figure 4. Plasma ^{45}Ca (-10 h) disappearance curves in calcitonin infused rats. ^{45}Ca injected 10 hours prior to start of infusion. Hormone dosage given in mU/g body weight/hour. All values expressed as percent of initial value. (Taken from Ref. 12.)

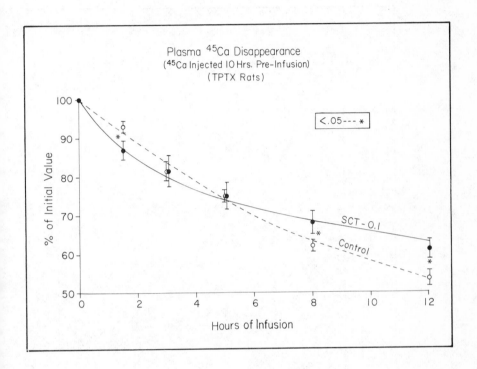

Figure 5. Plasma ^{45}Ca (-10 h) disappearance curves in calcitonin infused thyroparathyroidectomized rats. ^{45}Ca injected 10 hours prior to start of an infusion of 0.1 mU SCT/g body weight/hour. (Taken from Ref. 12.)

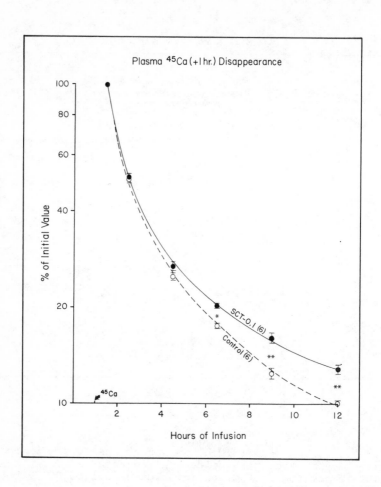

Figure 6. Plasma ^{45}Ca (+ 1 h) disappearance curves in calci-tonin-infused rats. ^{45}Ca was injected via intravenous catheter 1 hour after start of calcitonin infusion. Values expressed as percent of plasma sample obtained 1 hour later. Hormone dosage given in mU/g body weight/hour. * = p<0.025 ** = p<0.01 (Taken from Ref. 12.)

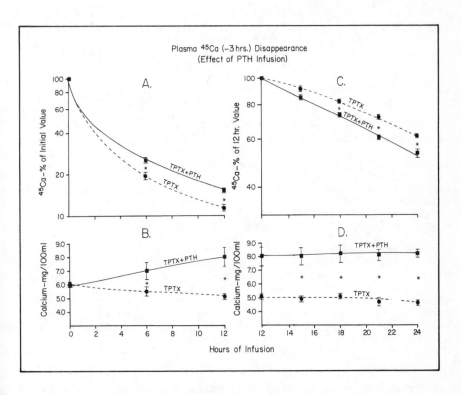

Figure 7. The effect of parathyroid infusion on plasma calcium and 45Ca (- 3 h) levels in thyroparathyroidectomized rats. In upper left panel, 45Ca values expressed as percent of pre-infusion plasma values. In upper right panel, 45Ca values expressed as percent of plasma values obtained after 12 hours of infusion. 45Ca injected 3 hours prior to start of infusion. Lower panels demonstrate plasma calcium values over the 24 hour infusion period. * = p <0.01. (Taken from Ref. 13.)

time in which plasma calcium levels are rising (lower left panel). After these concentrations stabilize (lower right panel) the rate of loss of ^{45}Ca from plasma becomes greater in PTH-infused rats (upper right panel).

We explain these data as follows: In the first phase of this biphasic ^{45}Ca response, calcium efflux from bone fluid is increased, returning a greater proportion of the ^{45}Ca entering bone fluid back to blood. This decreases the rate of net loss of the radionuclide from plasma. In the later stage, rates of both calcium efflux and influx are in equilibrium stabilizing the plasma calcium concentration at higher levels. Due to the elevated rate of cycling of calcium between blood and bone fluid, the diffusion of ^{45}Ca into bone is increased; thus, increasing its net rate of loss from plasma. The biphasic ^{45}Ca response to calcitonin is due to the reverse of the above process.

For our last series of ^{45}Ca tracer experiments, we would like to review our data on daily changes in plasma calcium and ^{45}Ca in rats maintained on a carefully controlled feeding schedule. Both plasma calcium concentrations and ^{45}Ca levels vary throughout the day in a cyclic manner determined by the feeding time of the rats. These results are summarized in Fig. 8. (14) The top panel summarizes data from normal rats, the bottom from parathyroidectomized animals. ^{45}Ca was injected at least one week before the cycling was monitored.

The drop in plasma calcium which occurs following the onset of feeding in normal rats is a phenomenon now under investigation. We believe it involves rapid changes in our calcium efflux system from bone fluid to plasma. It is probably produced through the involvement of gastrointestinal hormones. However, the role of the various hormones involved have not been clearly delineated. It is of interest to note that preliminary data indicate the same sequence occurs in human subjects under controlled conditions. Since this plasma calcium fall following feeding does not occur in parathyroidectomized rats (lower panel), it is tentatively assumed that in a normal rat a rapid drop in parathyroid secretion occurs at the time of feeding or its action on the calcium efflux system at the surface of bone is over-powered by other hormone activities. Though our evidence is insufficient, we favor the later possibility.

We would like to emphasize the plasma ^{45}Ca data in both panels. In normal rats, plasma ^{45}Ca (CPM/ml) values rose markedly during the fasting period, explained possibly by increased PTH activity. However, why is there a temporary rise in plasma ^{45}Ca levels at the start of the fasting period in rats without parathyroids? This occurs while plasma calcium concentrations are falling. A model explaining our concept is given in Fig. 9. (15) We assume that the calcium cycling process at the surface of bone is a basic process, and that the calcium entering bone fluid is mixed with that which is already there. The result is that some of the most recent

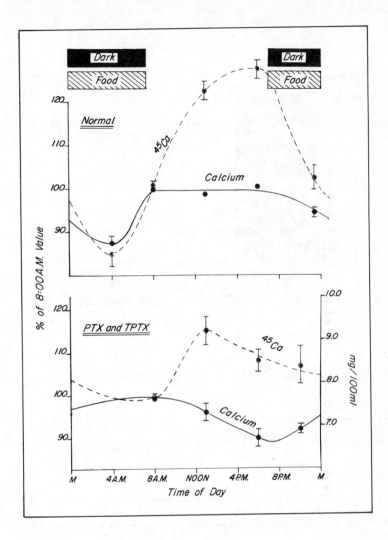

Figure 8. Plasma calcium and [45]Ca (>1 week) values during 24 hour period in rats maintained on controlled light and feeding periods. [45]Ca was injected at least one week before plasma sampling was started. Plasma [45]Ca values normalized to the 9 a.m. value each day to permit grouping of values. Top panel data are from normal rats; bottom panel represent average values from rats thyroparathyroidectomized for at least 1 week. (Taken from Refs. 14 and 15.)

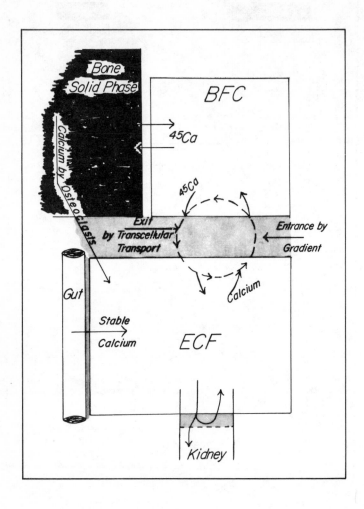

Figure 9. Diagrammatic model representing cycling of calcium and 45Ca between blood and fluid at the surfaces of bone. (Taken from Ref. 15.)

calcium to enter bone is that which is immediately returned to blood. In the PTX rat, as the source of unlabelled calcium decreases at the end of the feeding period, its entry into bone decreases, surface dilution of ^{45}Ca decreases but calcium efflux remains relatively constant. Therefore, it would be logical that at least temporarily, the actual amount of tagged calcium being returned to blood would be increased.

It is obvious that a concept such as that cannot rely solely on the interpretation of ^{45}Ca data. Other approaches to testing these hypotheses are in the literature and are being actively followed up. For example, there is no doubt that lining cells and osteocytes respond rapidly and characteristically to both parathyroid hormone and calcitonin. (16,17) We are extending these findings in our laboratory. Work in progress is also supporting a concept that calcium is stored on the surfaces of bone during feeding periods, which is readily available for use during fasting periods. We are beginning to be able to characterize these storage sites. Another important area is the role of phosphate in the action of PTH and calcitonin at the bone surfaces. Regretfully, time and space does not allow us to describe these relationships, but the role of phosphate must be important in any concept of calcium movements.

We would also be remiss if we did not identify what we feel are the two weakest aspects of our concepts. The first stems from the evidence that there is rapid extracellular movement of ions and large molecules between blood and bone fluids. This includes ions such as lanthanum, molecules such as horseradish perioxidase, and large organic entities known to synthesized in the liver. At the ultrastructural level it is easy to demonstrate that the channels between cells lining bone surfaces are open. These open channels between lining cells are required for our concept to be valid. However, if the channels are too large and uncontrolled, how can a calcium gradient between blood and bone fluid be maintained by a transcellular transport system yet to be identified? The lack of any good evidence for such a cellularly controlled transport system is the other uncertain aspect of our concepts. This is a troublesome point. However, even today, the method for transcellular transport of calcium across the intestinal mucosa is not thoroughly understood.

In conclusion, we have presented evidence that parathyroid hormone and calcitonin both influence plasma calcium concentrations by acting on cells lining the surfaces of bone and utilizing calcium supplies in bone fluid and on the surfaces of bone. We believe that under adequate exogenous calcium supplies and with the proper functioning of gastrointestinal hormones, parathyroid hormone, and calcitonin, this system can maintain plasma calcium concentrations during normal feeding and fasting conditions. There are other processes which protect the animal if the exogenous supply is restricted which can be best summarized using Fig. 10. (18) Parathyroid hormone has

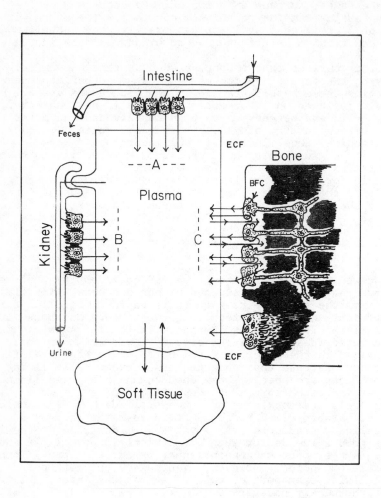

<u>Figure 10</u>. Diagrammatic model illustrating the role of
intestines, kidney and bone in the maintenance of plasma calcium concentrations. (Taken from Ref. 18.)

five major actions. We have concentrated on only one. The hormone also increases renal reabsorption of calcium. It stimulates 1 α hydroxylase activity for 25-OH Vitamin D3 in the kidney, therefore, indirectly increasing intestinal absorption of calcium. It also reduces renal tubular reabsorption of phosphate and thereby integrates phosphate into the process of calcium control in a manner to which we were only able to allude. The fifth action is its ability to simulate osteoclastic action. According to our concepts, this action under normal calcium supplies is to stimulate the bone remodelling process; namely, resorption followed by formation. This provides new morphological units governing calcium flux. Osteoclastic bone resorption is of increased importance in extended times of exogenous calcium deficiency. In such situations, under higher titers of parathyroud hormone, this process of bone destruction becomes the major source of calcium for the plasma calcium control processes. It is this concerted action of many processes which has given rise to the axiom, "Your body is going to maintain your plasma calcium levels even if it must destroy all your bone in attempting to do so".

References

1. Hastings, A.B. and Huggins, C.B. 1933. Experimental hypocalcemia. Proc. Soc. Exp. Biol. Med., 80, 458-59.

2. Copp, D.H. 1957. Calcium and phosphous metabolism. Am. J. Med., 22, 275.

3. Talmage, R.V., Elliott, J.R. and Erders, A.C. 1957. Parathyroid function as studied by continuous periotoneal lavage in neprectomized rats. Endocrinology, 61, 256-63.

4. McLean, E.C. and Urist, M.R. 1955. Bone. First Edition, Chicago Press, 77.

5. McLean, E.C. and Urist, M.R. 1961. Bone. Second Edition, Chicago Press, 124-26.

6. Talmage, R.V. and Elliott, J.R. 1958. Removal of calcium from bone as influenced by the parathyroids. Endocrinology, 62, 717-22.

7. Cooper, C.W., Yates, C.W. and Talmage, R.V. 1965. Some endogenous parathyroid hormone effects manifested by bone in vitro. Proc. Soc. Exp. Biol. Med., 119, 81-8.

8. Doty, S.B., Yates, C.W., Lotz, W.E., Kisceleski, W. and Talmage, R.V. 1965. Effect of short term alpha irradiation on parathyroid activity and osteoclast numbers. Proc. Soc. Exp. Biol. Med., 119, 77.

9. Arnold, J.S. and Jee, W.S.S. 1962. Pattern of long term skeletal remodelling revealed by radioautographic distribution of Pu[239] in dogs. Health Physics, 8, 705-8.

10. Rowland, R. 1966. Exchangeable bone calcium. Clin. Orthop. and Related Res., 49, 233-48.

11. Talmage, R.V., Doppelt, S.H. and Fondren, F.B. 1976. An interpretation of acute changes in plasma [45]Ca following parathyroid hormone administration to thyroparathyroidectomized rats. Calcif. Tiss. Res., 22, 117-28.

12. Grubb, S.A., Markham, T.C. and Talmage, R.V. 1977. Effect of calcitonin infusion on plasma concentrations of recently administered [45]Ca. Calcif. Tiss. Res., In Press.

13. Grubb, S.A., Edwards, G. and Talmage, R.V. 1977. Effect of endogenous and infused parathyroid hormone on plasma concentrations of recently administered [45]Ca. Calcif. Tiss. Res., In Press.

14. Talmage, R.V., Roycroft, J.H. and Anderson, J.J.B. 1975. Daily fluctuations in plasma calcium, phosphate, and their radionuclide concentrations in the rat. Calcif. Tiss. Res., 17, 91-02.

15. Talmage, R.V. 1975. Effect of fasting and parathyroid hormone injection on plasma ^{45}Ca concentrations in rats. Calcif. Tiss. Res., 17, 103-12.

16. Talmage, R.V., Matthews, J.L., Martin, J.H., Kennedy, J.W., Davis, W.L. and Roycroft, J.H. 1975. Calcitonin, phosphate and the osteocyte-osteoblast bone cell unit. Calcium-regulating hormones. (R.V. Talmage, M. Owen, and J.A. Parsons, eds.), Excerpta Medica Foundation, Amsterdam, 284-96.

17. Matthews, J.L., Talmage, R.V., and Doppelt, S.H. In Press 1978. Response of the osteocyte-lining cell complex to Parathyroid Hormone. Am J. Anatomy.

18. Talmage, R.V. and Meyer, R.A. 1976. The physiological role of parathyroid hormone. Handbook of physiology. (G.D. Aurbach, ed.), The Williams and Wilkins Company, Baltimore, Maryland, 7, 343-51.

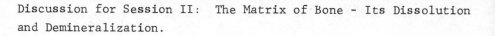

Discussion for Session II: The Matrix of Bone - Its Dissolution and Demineralization.

DR. MECHANIC: Dr. Raisz, we have been doing some work on bone organ culture and cell culture, and have found that collagenase-digestible protein may not be really collagen per se. We recently assayed a sample for cross-link analysis on the analyzer.   There was no hydroxylated proline, but yet there was collagenase-digestible protein.   So, I think one must be careful in assaying for prolylhydroxylase-2 for the production of collagen.   In other words, there might be some unhydroxylated proline in there.

DR. RAISZ: When one calculates the predicted amount of hydroxyproline from the amount of collagenase-digestible protein that we get here, and then analyzes the digest for hydroxyproline by column chromatography, one gets the predicted amount within 10 percent.

Now, there may be a 10 percent error; but we are talking about getting to collagen within 10 percent, not better than that with the collagenase method.   I think that kind of error is going to be there.

DR. MATTHEWS: Dr. Raisz, using your theory of antagonist resorption and formation, have you used glucagon?

DR. RAISZ: We have had no effect of glucagon on bone formation, although it does inhibit bone resorption.   The other inhibitor of bone resorption is calcitonin.   It also does not inhibit or stimulate collagen synthesis in this system.   Those are the only inhibitors we have used.

DR. TASHJIAN: Dr. Raisz, since Gaillard and Parsons apparently can stimulate bone formation in vitro as well as in vivo with the one-to-34 parathyroid hormone peptide, have you tried that, and have you succeeded?   Or, has anyone else been successful in stimulating bone formation with parathyroid hormone or related peptides?

DR. RAISZ: It is unfortunate that someone from that group isn't here to discuss it.   What was shown, as far as I can ascertain, was an increased turnover in the shaft, with a good number of osteoblasts with the low dose of one-to-34.   An absolute increase in the amount of collagen synthesized was not shown. Turnover increased.

This could be important. It may be that in the long bone, you can get this turnover phenomenon with very low doses of PTH. We have gone down to 0.1 nanogram, 100 picogram per mil, concentrations of both one-to-84 and one-to-34; in fact, we have gone below that, but we have never been able to see a consistent stimulation.

I don't think that doesn't mean it is there. The next thing we tried was intermittent application of PTH. Those experiments were also unsuccessful; but as you well know, these failures do not constitute evidence. They constitute failures.

I might say, though, that I think it would be unwise to give up the possibility that there is another factor besides PTH that is producing the osteoblastic proliferation in vivo. I think it is very premature to guess that is a direct effect of PTH.

DR. AVIOLI: Dr. Raisz, knowing that bone is not bathed constantly with a hormone at a certain level, have you or any of your group looked into a series of experiments where you actually have pulsed a hormone, or let it sit for a while, then pull it out, and then hit it with another hormone? I know it is a very difficult experimental design, but could you speak to that?

DR. RAISZ: We have done a few of those experiments. As you point out, they are very hard to do. There are two problems. Number one, once you put in the kinds of doses of hormones that we are putting in, there are both possible residual binding of the hormone left there, when you try to wash it off; and secondly, there may be fragments of the hormone which do something peculiar.

In any event, we have not been able to show any great differences. The most interesting thing about that intermittency phenomenon is insulin. Insulin takes a while to develop its effects, but then as quickly as you can take it away and measure collagen synthesis, it has gone back down. We think there must be something about insulin which needs fairly continuous pulses. Of course, we know that insulin in vivo comes out in pulses all day, but they are not very far apart.

DR. MINKIN: Dr. Raisz, is the bone collagen biosynthesis that you describe in this paper calcified or calcifiable collagen, or is this osteomalacic collagen?

DR. RAISZ: We have shown a great deal of calcium uptake in these tissues, but we have never been able to prove that which is newly synthesized as being calcified. We have the problem, which everyone has, that any tissue which calcifies could calcify for the wrong reasons. We can't prove, from measurements of calcium content, that it is calcifying. The calcium content does go up with insulin, but it might be something else.

The only way to prove it is morphologically. I can only say that in our control bones, we don't see calcification of the new matrix. We do not have the data on the insulin-treated as yet.

DR. MINKIN: Would that lead one to question the applicability of the hormone data in the organ culture system where we are faced with collagen biosynthesis that doesn't appear to be the same kind of collagen that is biosynthesized in vivo, which is calcifiable? Is there something different about the collagen?

DR. RAISZ: If we can show some difference between the in vivo collagen and the in-vitro collagen, we will tell you about it right away. Right now we can't see any difference. It is fully hydroxylated; it has cross-links, it has beta in it, as well as appropriate ratios of alpha-1 to alpha-2. We may be way off. There are things deposited at the calcification front which don't come from the osteoblasts at all, such as albumin and alpha-2 glycoproteins from the circulation.

All I can tell you about these osteoblasts is that they are morphologically healthy. They are making collagen which has the characteristics, by the criteria I just mentioned, of bone collagen.

DR. MINKIN: Do you know if they make type 3 collagen?

DR. RAISZ: We haven't any data on type 3. Our data on type 2 indicates that they do not make much.

DR PECK: I have two questions for Dr. Wong. The first relates to the possibility that PTH degradation may be going on in the presence of serum. Have you found any effect of PTH to be retained in the presence of serum, aside from the soluble collagen? In other words, is PTH effective in stimulating cyclic AMP formation, etc.?

DR. WONG: Yes. All of the previous results which we showed you were performed in the presence of serum.

DR. PECK: So PTH's effects on all other parameters that you have studied are retained.

DR. WONG: Yes; and even enhanced.

DR. PECK: And only the effect on collagen is lost; right. During the "chase period", was there a high concentration of non-radioactively-labeled proline in the medium?

DR. WONG: Yes; and in the rinse.

DR. PECK: What was the concentration?

DR. WONG: In the rinse, it was 1 millimolar and the chase, .1 millimolar.

DR. GOLDHABER: Dr. Wong, we have shown that if one uses

fetal calf serum with parathyroid hormone in our culture system, one does not get resorption. I refer to large amounts of serum. However, if one treats the fetal calf serum with charcoal, one then finds a positive effect with hormone. Therefore, I wonder whether your fetal calf serum is an adequate test of serum in general. I would suggest that you try some other sera, such as horse serum, for example.

DR. GAY: I wonder if trypsinization may not be destroying some of the PTH receptors that are known to be plasma membrane-situated.

DR. WONG: Trypsinization occurs six days previous, during the isolation procedure; and then the cells are never trypsinized again. We chose six days after initial seeding, because it appeared that the hormone response was highest at that time. Whatever receptor loss had occurred during the isolation procedure seemed to have been maximally repaired.

DR. AVIOLI: Dr. Wong, we always assume that if we are looking for the biological activity of PTH, we use the 1-34 fragment, because it has been shown to stimulate cyclic AMP and, through a variety of other biological assays, it is powerful. Have you, or has anyone that you know of, actually taken other fragments of PTH, which may be considered to be biologically inactive, using other criteria, and tested them in this system?

I ask this because of the work that is appearing from a variety of laboratories having to do with the metabolism of PTH by bone. Have you tried other fragments?

DR. WONG: No. We have stayed with the one-to-84.

DR. AVIOLI: Have you tried pieces of the 1-84 molecule?

DR. WONG: We have not. I don't know what that would tell us. We are not sure what the other pieces do; whether they bind to the cells at all, or whether they mask. We are still not sure what is happening in the biologically-active system that we have.

DR. COHN: Let me just make one additional comment. In some of the earlier measurements, not on the collagen work which Dr. Wong is talking about, but some of the earlier parameters such as citrate decarboxylation and hyaluronate synthesis, we were unable to distinguish any effects in our system between the one-to-34 fragment and the one-to-84.

Now, whether there are more subtle changes, such as are now being suggested, we really weren't looking; so we may have missed them. But grossly, they are the same.

DR. MUNDY: Dr. Wong, I found the last point that you were making on the summary slide fairly confusing, because you were talking, as I understand it, about a fix on collagen degradation in osteoblast-like cells, and tying this in some way with PTH-induced resorption.

Could you briefly clarify what you meant by that, please?

DR. WONG: We were simply saying that if the culture system that we are using is synonymous with what is happening in bone, then perhaps the effects of parathyroid hormone on bone formation are not mediated through a direct effect on collagen synthesis, but rather through a more rapid degradation of the collagen which is produced.

DR. WURTHIER: Dr. Talmage, do you think that maybe your factor on the surface might be this "gla" containing protein that Hauschka and Gallup are working on?

DR. TALMAGE: We think that there is something. The earlier work of Matthews which showed that when one gives calcitonin, one gets a complex form which mineralizes on sitting indicates that there is some type of inhibitor here which is able to hold the calcium at the surface of the bone without actually going into bone formation. But what it is, I don't know.

DR. WURTHIER: Certainly the "gla" protein as described meets many criteria that possibly could function in that capacity, with its marked ability to complex calcium and prevent the formation of hydroxyapatite.

DR. TALMAGE: Yes.

DR. MINKIN: Dr. Talmage, could you please explain the findings of the 83-year-old mentioned previously?

DR. TALMAGE: I thought my data probably did that. What I am saying is that this case was a very rare situation. Since most adenomas of parathyroid cause a major bone problem, what we possibly had here was a cyst rupturing to cause a sudden release of parathyroid hormone. If this lady had high levels of storage of calcium at the surface of the bone, she was able, with the parathyroid hormone and the storage, to temporarily raise the plasma calcium level without affecting bone. Obviously, this could not go on long. There is no way that she could maintain this high calcium level and not have bone damage.

But remember, she had these cysts which just recently broke. Apparantly, she was one who didn't excrete too much parathyroid hormone except when the cysts broke. When they broke, she released suddenly parathyroid hormone, and the calcium storage was sufficient to raise the plasma calcium level, and then it would come back down again.

Obviously, if she had kept this up, we would have had the typical situation where she would have had to call on bone and bone resorption to supply the calcium.

DR. SINGER: Dr. Talmage, in the acute rat experiments, did you look at any parameters of matrix resorption in these early changes? I am impressed that if one gives, say calcitonin, one can see very rapid changes, at least in hydroxyproline excretion or blood levels. If you are trying to dissociate simple exchange, or an exchange from an effect on bone resorption, I would wonder what changes would occur.

DR. TALMAGE: In the time frame that we are working, we get these changes in seven minutes. The reason we don't get them faster than seven minutes is because that is as fast as we can kill the rats and look at them. We could not expect, in that short time, to see any major changes in hydroxyproline content. Obviously, if one goes long enough with parathyroid hormone or calcitonin, one will get a change in these phenomena.

I would like to stress that the whole system is working together. Somehow, people may feel that I have deserted osteoclasts. I haven't. I am merely attempting to add another parameter and show that we have a cooperative system which, under a normal situation, doesn't really imply a major loss of bone just to maintain plasma calcium levels.

DR. TEITELBAUM: Dr. Talmage, I think your model is very appealing from an intellectual point of view. However, I would like you to comment on the fact that from a morphological point of view, the bone lining cells really don't look like pumps; and it is disturbing.

DR. TALMAGE: You may notice that I never talked about a "pump". This data which I presented today would just as well satisfy Newman's concept as mine, except possibly the recycling with parathyroid hormone and calcium-45. These cells could be reducing acids. But we feel it is the transport system, which we do not feel involves a metabolic ATP-ase pump.

Now, I think that when anybody asks me "How can you believe this when you have no proof of a calcium transport system"?; I merely ask him, "Well, why don't you tell me how calcium gets across the gut? If you can tell me how calcium gets across the gut, then I will tell you how it gets across these bone cells".

DR. TASHJIAN: Dr. Wong, I didn't catch the relationship between the dose of parathyroid hormone used in your experiments and the effects on bone cell collagen synthesis in relation to the effects that you observe in your laboratory on cyclic AMP metabolism.

DR. WONG: I did not show a dose response curve in this talk. All the data I showed was performed at 0.4 units, or 0.2 micrograms, per ml of PTH. We do have responses at lower doses; and all of the collagen work correlates very well with the previous work on citrate decarboxylation. There is total overlap.

DR. TASHJIAN: How about cyclic AMP?

DR. WONG: The same. The maximum dose is 0.4 micrograms per ml; and then it plateaus. The minimum that we can see an effect would be 0.02 micrograms per mil. This is using the one-to-84 bovine PTH.

DR. HEERSCHE: I have a question to both Dr. Raisz and Dr. Wong. If I understand their presentations correctly, I think that Dr.Raisz has measured collagen synthesis during a two-hour incorporation period, and has eliminated resorption from taking place on that particular collagen. He measures a decreased synthesis.

Now, Dr. Wong is showing us that when measuring collagen incorporation during that 90-minute period in her cells, she doesn't find any effect at all.

To me these two results seem contradictory, and I would like you to comment on that.

DR. RAISZ: I certainly can't argue with that. No, of course they are contradictory, but why they are contradictory is the point which has to be attacked. This is a workshop, and we have something here which may be an important point in the question of how parathyroid hormone works on various kinds of cells.

They are certainly different kinds of cells. I don't think anyone would say that the organ culture, in its first two, three, or four days out of the body, and the cell preparation of PT cells, six days cultured and then treated with hormones, are going to be the same cells.

The organ culture cell is clearly not the same as the in-vivo cell, which is responding to PTH. Each of these is going to show some differences in their response to PTH, depending on their collagen synthesis machinery, and also their level of collagen degradation machinery.

What I do think is true is that when you sum up all the in-vivo and in-vitro data, one of the things that PTH does in large doses is make osteoblasts stop looking like plump polygonal cells with oriented collagen production towards the bone surface. There are data, in vivo and in vitro, to make that a firm con-clusion.

Now, that phenomenon, in various culture systems, could lead to different things. For example, the collagen may be still synthesized but thrown out the other way, so that it can not be subject to degradation by surrounding fibroblastic cells. There is also the possibility that there is an intra-cellular system for rapid degradation as there is with lung collagen.

What we have been able to look at is total collagen synthesized and collagen fragments larger than 3,000 molecular weight. In our previous studies we found, when we pulse chase, that is all the collagen we can see. We can't see smaller material. But there may be, just as there is for glycoproteins and proteoglycans, some scrap material with a lot of collagen that is synthesized and rapidly degrading; that material which we can't see may be showing up in Dr. Wong's cells. There is a lot of "waste collagen synthesis". That material, until we know where it is involved, is going to give us large discrepancies in the different data. We have a lot of work to do to resolve this question.

DR. HEERSCHE: My second question relates to pool sizes. If I remember the variation correctly, PTH has no effect when the proline concentration is, let's say, one micromolar, or has even an effect on synthesis; when you use a proline concentration of one millimolar, you see these opposite effects.

How can one explain effects of medium proline concentration on intracellular pool sizes? Dr. Wong is apparently using 100 micromolar or so in her media. Could you please comment on the effects of pool sizes.

DR. RAISZ: That is a very important topic. There is a lot of data which shows that, acutely, PTH increases amino acid uptake in bone cells. This was shown by at least five or six people such as Feinerman, Rosenberg, and Adamson.

All of that data shows an increase in amino acid uptake. If we treat with PTH at a one micromolar tracer concentration, we get an increase in both CDP and NCP labeling, which we attribute to transport. This is, acutely, at three hours. If we raise to 1,000 micromolar, we get no effect.

Our effects of inhibition do not appear until six hours. At that time, we can still, in a tracer situation, see some increased amino acid uptake. I think that increased amino acid uptake-effect does persist, even when the cells may be altered in their collagen synthetic machinery, or their shape, or whatever it is that PTH does more slowly.

DR. WONG: In the cell culture system, also, without added proline, there appears to be more of an uptake of tritiated proline when the cells have been pre-exposed to parathyroid hormone. However, if one does the experiments with just carrier radioactive proline, one will see more radioactivie collagen in the presence of parathyroid hormone. If one chases that, however, one recovers proportionately less. If one adds the proline at 100 millimolar, one swamps out the system, apparently, and then one sees no effects of parathyroid hormone on uptake or synthesis.

DR. RAISZ: Could I just add that I think there may be a critical point here. 100 micromolar is roughly the blood level of proline. It was shown by the group at the NIH, and Jim Pong has subsequently expanded this, that endogenous pools are very substantial in the range of 100 micromolar and less. This may be something which is also changing during synthesis, during loading experiments, when you put in more proline.

What he has shown, however, is that this endogenous pool doesn't seem to increase or decrease very much when he loads the cells up with more proline.

I think in each system, one must look at what the endogenous proline is doing, the stuff that comes from ornithine and glutamine, which may be confusing some of these numbers.

DR. BRAND: May I break in on that? There was a paper, recently in the '77, American Journal of Physiology, where they actually did amino acid analysis on newborn, and then at hourly intervals, in rats. The newborn rat proline level in the serum is half a millimolar. I think that it is interesting to know because at 16 hours, it had dropped down to between 0.1 and 0.2 millimolar.

DR. RAISZ: Did they do fetal animals?

DR. PECK: They did prelactating, immediately taken newborns.

DR. RAISZ: I think that certainly reinforces the complexity of the problem.

DR. PECK: Yes. It has been known for many years that fetal serum amino acid levels are higher. This is probably due to a phenomenon of adaptation in the neonatal period which results in an acceleration of uptake, rather than any change in extracellular distribution. It refers not only to proline, but all amino acids that are transported by the "A" or sodium-dependent transport.

DR. MINKIN: I have a question for Dr. Wong. In your experiments, did you look to see whether calcitonin reversed the effect that you obtained with parathyroid hormone on degradation?

DR. WONG: There was no effect. The reason I didn't mention it is we have not been able to demonstrate any effect of calcitonin on any of the parameters measured in the PT cells.

DR. MINKIN: What I am referring to, and you may have misunderstood me, was specifically the effect of calcitonin on parathyroid hormone-treated PT cells.

DR. WONG: In terms of collagen synthesis?

DR. MINKIN: Yes. The organ culture experiments would indicate that in that more heterogeneous system, calcitonin can reverse the effects of parathyroid hormone.

DR. WONG: I am not sure about that.

DR. RAISZ: John Brand showed that the collagenase released in calcitonin-treated fetal rat calvaria was not decreased. John, is not that a correct statement?

DR. BRAND: Yes.

DR. RAISZ: So I think probably calcitonin certainly affects bone-resorbing cells; but some collagenolytic activity persists in these fetal cultures which is not inhibited by calcitonin.

DR. PECK: I have a question for Dr. Kleinman. Have you been able to show differences in bonding of cells in your system during different phases of the cell cycle? For example, could you inhibit proliferation in the osteogenic sarcoma cells and then show that during inhibition of DNA synthesis that they would attach?

Secondly is this similar to the binding of platelets to collagen?

DR. KLEINMAN: Let me answer the first question first. We haven't done those studies, but we suspect they are going to be very important. I forgot to mention with regard to the osteo-sarcoma cells that only the adherent cells produce tumors when we injected them back into the animals. The non-adherent did not. Further, we have taken tumors produced by the adherent cells and replated and cultured them and redone the experiment. It repeats itself. But, we didn't get enrichment. In other words, we took the tumors developed from the adherent cells and expected that we would see more adherence, but we didn't. We still saw only about 40 percent adherent. We suspect that the cell cycle may be involved, and that is our next series of experiments.

With regard to platelets, the story is incomplete or confusing at the moment. Platelets are supposed to specifically adhere, at least in terms of chick collagen, to CB-5, which is the peptide that contains carbohydrate. We see no activity in CB-5. Many people who look at platelet adherence to collagen can not explain why it works in the chick and doesn't work in another animal. There is no sequence-specific phenomena.

DR. KUETTNER: I have a question first to Dr. Raisz and then to Dr. Kleinman. First a comment: the work by Heuson on the survival rate of isolated mammary carcinoma cells showed that only insulin was capable of inducing survival of these cells, and only under these circumstances will these cells make what they call stroma. The stroma was composed of both collagen as well as whatever the other substance was called. I have a question specifically, now, with the insulin.

In your system, did you look for the turnover or the bio-synthesis of the carbohydrates stimulated, particularly the glycoseaminoglycans?

DR. RAISZ: It is obviously right on the top of our list when we know a little more about insulin.

Insulin still works in the presence of substantial amounts of serum, which is of interest to us. For example, if you have enough serum so you have a microunit of insulin present, and you then add another 150 microunits, you get substantial additional collagen synthesis without any effect on non-collagen protein. This is not just cell survival. We are talking about more differentiated functions.

DR. KUETTNER: My question to Dr. Kleinman: could you elaborate on your system? Number one, are you using fresh serum? Secondly, what is your current hypothesis with regard to fibronectin or the cell attachment factor, the whole system, with regard to interaction or inhibition of collagenase?

DR. KLEINMAN: We have used heat-inactivated serum and non-heat-inactivated serum. There is no difference in effect, because the protein that mediates the cell attachment is the LETS protein, which is stable with heat-inactivation.

As for my theory about this protein and collagenase, we are looking at a variety of cell types and tumor types. Our theory now is that this protein may block collagenase, if it binds to the collagen protein first. Obviously, if collagenase has already acted on the collagen chain, then the protein can't bind. The combination of this protein with collagenase may be to regulate certain cell matrix interactions.

I must preface all this by saying that we do have evidence that there are other factors elaborated by other cells. This protein is specific for fibroblasts. It is not found in other cells, or synthesized by other cells, for example, chondrocytes. However, there is some preliminary data out of our lab that if one places this protein on a growing culture, a limb bud culture for example, one can totally block chondrogenesis by adding as little as 20 micrograms per ml. What it is doing, we are not sure. Apparently it can control some aspect of differentiation in culture at extremely low levels.

DR. SCOFFIELD: Recently Ugella and Woodbury published a paper on the fetal calvaria of the rat, in which they pointed out that the entire calvaria contains only 20 percent osteoblasts. I wonder what implications this has in Dr. Raisz's and Dr. Wong's work, in terms of separating out bone cells as one would define osteoblasts, osteocytes, osteoclasts, and bone cells as being the cells present in fetal calvaria.

Also, I would like to make an observation which may be of interest to the work. If one looks at 15 to 19-day old fetal calvaria with an electron microscope, one finds that the fibroblastic cells contain large numbers of intracellular collagen fibers in vacuoles. They look identical to the photographs published some years ago in a study of resorbing karyogenic into S-granuloma, in which it was suggested that the fibroblasts themselves degrade the collagen, rather than relying on extraneous cells.

I wonder what implications that observation might have on the degradation of collagen in the systems you are using.

DR. WONG: In the preparative procedure that we use, we do six extractions. First of all, when we assay in terms of DNA what we have extracted versus what we have left behind, we have removed about 20 percent of the total starting DNA. Of that 20 percent, about a third are the cells which show CT or osteoclastic characteristics, and at least 60 to 70 percent would be the ones which show osteoblastic characteristics.

Now, I am talking about the actual number we get out before we put them in culture. They then undergo division at least three time within the six days before we do the experiments. Does that answer your question?

DR. SCOFFIELD: Yes, thank you.

DR. RAISZ: I think your second point is a very attractive one. When osteoblasts make collagen that wasn't deposited on new matrix in an orderly fashion, there is a fibroblastic population on the outside of the bone which can clearly degrade it. They may be as important for dealing with such collagen as they would be for collagen during resorption. If those cells are present or proliferate in any culture system, be it organ or cell, they are going to have an influence on the way collagen is laid down.

We have relied on autoradiography to detect where our collagen is being laid down. It is clear that a small percentage, as you point out, of osteoblasts are producing essentially all the collagen we see. There is very little in the way of extracellular deposition of grains, except in those active layers. The fact that we actually see them modulating from time to time in the culture further enhances our confidence that this is the major source of collagen being laid down. But we can't prove it by that method.

DR. KRANE: I have a couple of questions. One is that in parathyroid-induced inhibition of collagen synthesis, could that be overcome by indomethacin, for example?

The second question relates to part of the work that Dr. Wong was doing. When you are looking at collagen synthesis, you measure it only after pepsin; if you used a lathyrogen and then looked at the total procollagen synthesized, it may give you another clue.

It was shown by Lichtenstein and George Martin in their examination of cells that lacked the procollagen peptidase, that these cells synthesize much more collagen than do control cells. This can be easily shown, because you can get those cells from American Type Culture Association. They make more collagen, and a lot of it is procollagen. They thought in their paper published in Science a few years ago that the amino terminal piece actually got back into the cell and therefore acted in a feedback inhibitory fashion. It is also shown that if you take the purified alpha amino terminal piece, this could show a dose-dependent inhibition of collagen synthesis.

This may be a possible suggestion to you since the rates of collagen synthesis with your system were much more greatly suppressed than the rates of turnover. One of the things that serum would inhibit would be one of the peptidases that would inhibit procollagen cleavage, and therefore sort of unbreak collagen synthesis. This is one of the problems that one sees in a closed system of this kind.

DR. WONG: The pepsin was used only when we were preparing the collagen originally for gel electrophoresis. I do have profiles.

DR. RAISZ: We have only one experiment of indomethacin which failed to reverse. I might say that insulin also opposes but does not completely reverse the action of PTH.

The problem of endogenous prostaglandin synthesis in bone, which I think will become increasingly important, is probably a controlling factor. Indomethacin and the other substances we have are such uncertain inhibitors, but we have found we cannot get sufficient reversal at the usual concentrations of indomethacin in the system. We have to go to 10^{-5} molar. Others have been able to work with 10^{-7} and I think this is advantageous. Using both the RO and the indomethacin compounds, if we go just a little bit higher, we begin to see inhibition of collagen synthesis, perhaps due to their cyclic AMP effect. I think we are going to have to either get our system to respond to lower indomethacin or find another drug to unravel that problem.

DR. AVIOLI: There are two things that I have to come to grips with, Dr. Talmage. First some data and then some soft suggestions from observations of others.

I read your hypothesis as following: that the PTH must work on a cell at the surface, because you showed these direct immediate effects of PTH on a cell. So the phenomena that you speak of must be cell mediating.

If one makes a fast calculation about the amount of bone an 80-year-old woman should have in terms of bone mass and assumes that maybe she has one-third, and goes into the percent of that surface which is covered by cells, and then tries to appreciate the total circulating volume in terms of 60 percent or so of the body weight, it would be very difficult to generate a rise of 18 milligrams percent. One would have to incriminate a cell response. I would imagine that the only cell that would be responding would be, in that case, maybe an osteocyte or something deeper in bone.

Number two, some data which are of interest: there are patients with a disease called Marble Bone disease, or osteopetrosis. To my knowledge, they have no problems in the day-to-day regulation of serum calcium because they don't tend toward hypocalcemia. But I do know, as others have published, that if you infuse them with EDTA, and drop their serum calcium, and then wait for the response, namely, the response of the calcium toward normal which supposedly is PTH-induced, it takes quite a long time for their serum calciums to return to normal.

This has been interpreted by others in the past that the deep bone is not responding to PTH in this disease because it is diseased. Now, I am not saying you are right or wrong, but I am a little confused.

DR. TALMAGE: All I can tell you is that the trabecular bone our pathologists looked at was in pretty good shape. The other point I would like to suggest is the point which we already have discussed with you and Dr. Teitelbaum. In the 85-year-old woman, probably every surface of bone is covered with cells. Therefore, the osteoid is a site where we could be storing calcium. We don't have to limit it by the old-fashioned data that only a certain percentage of the bone is covered with cells. There is plenty of place to store calcium in the bone fluid, even in an 85-year-old woman, on the bone surfaces.

DR. AVIOLI: They wouldn't be active osteoblasts though.

DR. TALMAGE: The big problem is when you say "active osteoblasts", you usually refer to osteoblasts that are synthesizing collagen. We are talking about active cells; viable cells. They are not synthesizing collagen.

DR. CANTEBURY: Dr. Raisz, I am interested in your effects with the 24-25 and 25-hydroxy in your cultures on osteoblastic activity. I assume that you did these over a wide dose range.

DR. RAISZ: Yes.

DR. CANTERBURY: Have you seen any effects in vivo by pre-treating in vivo and then looking at bone for osteoblasts?

DR. RAISZ: We have not done the in vivo experiments, and I don't know of any. There are some effects of 24-25 on cartilage which have been shown by the French group, but their 1-25 apparently was also effective as a stimulus for cartilage growth

The one point I would make is that 25-hydroxy is a perfectl good bone resorber, only a thousand times less potent, than 1-25 Yet over a more than thousand-fold, a hundred-thousand fold range of doses, we have gone above the 10^{-7} indicated there, we haven't seen any consistent inhibition of bone formation with 25.

So there may be a dissociation. It is possible that 1-25 has a greater osteoblastic inhibitory effect, equal to its bone resorptive effect, at the same dose response. The dose response curves are parallel, whereas 25 may show a dissociation. If tha is true, that would make 25, in some sense, at least, not an anti-bone growth hormone. However, those data need more work.

DR. MARKS: Dr. Wong, with regard to the PTH-dependent

collagen degradation, do you have any evidence as to whether it is occurring intracellularly or extracellularly?

DR. WONG: Preliminary experiments done over a very short period of time suggest that exogenous collagen added to the culture is not broken down. However, the incubation was only for six hours. I feel before we can make a statement on this, it should be repeated for longer periods.

DR. KLEIN: Dr. Raisz, have you looked at bones where you prelabeled with calcium-45 to see if there is a release of calcium-45 at the time there is inhibition of collagen synthesis?

DR. RAISZ: Most of these experiments were done with bones that were left over from the resorption system, and already had calcium-45 in them. In those circumstances, there was usually bone resorption going along with PTH inhibition of bone formation. But percentagewise, in rat calvaria, which is a very interesting thing to me, as opposed to mouse calvaria, the rates of resorption are much lower. I think others have had the same observation.

With mouse calvaria, you can get 25 to 45 percent of the bone to resorb, in a few days. We have never seen more than 10 percent resorption in a rat calvaria around the perinatal period. They apparently have less bone resorptive precursors, so that the amount of resorption has never been great enough to account for. We have never lost enough by resorption to account for the decrease in formation.

DR. KLEIN: What I mean is, would you get a flare of release of calcium-45 at the time you were getting inhibition of the collagen?

DR. RAISZ: Oh. As a result of the inhibition of formation, you could well get that. It hasn't been large, from what I just said. We couldn't tell whether the ^{45}Ca we see is from osteoclastic resorption or prevention of osteoblastic deposition, but it is only a few percent difference; 5 percent or so of total calcium.

DR. WERB: I have a couple of questions. First of all, I think the finding that cells bind to collagen makes them happier, or spread better, is very important. The question I have is: does binding of cells to collagen make them synthesize collagen better?

DR. KLEINMAN: I haven't done that study. Dr. Abbay tried it, and I believe there was some stimulation, but not a tremendous amount.

There is one situation which I would like to mention, not in terms of collagen, but in terms of differentiation, and that is in the muscle system. Hauschka has found that if one collagen-coats plates one can get muscles differentiating in

culture, whereas if one doesn't, they won't. He also finds that
the specific molecule that is active for cell attachment is the
peptide. When he coats the plate with that peptide, it is the
peptide that works for the stimulation.

So collagen in culture has a growth-promoting effect on
many cells, and it can promote differentiation of some cells.

DR. WONG: I have coated plates with collagen and not gotten
any reproducible increase in collagen synthesis in the cells
which were then layered on top. However, what I did find was if
I took commercially-prepared collagen and put it in a plate and
then added the cells, there was a stimulation. When I washed it,
there wasn't any. This may relate to the binding protein that
Dr. Kleinman has discussed.

DR. RAISZ: We have the same negative results. I think
they should all be used as a spur to find out why it didn't work,
because it ought to. I think you are right.

Fibronectin may not be the entire answer, because we had
negative results with serum present. Is it fair for me to ask
Dr. Kleinman a question?

All of these things are supposed to come from cells. Yet
you get most of your effects from serum. Do you think that
these things are coming from cells via serum, or do you think
that most of the action in biology is by the cell making its own
attachment proteins to attach to its own adjacent piece of
collagen?

DR. KLEINMAN: It is purely speculative for an in-vivo
situation. Since these cells do make this protein, what one
sees is what is made by the cell in that particular tissue or
locus,rather than what is present in the serum. We do have
evidence to suggest that there are different proteins, i.e.
attachment proteins, for different types of cells and different
mechanisms. So it would seem to be a cell-specific phenomenon.

DR. WERB: The other question I have for Dr. Kleinman is
that there has now been a second revival of interest in proteins
that are present in serum.

The first was about in the '50s; and many proteins were
described then that were supposed to be involved in attachment
of cells to glass or plastic. One of them was described by Park
and Lieberman; it is either fetuin or compounds which contami-
nate fetuin preparations which are supposed to make cells attach.
Apropos that, when you iodinate cells which were in the presence
of serum, what you find is not a great preponderance of a
LETS-like protein, I mean a high molecular weight protein. But
you see everywhere a 40,000-ish molecular weight iodinatable
protein. What is the contribution of other proteins from serum
or plasma for cell attachment to glass and to collagen?

DR. KLEINMAN: We call the large protein, the 200,00 M.W.,

"LETS", and then there is another protein called "SMETS", which is a small molecular weight, external sensitive protein.

We also see in different stages of, for example, transformation increases and decreases of certain cell surface proteins. Isolating these proteins and looking for their specific function in cell attachment has not been done. Klieb has isolated a protein synthesized by hepatocytes that will cause hepatocytes to specifically adhere to collagen. Whether it works on other cell types or not, I don't know, but it is a low, less than 100,000, molecular weight, protein.

There is quite a bit of evidence to suggest other proteins, other phenomena. I can use the purified LETS protein on some cells, and it inhibits cell attachment. But what the protein is that the cell wants to insert in this site we don't know yet, other than the Klieb factor.

I would like to emphasize that in terms of cell attachment, this particular aspect is probably one small portion of an enormous complex mechanism. I have some evidence for a factor that only binds to Type IV collagen; but I can't say more than that.

DR. TASHJIAN: Is there unanimity about the effects of parathyroid hormone on collagen metabolism in bone or bone cells? It seems that we have heard from Dr. Wong that there is no effect of parathyroid hormone on short-term pulse labeling of collagen in bone cells _in vitro_.

Dr. Raisz talks about inhibition of collagen synthesis using techniques of which Dr. Mechanic has questioned the validity. Then there are effects on proline uptake. So what is the picture? Do we come to the conclusion that there are effects of parathyroid hormone on synthesis rates _per se_, only on degradation rates, or only on uptake, or some complex combination of all of those things?

DR. RAISZ: I think the first thing we need to decide is that we can't come to a final conclusion. There is perfectly good evidence for all three. I think the one that is firmest is the effect on amino acid uptake. That has been reproduced without anybody denying it, as far as I know.

I think the inhibition of collagen synthesis, and Dr. Mechanic is perfectly right to question the methodology, but if you want, I will show the slide. The hydroxylation of that material is the calculated hydroxylation. It is collagen, and we can show exactly the same thing with hydroxyproline measurements, with short-term pulses, and we can show morphologic changes in osteoblasts.

We have, we think, every reason to believe that these changes fit decreased collagen synthesis machinery. That doesn't rule out the other possibilities. I don't think it is likely that PTH is going to have only one effect on osteoblasts and their precursors. I think it is probably going to have three, or four, or five, or six.

Also, there is the very important argument that all of these data, every one of them as far as I know, was done at something between 100 and 1,000 times the blood level of PTH. That is something we have to face.

DR. COHN: May I emphasize something that Dr. Raisz said, and try to bring a little clarity into what may have been more confusion than I think anybody really intended.

Dr. Raisz, after all, is working in a system which has both osteoclasts and osteoblasts coexisting side by side, and exhibiting their unique hormonally-sensitive responses simultaneously. He is measuring a total effect, an averaged effect, in the tissue.

What we have been trying to do, Dr. Wong and myself, is to sort out the specific effects. Wong was talking about effects observed in predominantly one type of cell. Hopefully, most of the osteoclastic or CT-type cells, as we have been terming them, have been removed from the equation, from the system.

Now, of course there is an effect of parathyroid hormone on collagen, net collagen synthesis, or at least formation, because you can show very niftily that there is less collagen there and bone resorbs. And in fact the CT cells, as Luben showed with the rest of us, when you take those cells and you lay them on top of a bone and add parathyroid hormone, you get the bone to resorb and the collagen to come into solution.

So there really isn't much problem in trying to fit these data together. Raisz made a very important point: the differences are pointing the way to the kind of experiment that ought to be done to try to explain the overall hormonal effects on the various cell types in bone in terms of their specific regulation, differentiation, and change.

DR. TASHJIAN: Dr. Cohn, I would raise the question that your two systems raise more problems, because I would think that your cells are the ones that are likely to be the collagen-synthetic cells; the osteoblast-like cells. Therefore, I would think your results would set up a situation where you would be more likely to see an effect of parathyroid hormone on inhibiting synthesis, and you don't see it. so that seems odd to me.

DR. COHN: Well, we would like you to believe our results.

DR. WONG: I think that we have to keep in mind, first of all, that the organ culture system is not the same as the cell culture system. Dr. Raisz showed autoradiographically that he did not get collagen synthesized generally throughout the entire bone, even in places where osteoblasts were present.

Our system is obviously an artificial system, even more

artificial than the culture system. The point is that the cells
are probably pretty well synchronized when we use them. I think
you have to keep in mind that there may be effects of cell cycle.
It may be that at some time the cells react one way to the
hormone and at another time, maybe they start degrading.

At the moment, what our results point to is that we see
effects that say hormone exerts its decrease in collagen through
degradation. This does not mean that within the organ culture
or in vivo, there are not other effects.

We don't claim to have all of the osteoblasts from the bone.
Maybe there are sub-populations, and within the bone itself, one
may be seeing the activities of one kind versus another. I think
these are problems for the future.

DR. TALMAGE: Some of us are actually working in vivo. Not
too long ago, working with Gene Russell, we studied the effects of
endogenous parathyroid hormone on decreased glycine uptake in
collagen. One of the things that we discovered was that one
could obviously inhibit with endogenous parathyroid hormone the
uptake of extractable tritiated proline and tritiated hydroxyproline with endogenous parathyroid hormone.

But we also found we could do it by just raising the calcium
level of the blood. If we increased the calcium level above
normal, we got the same type of inhibition. I wonder if, in
vitro, one ever worried about how much of this was being done by
parathyroid hormone and how much was being done by calcium
entering the cell.

DR. RAISZ: Your "entering the cell" is the key issue. As
far as extracellular calcium concentration, collagen synthesis
in our system is stable over a wide range of extracellular calcium concentrations, but obviously, PTH might enhance entry; and
maybe in the whole animal, calcium entry might be different.

I don't think it is worth going through it, but the list of
evidences that the osteoblast is a target cell for PTH is very,
very long. I hope that we are not going to come away with the
idea that it is not. I think the evidence shows it is a direct
target cell for PTH. What is still needed, of course, is to
show that through receptor work, which I do not think that anyone has done.

DR. SAKAMOTO: Recently we have seen that a commercial preparation of fetuin inhibits mouse bone collagenase. If we use
a more purified fetuin, it doesn't. These are relevant findings
to the study reported by Dr. Kleinman, today.

I have two questions. One is, have you ever characterized
the cell attachment protein in terms of a possible relation to
fetuin-like protein? Secondly, how strong is the binding of that
cell attachment protein to the collagen?

DR. KLEINMAN: To your first question, we have never looked

at fetuin. The second question's answer is that the binding would be considered very strong. It requires 8 molar urea or 1 molar potassium bromide to release the protein.

SESSION III

THE ROLE OF MICROBES, MEDIATORS, AND
MONONUCLEAR CELLS IN LOCALIZED BONE LOSS.

Partial Characterization of a Bone Resorptive Factor from
Actinomyces Viscosus

E. Hausmann, B.C. Nair, M. Reed and M.J. Levine

Department of Oral Biology, School of Dentistry
State University of New York at Buffalo,
Buffalo, NY 14226

A relationship between periodontal bone loss and microbial
deposits on the surface of teeth has been well documented in
humans (1) and animals. (2,3) Interestingly, in periodontal
disease, bacteria rarely invade the diseased tissue. (4)
It can be inferred therefore that plaque organisms release products which gain entrance to the periodontal tissues and act
on bone progenitor cells to differentiate into osteoclasts
which resorb the alveolar bone. The possibility for such a
mechanism has been reinforced by the findings that lipopolysaccharides (5,6) and lipoteichoic (7) acids obtained from
bacteria of dental plaque origin stimulate osteoclastic resorption of fetal bones in organ culture. Actinomyces viscosus
isolated from humans has been shown to result in marked plaque
formation and alveolar bone loss in monoinfected, gnotobiotic
rodents. (8) Recently two strains of Actinomyces viscosus have
been described, T14V and its spontaneously occurring avirulent
mutant T14AV. (9) Both produce plaque deposits when inoculated
into gnotobiotic rats but only the T14V strain produces alveolar
bone loss.

This report describes the partial characterization of a
factor obtained from three strains of Actinomyces viscosus,
which stimulates resorption of fetal bones in organ cultures.

Materials and Methods:

Actinomyces viscosus (ATCC 19246, T14V, T14AV) were grown
in Trypticase soy broth for 72 h in batch cultures of up to 20
liters. The purity of the cultures was checked by phase microscopy and gram staining. The cultures were harvested by
centrifugation and the resultant pellets were disrupted by using
a Heat Systems Sonifier, Model W185 (Branson Ultrasonics,
Plainview, N.Y.). The temperature was maintained below 10°C
during sonication. Suspensions of bacteria at a concentration
of 100 mg (wet weight)/ml in 0.005M phosphate, pH 7.2 were
sonicated until more than 95% breakage of microorganisms had
occurred as determined by phase contrast microscopy. The
sonicates were centrifuged at 12,000 x g for 30 minutes at 4°C
and the sonicate-supernatants dialysed and lyophilized. Portions of lyophilized sonicate-supernatants were dissolved in
0.5M phosphate buffer, pH 7.4 at a concentration of 30 µg/ml,

boiled for 30 minutes, dialysed against the same medium used for bone organ culture and tested for the release of ^{45}Ca from prelabeled bones. Another sample of lyophilized sonicate-supernatant was suspended at a concentration of 20 mg/ml in a solution containing 2 mg/ml, pronase, 0.05M Tris, pH 8: 0.5M CaCl$_2$; and incubated for 24 hrs at 37°C. The incubation mixture was dialysed against media used for bone organ culture. The volume of solution was adjusted to a sonicate-supernatant concentration of 30 µg/ml disregarding any effect on pronase digestion. The concentration of pronase in this solution was 1.5 µg/ml which does not affect ^{45}Ca release from prelabeled bones. Aliquots of lyophilized sonicate-supernatant were suspended in water at a concentration of 1 mg/ml and extracted with an equal volume of phenol. The aqueous phase of the phenol extracts were extensively dialysed.

The quantitative bioassay for measuring bone resorption has been described in detail previously by Raisz. (10,11) Sprague-Dawley rats (Holtzman) were injected with 400 µCi of ^{45}CaCl on the 18th day of pregnancy and sacrificed one day later. The fetal radii and ulnae after removal of the cartilaginous ends were explanted as pairs for organ culture. All bones were precultured in control media for 24 h in order to remove most of the exchangeable ^{45}Ca. After 48 h of culture, samples of media were prepared for liquid scintillation counting of ^{45}Ca. The amount of ^{45}Ca released from the bones during culture were expressed as a ratio of the ^{45}Ca released by contra-lateral members of a pair of radii or ulnae. Bone resorbing activity was considered to be present when the treated-to-control ratio was greater than 1.00 (p<0.05).

Results and Discussion:

When lyophilized sonicate supernatant from Actinomyces viscosus of strains, ATCC 19246, T14V or T14AV at a concentration of 30 µg/ml was added to prelabeled fetal bones in culture significant release of ^{45}Ca into the media was observed with all preparations (Table I). The presence of this factor does not explain the difference in the pathogenicity of the T14V and T14AV strains.

The ability to stimulate ^{45}Ca release by sonicate-supernatants is not influenced by boiling (Table II) or by pronase digestion (Table III). Lyophilized preparations of sonified-supernatants were dissolved in water and extracted with phenol. Comparable bone resorptive activity was observed in each of the aqueous phases derived from ATCC 19246, T14V and T14AV (Table IV). On the order of 60 percent of the composition of the sonified-supernatants can be accounted for by protein and 10 percent by carbohydrate. The aqueous phase on phenol extraction was markedly enriched in carbohydrate (Table V). For this reason the dose-response relationship of bone resorptive activity before and after phenol extraction was compared on the basis of carbohydrate concentration. When so compared, the bone resorptive activity of the sonified-supernatant preparation and the aqueous phase on phenol extraction had similar bone resorptive

Table I

Effect of Actinomyces viscosus, Sonicate Supernatants
on ^{45}Ca Release from Fetal Rat Bones in Organ Culture

Source	^{45}Ca Release Ratio (24 to 72 hrs.)
A. vis., ATCC 19246	
lot 1	2.33+0.27*
lot 2	2.94+0.25*
A. vis., T14V	2.24+0.30*
A. vis., T14AV	1.86+0.21*

30 µg (lyophilized material)/ml of sonicate supernatant used in each experiment.
^{45}Ca release ratios are mean $\pm$ SE for four pairs of
cultures in each experiment.
*p<0.05; p values based on a difference of a ^{45}Ca
release ratio from 1.0.

Table II

Effect of Boiling Sonicate Supernatants
from Actinomyces viscosus (ATCC 19246) on ^{45}Ca Release
from Fetal Rat Bones in Organ Culture

Addition	^{45}Ca Release Ratio (24 to 72 hrs.)	
	boiled	unboiled
Sonicate Supernatant, expt. 1	1.90+0.20*	1.92+0.31*
Sonicate Supernatant, expt. 2	1.97+0.34*	3.34+0.37*

30 µg (lyophilized material)/ml of sonicate supernatant used in each experiment.
^{45}Ca release ratios are mean $\pm$ SE for four pairs of
cultures in each experiment.
*p<0.05; p values based on a difference of a ^{45}Ca
release ratio from 1.0.

Table III

Effect of Pronase Digestion of Sonicate Supernatants
from Actinomyces viscosus (ATCC 19246) on ^{45}Ca Release
from Fetal Bones in Organ Culture

	^{45}Ca Release Ratio (24 to 72 hrs.)	
	pronase digested	undigested
Supernatant Sonicate	2.98+0.68*	3.18+0.86*

In digestion mixture the concentrations of supernatant
sonicate and pronase are 20 mg/ml and 200 µg/ml respectively.
In bone culture incubation medium pronase conc. is 0.3 µg/ml
and supernatant sonicate concentration is 30 µg/ml or its
equivalent.
^{45}Ca release ratios are mean $\pm$ SE for pairs of six pairs
of cultures in each experiment.
*$p < 0.05$; p values based on a difference of a ^{45}Ca release
ratio from 1.0.

Table IV

Effect of Phenol Extraction (Aqueous Phase) from
Actinomyces viscosus, Sonicate Supernatants on
^{45}Ca Release from Fetal Rat Bones in Organ Culture

Source	^{45}Ca Release Ratio (24 to 72 hrs.)
ATCC 19246	2.85+0.48*
T14V	2.86+0.35*
T14AV	3.19+0.28*

30 µg (anthrone-carbohydrate)/ml of aqueous phase
used in each experiment.
^{45}Ca release ratios are mean $\pm$ SE for four pairs
of cultures in each experiment.
*$p < 0.05$; p values based on a difference of a ^{45}Ca
release ratio from 1.0.

Table V

Carbohydrate and Protein Composition of Fractions
from _Actinomyces viscosus_ with Bone Resorptive Activity

Source	Fraction	Protein[a]		Carbohydrate[b]	
		μg/mg	μg/ml	μg/mg	μg/ml
ATCC 19246	Sonicate supernatant	672		112	
T14V	Sonicate supernatant	564		105	
T14AV	Sonicate supernatant	570		84	
ATCC 19246	Aqueous phase; phenol extraction		0		91
T14V	Aqueous phase; phenol extraction		17		175
T14AV	Aqueous phase; phenol extraction		150		270

a) protein by Lowry method
b) carbohydrate with anthrone reagent

activities (Fig. 1). Sonified-supernatants and aqueous extracts on phenol extraction from the T14V strain were characterized by immunoelectrophoresis with antisera to sonicate-supernatant and to whole bacteria (Fig. 2). The multitude of precipitin arcs obtained with each antiserum reflects the heterogeneity of the sonified-supernatants. When tested against the antiserum to the whole bacteria a very pronounced electronegative band was observed. This was the only precipitin arc observed in the phenol extracts. In contrast, this same precipitin arc was not observed in similar preparations from T14AV. These results suggest that the bone resorptive factor observed by us is different from the electronegative antigen. Preliminary gas chromatographic analysis did not detect the presence of glycerol or ribitol. Therefore lipoteichoic acid (12) does not seem to be responsible for the bone resorptive activity observed.

While this study was in progress another report (13) appeared on bone resorptive activity in the culture media on T14V.

Summary: Fractions with bone resorptive activity have been prepared with sonicate-supernatants from the following Actinomyces viscosus strains: ATCC 19246, T14V and T14AV. The activity is resistant to boiling and to pronase digestion. Aqueous extracts obtained on phenol extraction are enriched in carbohydrate but contain little if any protein. Bone resorptive activity is retained in these fractions. Even though the T14V and T14AV strains differ markedly in their potential to cause alveolar bone loss in monoinfected rodents, they do not differ in their content of bone resorptive factor.

This research was supported by grant DE-01932 from the National Institute of Dental Research.

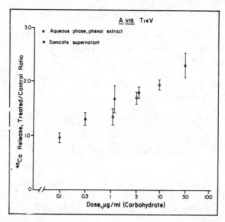

Figure 1.   Dose-response relationship for treatment of cultured
bones with preparations from A. viscosus T14V as
measured by ratio of ^{45}Ca released by paired control
bones during 48 h of incubation after 24 h or pre-
incubation.   Each point represents mean $\pm$ SE of six
pairs of cultures.

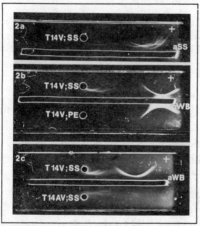

Figure 2.   Immunoelectrophoresis of fractions of A. viscosus
T14 and T14AV.
a.   Well contains sonicate-supernatant of T14 and
trough contains antiserum against sonicate-supernatant of ATCC 19246.
b.   Upper well contains sonicate-supernatant of T14
and lower well contains aqueous phase (phenol
extraction) of sonicate-supernatant of T14.
Trough contains antiserum against whole bacteria
of ATCC 19246.
c.   Upper well contains sonicate-supernatant of T14
and lower well contains sonicate-supernatant of
T14AV.   Trough contains antiserum against whole
bacteria of ATCC 19246.

References

1. Schei, O., Waerhaug, J., Lovdal, A., Arno, A. 1950. Alveolar bone loss as related to oral hygiene and age. J. Periodont. 30: 7-16.

2. Lindhe, J., Hamp, S.-E., Löe, H. 1973. Experimental periodontitis in the beagle dog. J. Periodont. Res. 8: 1-10.

3. Garant, P.R. 1976. Light and electron microscopic observations of osteoclastic alveolar bone resorption in rats monoinfected with Actinomyces naeslundii. J. Periodont. 47: 717-723.

4. Freedman, H.L., Listagarten, M.A., Taichman, N.S. 1968. Electron microscopic features of chronically inflamed human gingiva. J. Periodont. Res. 3: 313-327.

5. Hausmann, E., Weinfeld, N., Miller, W.A. 1972. Effects of lipopolysaccharides on bone resorption in tissue culture. Calcif. Tiss. Res. 9: 272-282.

6. Rowe, D.J., Hausmann, E. 1977. Quantitative analyses of osteoclast changes in resorbing bone organ cultures. Calcif. Tiss. Res. 23: 283-289.

7. Hausmann, E., Lüderitz, O., Knox, K., Weinfeld, N. 1975. Structural requirements for bone resorption by endotoxin and lipoteichoic acid. J. Dent. Res. 54: Special Issue B, B94-B99.

8. Socransky, S.S., Hubersak, C., Propas, D. 1970. Induction of periodontal destruction in gnotobiotic rats by human oral strains of Actinomyces naeslundii. Arch oral Biol. 15: 993-995.

9. Hammond, B.F., Steel, C.F., Peindl, K.S. 1976. Antigens and surface components associated with virulence of Actinomyces viscosus. J. dent. Res. 55: Special Issue A., A19-A25

10. Raisz, L.G. 1965. Bone resorption in tissue culture. Factors influencing the response to parathyroid hormone. J. clin. Invest. 44: 103-116.

11. Raisz, L.G., Niemann, I 1969. Effects of phosphate, calcium, magnesium on bone resorption and hormonal responses in tissue culture. Endocrinology 85: 446-456.

12. Wicken, A.J., Knox, K.W. 1975. Lipoteichoic acids: A new class of bacterial antigen. Science 187: 1161-1167.

13. Trummel, C.L., Past, M.J., Cisar, J.O. 1977. A stimulator of bone resorption produced by Actinomyces viscosus. J. dent. Res. 56: Special Issue B, B156.

Bone-Resorbing Activity in Serum Albumin.

P.Stern, S.Chen and D.Kahn.

Department of Pharmacology, Northwestern University,
Chicago, ILL 60611

The studies to be described were not originally undertaken
in an attempt to more fully understand the etiology of local
bone resorption. If they ultimately do so, it will be an
example of serendipity.

A number of years ago we attempted to use chemically defined media for studies of bone resorption in order to examine
the biochemical changes under controlled conditions (1). It
was soon found that these defined media were inadequate, not
only for peptide hormones such as PTH (1) but also for vitamin
D metabolites (2). In the course of searching for a protein
which would restore the bone-resorbing effect of PTH, we found
that some serum albumins stimulated bone resorption in a reproducible, dose-dependent manner (1,3). Different lots of
fraction V bovine serum albumin (BSA) varied in potency.
Crystalline bovine serum albumins were generally less active,
but not always devoid of activity. The bone-resorbing activity
of the albumin was found to be removed by activated charcoal
treatment or boiling, but not by heating at 55° for 30 minutes
(3). The activity was dialyzable and was not separated from
albumin by Sephadex chromatography.

We have recently (4,5) found that column or batch chromatography of the albumin on DEAE-Sephadex permits us to separate
a more potent bone-resorbing substance (brA) from the bulk of
the albumin. For batch preparation, 1.5 gm of albumin is dissolved in 5ml of 0.09M NaCl in 0.1M Tris buffer, pH 8.35. This
is added to 8gm of DEAE-Sephadex A-50 which was previously
equilibrated for 24 hr at 4°C with the same buffer. After
addition of the albumin, another 100 ml of buffer is added and
the mixture is shaken for 1 minute and centrifuged. The
extraction procedure is repeated 6 times. When this was done
with Pentex lot 177 bovine serum albumin fraction V, 2 to 10%
of the dry weight of the albumin was recovered in pooled supernatants. The material was 10-30 times more active than the
albumin from which it was derived. Some further increase in
activity was obtained with $(NH_4)_2SO_4$ fractionation or $CHCl_3$:
CH_3OH extraction of the brA (4,5).

Comparision of the stability of bone-resorbing activities
in the original albumin and of the brA is shown in Table 1.

Table 1. Characteristics of the bone-resorbing activity of BSA and brA

		original albumin (3)	brA(4,5)
a)	long term stability of dry material at $-20°C$	stable for > 1 year	activity declines within weeks
b)	stability:30 min. @ 55°C*	stable	stable
c)	stability:10 min. @ 100°C**	variable, sometimes loses activity	stable
d)	16 hr. protease treatment	activity lost	activity lost

* in water bath

We have compared (Table 2) the effects of a series of treatments on the bone resorption produced by BSA, brA and PTH.

On the basis of the available data, brA seems to be different from known bone resorbing substances. The fact that the activity in the residual fraction is not diminished but is actually enhanced by $CHCl_3$: CH_3OH extraction suggests that it is not due to substances such as vitamin D metabolites, fatty acids, or prostaglandins which should be soluble in the organic solvents. The heat stability of brA would indicate that it is not OAF (15) or complement (16). On the basis of chemical characteristics, the bone resorber seems most like PTH, being non-dialyzable, fairly heat stable (17) and probably protein in nature. However it differs from PTH in being susceptible to inhibition by indomethacin and on the basis of its concentration in serum. The current lot of albumin, which is a representative one, produced resorption at a concentration of 3 mg/ml. Since the concentration of albumin in serum would be 30-40 mg/ml, the bone resorber would seem to be active in vitro at physiologic concentrations. PTH, in contrast, has not been shown to be capable of eliciting bone resorption at concentrations (18) present in serum. Concentrations approximately ten times greater than the normal serum levels of PTH are required to produce resorption in vitro (12,19,20).

Table 2.   Effects of various treatments on the bone-resorbing
           effects of BSA, brA and PTH

	albumin	brA	PTH
a) calcitonin, 1µg/ml	blocks (3)	blocks (4,5)	blocks (6,7)
b) glucagon, 1µg/ml	blocks (3)	blocks (4,5)	blocks (8)
c) dexamethasone, 10^{-7}M	blocks (3)	blocks (4,5)	blocks (9,10)
d) phosphate, 3mM	not tested	blocks (4,5)	blocks (11)
e) pH 7.5	blocks (3)	not tested	blocks (12)
f) actinomycin-D	blocks* (3)	blocks** (4,5,)	blocks (13)
g) indomethacin, 10^{-7}-10^{-5}M	inhibits partially	inhibits partially	no effect (14)

———————————

* .04 µg/ml, ** .02 µg/ml

References

1. Stern, P.H. and Raisz, L.G. (1967) Exp. Cell Res. 46, 106-120.

2. Trummel, C. (1974) Ph.D. Thesis, Univ. of Rochester.

3. Stern, P.H. (1971) Calc. Tiss. Res. 7, 67-75.

4. Stern, P.H., Miller, J. and Blair, T. (1977) Fed. Proc. 36, 985.

5. Stern, P.H. and Miller, J. Calc. Tiss. Res., in press.

6. Friedman,J., Raisz, L.G. (1965) Science 150, 1465-1467.

7. Aliapoulious, M.A., Goldhaber, P. and Munson, P.L. (1966) Science 151, 330-331.

8. Stern, P.H. and Bell, N.H. (1970) Endocrinology 87, 111-117.

9. Stern, P.H. (1969) J. Pharm. Exp. Therap. 168, 211 -217.

10. Raisz, L.G., Trummel, C.L., Wener, J.A. and Simmons, H. (1972) Endocrinology 90, 961-967.

11. Raisz, L.G. and Niemann, I. (1969) Endocrinology 85, 446-452.

12. Raisz, L.G. (1965) J. Clin. Invest. 44, 103-116.

13. Raisz, L.G. (1965) Proc. Soc. Exp. Biol. 119, 614-617.

14. Goldhaber, P., Rabadjija, L., Beyer, W.R. and Kornhauser, A. (1973) J. Amer. Dent. Assn. 87, 1027-1033.

15. Luben, R.A., Mundy, G.R., Trummel, C.L. and Raisz, L.G. (1974) J. Clin. Invest. 53, 1473-1480.

16. Barrett, J.T. Textbook of Immunology 2nd ed. (1974), Mosby, St. Louis.

17. Raisz, L.G. personal communication.

18. Habener, J.F., Powell, D., Murray, T.M., Mayer, G.P. and Potts, J.T., Jr. (1971) Proc. Nat.Acad. Sci., U.S. 68, 2986-2991.

19. Reynolds,J.J. and Dingle, J.T. (1970) Calc. Tiss. Res. 4, 339-349.

20. Zanielli, J.M., Lea, D.J. and Nisbet, J.A. (1969) J. Endoc. 44, 33-46.

Regulation of Osteoclast-Activating Factor (OAF)-Stimulated Bone Resorption In Vitro with an Inhibitor of Collagenase.

John E. Horton[1], Frederick H. Wezeman[2], and Klaus E. Kuettner[3]

[1]Departments of Microbiology and of Immunology, USA Institute of Dental Research, Walter Reed Army Medical Center, Washington, D.C. 20012 (present address: Department of Periodontology, Harvard School of Dental Medicine, Boston MA 02115); [2]Department of Pathology, Michael Reese Hospital and Medical Center, Chicago, IL 60616; [3]Department of Orthopedic Surgery and of Biochemistry, Rush Medical College and Rush College of Health Sciences, Chicago, IL 60612.

INTRODUCTION

Investigations to define mechanisms regulating the activity of osteoclasts in both physiologic and pathologic states have generally centered on the effects and homeostatic control of systemic hormones and inorganic ions (1). While such approaches have elucidated much knowledge concerning responses of skeletal tissue in generalized metabolic bone disease, little is known of the pathogenesis of localized disorders of bone. However, recent reports suggest that specific biologic molecules capable of stimulating osteoclastic activity may exist at the local site of disease or injury independent of a generalized skeletal effect (2-9). These findings could explain the lack of clinical systemic evidence for regulation of these cells in bone loss associated with inflammatory states.

In inflammatory reactions, numerous lymphocytic cell populations operate and interact. Such cells are capable of elaborating biologically-active effector molecules called lymphokines (10, 11). Some of these mediators are believed responsible for amplifying the reactive events in such localized connective tissue diseases as periodontal disease and rheumatoid arthritis. One of these lymphokines was detected by us as being effective in stimulating the activity of osteoclasts in vitro resulting in the enhanced loss of bone (8, 12).

We initially demonstrated that osteoclasts could be stimulated in vitro by a biologic mediator detected in culture fluids of activated human lymphocytes (8). This "osteoclast-activating factor" (OAF) was elaborated following stimulation with mitogen or dental plaque antigenic material by cultured leukocytes from subjects with periodontal disease. Cultured leukocytes from subjects without disease were unresponsive to the antigenic material and did not produce OAF. Further investigations have revealed that bone resorbing activity with the characteristics of OAF is found in stimulated cultures enriched in T-cell or B-cell lymphocytes (13), cultures of bone marrow aspirates from patients with myeloma (14), as well as newly-established T-cell, B-cell and myeloma murine cell lines (15) and continuous cell lines from other hematologic neoplasms (16).

Eroded areas called Howship's lacunae are accepted as histologic evidence of the resorption and penetration by osteoclasts
into matured bone tissue. Erosion of bone is also known to occur
by invading endothelial and tumor cells. By defining invasion as
the interpenetration of a cell or tissue into adjacent tissues
combined with the destruction of the matrix of the invaded tissue, osteoclasts may be interpreted as being "invasive" cells.
In contrast, uncalcified cartilage often lies adjacent to bone
and resists erosion and invasion by multinucleated cells, endothelial and vascular elements, and tumor cells. As suggested in
our other studies, this resistance to penetration may well be due
to material present within the cartilage matrix (17, 18). Indeed, we found that poorly vascularized tissues such as
cartilage, blood vessel walls and dentin contain a low molecular
weight inhibitor of proteolytic activity (19-21). Extracts derived from cartilage were subsequently found to suppress endothelial but not fibroblast cell proliferation and to inhibit the
collagenolytic activity derived from fibroblasts as well as endothelial, osteosarcoma, and mammary carcinoma cells in culture
(22-24).

The function of osteoclasts is to attach to and resorb bone
through a coupled process of demineralization and degradation of
matrix collagen. Since osteoclasts share the characteristics of
collagen degradation with the above-named cells, and since collagenase has been demonstrated in the resorptive events of bone
collagen by osteoclasts (25), we tested our cartilage-derived
collagenolytic inhibitor on OAF-stimulated bones in vitro and
found that it reversibly inhibited osteoclastic resorption of
bone. Since this collagenase-inhibitor-enriched material modulates the activity of osteoclasts in addition to the above-
mentioned cellular processes, we have tentatively named it
"anti-invasion factor" (AIF).

MATERIALS AND METHODS

Preparation of Osteoclast-Activating Factor (OAF): Human
mononuclear cells (MNL) were fractionated from peripheral blood
leukocytes by isopycnic gradient separation of leukocyte-rich
plasma (12, 26). The cells were suspended at 2×10^6 viable
cells/ml in modified RPMI 1640 (Microbiological Assoc.) supplemented with 0.5% heat-inactivated autologous plasma, 1 mM L-
glutamine, 100 units penicillin and 100 μg streptomycin/ml (Flow
Labs). Replicate cultures were incubated in an humidified
atmosphere of 5% CO_2 in air at 37°C for 48 hr or 72 hr. MNL
cultures were either unstimulated or exposed to 2.0 μg/ml of
phytohemagglutinin (PHA, batch E316/Q1; Burroughs Wellcome).
To inhibit the possible production of prostaglandin by MNL,
indomethacin (kindly provided by Dr. Davis P. Jacobus, Merck,
Sharp & Dhome Research Labs) was dissolved in ethanol, tested at
final concentrations ranging from 10^{-9} to 10^{-5} M, and subsequently
added to MNL cultures at a final concentration of 5×10^{-5} M at
the onset of incubation. For comparative purposes, some cultures in these experiments acted as control and received
identical quantities of the diluent ethanol alone. DNA synthesis by the cultured MNL was determined by adding 1 μCi of

tritiated thymidine (TdR^{3}H, sp. act, 6 Ci/mM; Schwarz-Mann) to 6 or more replicate cultures of sedimented cells after aspiration of the culture fluid. The counts per minute (cpm) of cell-incorporated radioactivity in trichloroacetic acid-insoluble material was assayed using a scintillation spectrometer (model 3385; Packard Insts. Corps.). The analysis of variance was used to determine the statistical significance of the data (27).

Supernatant culture fluids to be used in the bone assay were aspirated and appropriately pooled from stimulated and unstimulated cultures of sedimented MNL. PHA was added to supernatant fluids from unstimulated cultures in amount equal to that added at the onset of incubation to stimulated cultures. The fluids were separately filtered through 0.22-μ pore-size membranes (Millipore Corp.) and stored frozen at -70°C for up to two months prior to use.

Preparation of the Cartilage-Derived Trypsin-Inhibitor with Collagenolytic Specificity (AIF): Slices of fresh bovine nasal septa cartilage were extracted with 1 M NaCl or 1 M guanidium hydrochloride (pH 5.8) for 48 hr at 4°C. After decantation the salt concentration was raised to 3 M and ultrafiltered under dissociative conditions at 4°C through a XM-50 filter membrane (M.W. cut-off of 50,000 Daltons; Amicon Corp.). The material was then concentrated and dialyzed into physiologic phosphate buffered saline (0.15M NaCl) with a UM-2 filter membrane (M.W. cut-off of 2,000 Daltons; Amicon Corp.) to yield a final concentration of 5 mg protein/ml. One hundred grams of cartilage yielded approximately 4 mg. Chemical analyses revealed that this material contained 95% protein; less than 0.5% uronic acid, indicating the absence of collagenous proteins; and approximately 1% hexosamine. Electrophoretically the proteins migrated as cationic proteins on cellulose acetate (pH 8.4) and in polyacrylamide gels (pH 7.4). Two of these proteins have been purified and identified: one is cartilage lysozyme, and the other a low molecular weight protein which acts not only as a trypsin inhibitor but specifically inhibits collagenases (21,22, 28).

Assay for Bone Resorption: The organ culture technique which measures the resorption of bone explants has been described (29). Paired shafts of the radius and ulna from 19-day-old rat fetuses, radiolabelled by injection of the mother with 250 μCi of ^{45}Calcium (^{45}Ca; sp. act. 25 Ci/g Ca; New England Nuclear) on the previous day, were incubated at 37°C in an humidified atmosphere of 5% CO_2 in air in 0.25 ml of BGJ$_b$ (GIBCO) supplemented with 1 mg/ml bovine serum albumin (BSA, fraction V; Pentex Miles Labs.), 1 mM L-glutamine, 100 units penicillin and 100μg streptomycin/ml (Flow Labs). The bone shafts were placed in test and control medium and cultured for up to 144 hr with appropriate transfer into fresh test and control medium each 48 hr. In selected experiments, the bone shafts were cultured in medium only for an initial 18-24 hr period which served to remove exchangeable ^{45}Ca and then transferred to test and control medium for up to 120 hr with one change into fresh medium at 48 hr. In all experiments, each cultured bone explant when transferred from one culture vessel to another was rinsed for 30 second in culture medium without additives.

OAF-containing test and control MNL culture fluids were diluted 1:2 in the bone culture medium. Three proteolytic inhibitors, 1) soybean trypsin-inhibitor (crystallized 5x; Nutritional Biochemical Corp.), 2) bovine trypsin-kallikrein-inhibitor (Trasylol[R]; aprotein; kindly supplied by Dr. E. Truscheit,Bayer,A. G.), and 3) AIF, the cartilage-derived material enriched in an inhibitor of collagenase, were diluted in culture medium and added to bone cultures at a final concentration of 300 µg protein/ml. Control fluids with and without additives were tested also for their effects in the bone resorption assay against undiluted culture medium. In some experiments, indomethacin dissolved in ethanol was added to the bone cultures at a final concentration of 5×10^{-5} M at the onset of the experiment and again when the bones were transferred. Control cultures in these experiments received identical quantities of the diluent ethanol alone.

The degree of bone resorption in each culture was measured using liquid scintillation spectrometry to determine the amount of ^{45}Ca released into the culture fluid during each culture period and also that which remained in the bones at termination of the experimental period. The data are expressed as the mean percent of radioactivity released from four pairs of cultured bones and also as the mean ratio of treated to control cultures for four pairs of bones. The Students' "t" test was used to determine the statistical significance of the data (27).

Preparation of Cultured Bones for Morphology and Quantitative Histometry: Bone cell morphology and quantitative histometry was determined from light and electron microscopic sections of cultured bones selected from representative periods during experiments. Bones from culture were fixed in 2.5% gluteraldehyde in 0.1M cacodylate buffer, pH 7.4. The undecalcified specimens were then rinsed in cacodylate buffer containing 3% sucrose and postfixed in 2% OsO_4 in 0.2 M collidine buffer. Specimens were then dehydrated in graded alcohols and embedded in Epon 812 for longitudinal sectioning. Sections 3.0 µm thick were stained with borate-toluidine blue and observed under light microscopy for quantitative histometry. Other bones were routinely processed, embedded in paraffin or plastic, and stained with hematoxylin and eosin for observation by light microscopy. Quantitative data were obtained by examining six total midsagittal sections from each bone shaft without knowledge of slide identification after the method of Rowe and Hausmann (30). Osteoclasts were identified by their large size, multiple nuclei and other cytoplasmic organellar features. Cell and nuclear counts of osteoclasts were determined from the total number of cells in adjacent midsagittal sections from both experimental and control bones. Counts were averaged from six midsagittal sections and expressed as the mean plus or minus the standard error. Statistical significance of the data was determined using the Students' "t" test (27).

For electron microscopic observations, Ultrathin Epon 812 sections of bone specimens were placed on parlodian-coated 150 mesh copper grids and stained with 5% uranyl acetate and 2% lead citrate. A Phillips 300 electron microscope was used to examine the tissues.

RESULTS

Generation of OAF Activity: Consistent with our previous reports, the bone resorbing activity OAF was routinely elaborated in mitogen-stimulated cultures of MNL, while none could be detected in control fluids from unstimulated MNL and bones cultured in medium alone (data not shown) (12, 13).

To exclude the possible contamination of OAF-containing fluids with prostaglandins, indomethacin, a known inhibitor of prostaglandin synthesis, was added to cultured MNL. Additions of this agent in concentrations from 10^{-9} to 10^{-5} M did not impair the reactivity of mitogen-stimulated MNL nor their ability to generate OAF activity (representative experiment shown in Table 1). Furthermore, as previously reported, additions of indomethacin to the bone organ cultures failed to suppress the effect of pre-formed OAF activity (31).

Effect of Proteinase Inhibitors on OAF-Stimulated Bone Cultures:

Osteoclastic bone resorption results in demineralization and dissolution of matrix collagen. Proteolytic enzymes, specifically collagenase, are required to digest the collagen molecule. We therefore tested the effect of blocking proteolytic activity with specific proteinase inhibitors in OAF-stimulated bone cultures.

The two proteinase trypsin-inhibitors, soybean trypsin-inhibitor and Trasylol[R], were each added at culture onset and on bone transfer at 48 hr at eight different concentrations up to a maximum final concentration of 400 µg/ml to OAF-stimulated and unstimulated fetal rat bone cultures (Table 2). Neither inhibitor suppressed the amount of ^{45}Ca released from cultured bones stimulated with the bone resorber OAF nor from cultures of bones receiving unstimulated MNL culture fluids.

We also tested the cartilage-derived proteinase inhibitor with known specificity toward collagenase, AIF (Table 3). Additions of AIF completely blocked the effect of OAF stimulation in the bone cultures when compared in ratio with control bone cultures. Furthermore, this cartilaginous extract was so potent that bones transferred twice into fresh OAF-containing medium could not overcome additions of this inhibitor even up to 144 hr of culture. However, the mean percent (6%) of ^{45}Ca released by control bones cultured with additions of this cartilage-derived inhibitor was also significantly reduced when compared with control bones cultured in the absence of this agent (19%).

Table 1

Failure of Indomethacin to Inhibit the Generation in MNL Cultures and Activity in Bone Explants of OAF

MNL Culture Stimulant	Indomethacin Additions[1]	Mean cpm ± S.E. of TdR ^{3}H Incorporated by MNL Cultures	120 Hr, ^{45}Ca-Release by Fetal Bone Cultures (Treated/Control Ratio ± S.E.)
None	None	925 ± 101	1.03 ± 0.02
PHA		151,477 ± 6,932[2]	3.25 ± 0.22[3]
None	MNL Cultures	1,057 ± 155	0.98 ± 0.04
PHA		166,383 ± 8,772[2]	3.42 ± 0.29[3]
None	Bone Cultures	(925 ± 101)[4]	1.01 ± 0.03
PHA		(151,477 ± 6,932)[4]	3.56 ± 0.33[3]

[1] Indomethacin was added to either cultures of MNL or bone explants at a final concentration of 5 x 10^{-5} M.

[2] Significantly different from respective unstimulated cultures, p<0.01, but not significantly different from each other.

[3] Signigicantly different from the value of 1.0, p<0.01, but not significantly different from each other.

[4] Supernatant fluids without additions of Indomethacin to MNL cultures.

Table 2

Failure of Soybean Trypsin-Inhibitor and Trasylol^R to

Suppress OAF-Stimulated Bone Resorption In Vitro

Culture Stimulant	Inhibitor[1]	120 Hr, Mean Percent ± S.E. of ^{45}Ca Released from Fetal Bones
None	None	18.51 ± 1.03
OAF		51.10 ± 4.15[2]
None	Soybean Trypsin Inhibitor	19.70 ± 1.19
OAF		52.97 ± 3.98[2]
None	None	21.65 ± 1.93
OAF		63.52 ± 5.01[3]
None	Trasylol^R	23.52 ± 2.11
OAF		62.78 ± 4.25[3]

[1] Soybean trypsin-inhibitor and Trasylol^R were added at a final concentration of 400 μg/ml to bone cultures at onset of incubation and on transfer at 48 hr.

[2] Significantly different from respective control cultures, p<0.01, but not significantly different from each other.

[3] Significantly different from respective control cultures, p<0.01, but not significantly different from each other.

Table 3

Effect of AIF on OAF-Stimulated Bone Resorption In Vitro

144-Hr, ^{45}Ca-Release of Treated and Control Cultures

Inhibitor[1]	Mean Percent $\pm$ S.E.		Mean Ratio $\pm$ S.E.
	Treated Cultures	Control Cultures	
Absent	51.19 $\pm$ 4.78[2]	19.54 $\pm$ 1.20[2]	2.67 $\pm$ 0.44[2,3]
Present	6.64 $\pm$ 0.71	6.10 $\pm$ 0.69	1.08 $\pm$ 0.02

[1]AIF and OAF were added at onset of incubation and at each 48 hr transfer.

[2]Significantly different from respective values obtained from bones cultured in the presence of inhibitor, $p < 0.01$.

[3]Differs significantly from the value of 1.0, $p < 0.01$.

To determine whether this blockade of osteoclast activity was permanent or reversible, we cultured three groups of OAF-stimulated bone explants and their controls with and without additions of AIF and separately measured the amount of ^{45}Ca released during each of three 48-hr incubation periods (Table 4). The first group of bones was cultured and transferred at 48 hr intervals in OAF-containing and control culture fluids only. OAF-stimulated bones released 24% of ^{45}Ca during the first 48 hr incubation and comparable amounts during each subsequent 48 hr culture period. Unstimulated bone cultures released only 13% of ^{45}Ca during the first 48 hr and a lesser amount during each subsequent 48 hr period.

The second group of bones was identically cultured with the exception that all cultures also received additions of AIF at the onset of incubation. Each bone was then transferred 48 hr and 96 hr later into its appropriate culture fluid devoid of AIF. In contrast to the first group, bones receiving additions of the cartilage-derived inhibitor released only 3% of ^{45}Ca during the first 48 hr. However, when these bones were rinsed and transferred to their appropriate culture medium without further addition of AIF, increased release of ^{45}Ca occurred. In OAF-stimulated bones, the increase was approximately 3-fold greater within 48 hr and then doubled during the subsequent 48-hr period of culture. Also, the amount of ^{45}Ca released by control cultures devoid of AIF doubled during the second 48-hr period of incubation but then lessened during the final 48-hr period of incubation. It should be noted that OAF-stimulated bones released over 28% of their ^{45}Ca once the culture medium was devoid of AIF, while only 3% could be released in its presence.

The third group of bones was also cultured and transferred each 48 hr in OAF-containing and control culture fluids, but received additions of AIF only upon transfer to their respective fresh medium at 48 hr and 96 hr culture periods. The amounts of ^{45}Ca released during the first 48 hr in OAF-stimulated and control cultures were comparable to those values seen at 48 hr in the first group of bones. However, when these bones were subsequently transferred to approprite medium containing AIF, ^{45}Ca-release was dramatically reduced. Less than 5% of the radiolabelled bone calcium could be released with continued OAF-stimulation during the second 48-hr incubation and recovery from this suppression failed to occur even after 96 hr of culture. A similar blockade of ^{45}Ca-release occurred in control bone cultures which received additions of AIF.

Effect of OAF and AIF on Osteoclast Morphology: Using light microscopy, counts of osteoclasts and osteoclast nuclei per cell in total midsagittal sections from both control and experimental groups reflected the ^{45}Ca-release data (Table 5). The singular presence of OAF during the first 48 hr period of culture resulted in a marked increase in the size and number of osteoclasts, and each osteoclast also manifested greater numbers of nuclear profiles. In explants cultured in the presence of both OAF and

Table 4

Effect of Additions and Removal of AIF on OAF-Stimulated Bone Resorption In Vitro

Bone Culture Stimulant	Duration Inhibitor Present (Hr)	Mean Percent $\pm$ S.E. of ^{45}Ca-Released each 48-Hr Interval from Cultured Fetal Rat Bones		
		0-48 Hr	49-96 Hr	97-144 Hr
None	None	13.44 ± 0.71	6.28 ± 0.92	6.89 ± 1.06
OAF		24.63 ± 2.65[1]	23.61 ± 2.29[1]	26.36 ± 2.19[1]
None	0-48	3.05 ± 0.44	6.28 ± 0.54	3.65 ± 0.42
OAF		3.38 ± 0.16	9.40 ± 0.82[2]	18.61 ± 1.75[1]
None	49-144	13.52 ± 0.51	2.83 ± 0.35	1.97 ± 0.39
OAF		21.67 ± 2.26[1]	4.34 ± 0.93	3.10 ± 0.88

[1] Significantly different from respective control culture, $p < 0.01$.

[2] Significantly different from respective control culture, $p < 0.05$.

Table 5

Quantitative Histometric Observations of the Effect of OAF With and Without the Presence of AIF on Osteoclasts in Cultured Fetal Rat Bones

Additives	Mean No. of Osteoclasts Per Total Midsagittal Section[1]	Mean No. of Nuclei Per Osteoclast[1]
None	7.4 ± 0.21[2]	4.1 ± 0.10[2]
OAF	15.8 ± 0.36[3]	7.5 ± 0.25[3]
OAF + AIF	9.5 ± 0.16[2,3]	5.5 ± 0.15[2,3]

[1] Values were collected and averaged from the total number of osteoclasts and their nuclei in 6 midsagittal sections of each 48 hr cultured bone and are expressed as the mean $\pm$ S.E.

[2] Significantly different from OAF-Stimulated bones, $p < 0.01$.

[3] Significantly different from control bones, $p < 0.01$.

AIF, the observed number of osteoclasts was significantly decreased, as was the number of nuclear profiles per osteoclast.

As observed with the electron microscope, control osteoclasts revealed morphological characteristics consistent with
previous reports for these cells (32-34) (Fig. 1). The osteoclasts reflected minimal resorptive activity by attachment to
bone surfaces and some evidence for ruffled borders. Such cells
were without swollen mitochondria, extensive cytoplasmic vacuolations, and gave no evidence for augmented dense bodies. However, osteoclasts stimulted by OAF developed expanded ruffled
borders and clear zones (Fig. 2). Adjacent spicules of bone
were extensively resorbed. Not infrequently viable OAF-stimulated osteoclasts were observed with more than one ruffled border
region. Invaginations from the ruffled border region extended
deep into the cytoplasm of these OAF-stimulated cells. Mineralized debris was present both within the ruffled border region and
in the subjacent vacuolar apparatus. Swollen mitochondria and
swollen peri-nuclear Golgi fields (35) were also noted within
these OAF-stimulted cells at 48 hr of culture. In contrast,
significant morphological differences were observed in bones
cultured in the presence of OAF plus AIF (Fig. 3). Microscopically, the total cellularity of the cultured bones was increased.
Viable osteoclasts were observed adjacent to spicules of bone
but their cell membranes were distinctly separated from bone
surfaces (Fig 3-A). No evidence could be found in these cells
for ruffled borders or clear zones. Additionally, these osteoclasts were decreased in size and their cytoplasm contained
fewer vacuoles and mitochondria (Fig 3-B). However, these cells
could be clearly identified as osteoclasts on the basis of their
multinuclearity and other cytoplasmic characteristics. Indica-
tions of cellular damage were not observed.

DISCUSSION

The skeleton provides to the organism support as well as an
accessible reservoir of minerals to regulate concentrations of
blood electrolytes. These functions, while distinct, are intimately related through the activity of bone cells. In general,
cellular responses of bone to endocrinological disorders affect
both skeletal and mineral metabolism to manifest as generalized
bone disease, while in contrast responses to adjacent infection
and inflammation are often seen only as skeletal defects mani-
festing as a localized disorder of bone. Our current investigations have centered on the activity and regulation of the
biologically-active lymphokine OAF which is believed responsible
for the stimulation of osteoclasts in localized bone disorders
associated with chronic inflammatory states.

OAF is a unique biologic stimulator of osteoclasts in vitro
and is chemically distinct from other known bone resorbing
agents (36). The potency of this factor in stimulating osteoclasts in vitro has been found comparable with parathyroid
hormone (PTH) (31). Neither the production nor expression of
this lymphokine requires mediation by prostaglandins, since

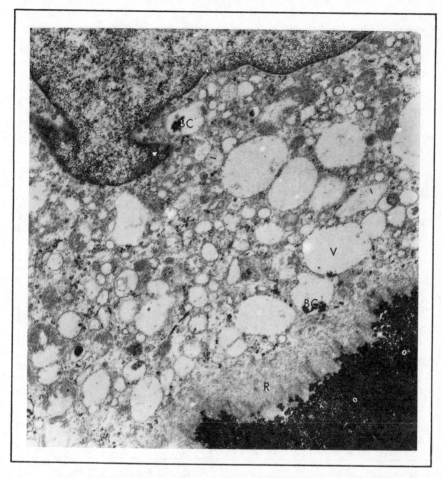

Figure 1 - Osteoclasts of control 48-hr bone cultures reveal moderate
development of ruffled border regions (R) and vacuolations (V). The
disrupted bone surface and free bone crystals within vacuoles (BC)
give evidence of resorptive activity.   X 33,576.

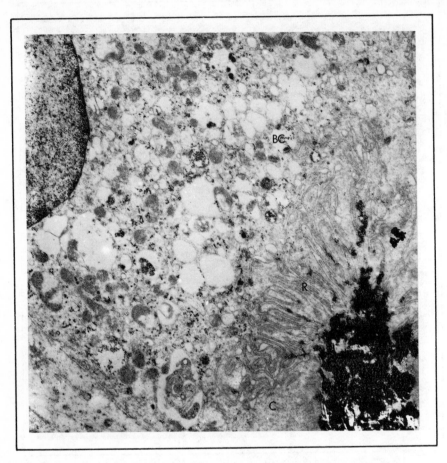

Figure 2 - Osteoclasts of 48-hr OAF-stimulated bone cultures reveal extensive development of the ruffled border region (R) and clear zone areas (C). Extensive ruffled border channels and their channel expansions are associated with significant disruption of the bone surface and free bone crystals (BC) within subjacent vacuoles. X 17,590.

Figure 3 - Osteoclasts of 48-hr bone cultures which contained both OAF and AIF reveal altered morphology indicative of inhibition of osteoclast function. Figure 3-A shows a portion of an osteoclast which had no ruffled borders and was separated from the bone surface. Note the high nuclear-cytoplasmic ratio, reduced vacuolation, and undisturbed bone surface. X 24, 622. Figure 3-B shows a portion of an osteoclast separated from the disturbed bone surface. Mitochondria are swollen and numerous vacuoles and free ribosomes are present but ruffled borders are absent. N=nuclei. X 16,240.

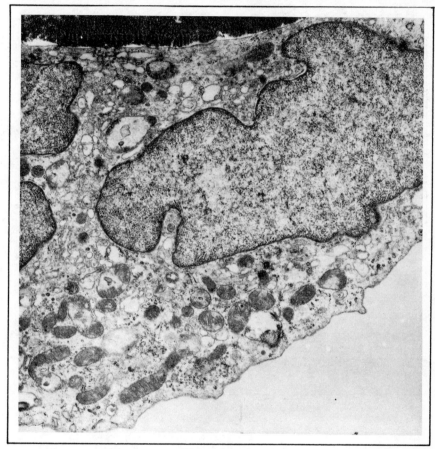

Figure 3-A

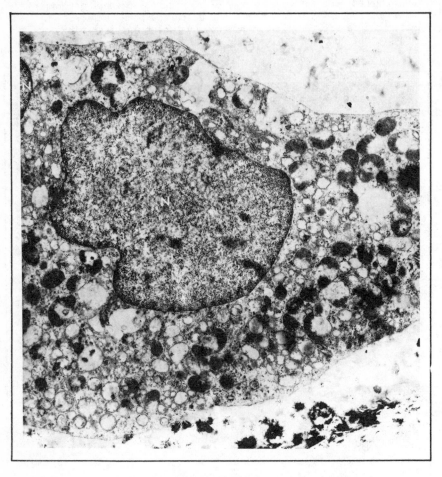

Figure 3-B

additions of indomethacin to stimulated MNL, as shown herein, and to bone cultures (31) are without effect.

While the bioassay system used to determine bone resorption measures the release of previously incorporated ^{45}Ca, osteoclastic activity in these cultured bones results in loss of both mineral and organic matrix components (37). Current concepts allow the conclusion that under physiologic conditions a highly specialized enzyme, collagenase, initiates the degradation of the major structural protein of bone, collagen, by a specific cleavage into two fragments which are then further degraded by other non-specific proteases. It has been implicated and recently documented that during PTH-stimulated osteoclastic bone resorption collagenase activity can be harvested from the bone culture medium (25, 38-41). Our reports that the lymphocyte factor, OAF, also stimulates osteoclastic bone resorption suggests that collagenase production would also be stimulated by this mediator. This concept is not without precedent since Dayer et al reported that a factor released by human lymphocytes in vitro markedly stimulated collagenase production by cultured rheumatoid synovial cells (42). Further, preliminary data in our laboratories indicate that in the system described herein, collagenase activity can also be detected in the culture medium. We therefore decided to test in the bone culture system the effect of our cartilage-derived material enriched in a trypsin-inhibitor which acts as a specific collagenolytic inhibitor and which we have termed "AIF" (43). We also tested two other trypsin inhibitors devoid of specificity toward collagenase in this comparative study. The first, soybean-trypsin inhibitor, is a plant-derived polypeptide which stoichiometrically inhibits trypsin and to a lesser extent chymotrypsin (44). Inhibitory activity is also directed towards thrombin, plasmin, and leukocytic proteases. The other was Trasylol^R, the trypsin-kallikrein inhibitor, which is obtained from bovine lung and is identical with the pancreatic trypsin inhibitor described by Kunitz (44-46). Trasylol^R inhibits proteases with proteolytic and esterolytic activity. Included in this group are trypsin, chymotrypsin, the kinogenases, plasmin, plasmin activator, plasma factors active in pre-coagulation, and tissue and leukocytic proteinases. In other experiments we have tested each for their ability to inhibit collagenolytic activity from normal human skin and human hypertrophic scar tissue and found that even at high concentrations they showed only minimal effect (22, 47).

Our inability to influence osteoclastic resorption using the non-collagenolytic trypsin-inhibitors of proteolysis was not surprising, since the collagen molucule is relatively resistant to proteolytic activity until it is specifically cleaved by the enzyme collagenase (48). However, the dramatic sequence of events which occurred using AIF was unexpected. This inhibitor prevented osteoclastic resorption in both OAF-stimulated and control bones which was completely blocked throughout six days of culture and from which there was no "escape" (49). Suppression of the activity of these cells was confirmed histologically in addition to large reductions in amounts of ^{45}Ca released from such cultured bones.

Further experiments revealed that the AIF material was neither toxic to the cells nor were their responses destroyed. Osteoclasts in both OAF-stimulated and unstimulated bones cultured in the presence of AIF for 48 hr were completely unresponsive in their ability to release ^{45}Ca. However, upon transferring such inhibited bones to OAF-containing and control medium devoid of AIF, osteoclastic bone resorption was once again found to recur with increased release of the ^{45}Ca. The biologic potency of AIF is indicated by its ability to completely inhibit OAF-stimulated osteoclastic resorption which had already progressed for 48 hr.

Morphologic and quantitative histometric studies on osteoclasts within these cultured bones reflect the biologic effects of OAF-stimulation and AIF-suppression. The cellular architecture of the osteoclast engaged in active bone resorption includes specific structural characteristics which implicate its function (32-34, 50). Essential to a histologic assessment of cellular activity is an intimate contact with a bony calcified matrix. Other associated morphological features are the presence of a ruffled border with adjacent clear zones, multinucleation, and expanded vacuolations to include dense bodies, and numerous mitochondria. The degree of irregularity of the adjacent bone surface reflects the resorptive activity and results in the appearance of bone debris, mineral material, and collagen in the extracellular space between the bone surface and ruffled border as well as within the expanded channels and vacuoles of that zone (33). Other "populations" of osteoclasts give minimal evidence of resorptive activity. They are present on or near bone surfaces and are not associated with an obvious disturbance of the subjacent bone surfaces (33). These morphological criteria of relatively active and less active (inactive) states of the osteoclast are interpreted as expressions of the normal range of morphological characteristics for this population of cells. Thus, alterations in osteoclast morphology are the basis upon which osteoclastic functions are assessed with hormonal, chemical and other biologically-active molecules such as OAF.

The increased size, number and nucleation of active osteoclasts in this investigation gave ample structural evidence of the extensive resorptive capability of the OAF-stimulated osteoclast as reflected in the degree of expansion of the ruffled border region of all osteoclasts observed. The presence of AIF in these cultures was always capable of inhibiting the egress of ^{45}Ca from these bones. The morphological expression of this inhibition was separation of osteoclasts from the bone surfaces with loss of ruffled border and a reduction in the extent of ruffled border size in those few cells observed to be still in contact with bone. Removal of the collagenolytic inhibitor resulted in a resumption of resorption and was reflected in the re-establishment of contact by morphologically-active osteoclasts with the bone surfaces. A striking parallel in this regulation of osteoclasts can be drawn from observations of the effects of PTH and calcitonin (CT) on such cell-mediated resorption. Available evidence indicates that these homeostatic hormones act on the same cell (51). Inhibition by CT of PTH-stimulated osteoclastic resorption has been demonstrated to affect the relationship of these cells to bone surfaces (34, 49, 52-54). Concomitantly, the change in organellar features characteristic of the active resorptive state and the separation of the osteoclast from the bone surface (55) were reversible events and parallel the observations in the present investigation wherein the effects of OAF and AIF equate morphologically to the respective effects of PTH and CT.

The data presented here support our theory that cell-mediated resorption of bone, either by osteoclasts or by tumor cells (56, 57), is directly related to the release of collagenase by the cells effecting resorption. Inhibitors of other neutral proteases in our in vitro system did not block osteoclastic activity. This selectivity of a collagenase inhibitor on osteoclastic activity may therefore be a model for a local regulatory system for bone matrix removal. This concept is supported by the findings of Sellers et al that bones in culture synthesize an inhibitor of collagenase (58). Contrary to AIF, however, this inhibitor can be degraded by trypsin and chymotrypsin.

Our morphologic observations revealed that active osteoclasts lie on bone surfaces and AIF-inhibited osteoclasts are removed from bone surfaces with loss of ruffled border and other cytoplasmic alterations. This suggests to us that alterations of osteoclast plasma membrane occur in the presence of AIF. Since AIF may prove to selectively act on the collagenase molecule, we further suggest that this enzyme activity is an integral part of the cell membrane. Validity for this concept is forwarded from investigations in other systems in which invasive tumor cell membranes appear to be in direct contact with connective tissue collagen fibers during the process of collagenolysis (59-63). Further, Rose and Robertson recently provided indirect evidence that the collagenolytic activity of gingival fibroblasts derived from patients with periodontal disease is cell membrane-bound and acts only when the cell membrane contacts the collagen fibrils, but remains on the cell membrane after collagen destruction rather than being released into extracellular spaces (64). Our observations permit the hypothesis that the same phenomenon may be true with respect to osteoclasts. Therefore, local tissue-specific collagenase inhibitors may well be critical regulators in modulating the expression of osteoclastic activity through control of cell surface components.

SUMMARY

The regulation of osteoclastic activity is exemplified in the growth and development of long bones, fracture repair, periodontal disease, and rheumatoid arthritis. These states exist independent of a generalized skeletal response or disruption in systemic mineral metabolism which suggests that specific biologic molecules exist at such local sites to control cellular responses.

We previously established that osteoclasts could be stimulated to resorb bone in vitro by a product elaborated by activated lymphocytes and have suggested a role for this "osteoclast-activating factor" (OAF) in localized disorders of bone.

We now have detected a cartilage-derived trypsin-inhibitor with specificity toward collagenase which inhibits osteoclastic activity. This inhibitor not only prevents the invasive resorption of bone by osteoclasts in vitro, but also results in morphological characteristics indicative of cell inactivity to include the separation by these cells from bone surfaces. The inhibitory activity of this "anti-invasion factor" (AIF) appears more potent than calcitonin (CT) in that the suppression of osteoclastic activity could not be overcome by OAF when AIF was present. However, this blockage of osteoclastic activity by AIF was reversible, since osteoclasts could be subsequently stimulated with OAF when AIF was removed from bones previously cultured in the simultaneous presence of OAF and AIF. We also found the effects of OAF and AIF on osteoclasts to equate morphologically to the respective effects of PTH and CT.

Our studies indicate that osteoclastic activity in vitro may be regulated with the biologic molecules, OAF and AIF. Our results further suggest that the specific inhibition of collagenase modulates the activity of osteoclasts, and demonstrate that bone cell activities may be controlled locally in part by tissue-specific enzyme regulators. Finally, the coupled effects of OAF and AIF on osteoclast activity may well explain mechanisms involved in localized disorders of bone loss.

ACKNOWLEGEMENT

We gratefully acknowledge the expert technical assistance of Vicki J. Wyan, Susan D. Jenkins, Hilda Sanders, Richard Croxen, Alice Croxen and Marjorie Chow; and the secretarial assistance of Cathlyn Hill and Mary Nelson.

This work was supported in part by NIH-NIDR Interagency Agreement Y01-DE-60025, and grants NIH-GRS-5476; NIH-AM-09132, and NIH-CA-21566.

ABBREVIATIONS

AIF, anti-invasion factor; ^{45}Ca, calcium-45; CT, calcitonin; MNL, mononuclear leukocytes; OAF, osteoclast-activating factor; PHA, phytohemagglutinin; PTH, parathyroid hormone.

REFERENCES

1. Rasmussen, H. and Bordier, P. 1974. The Physiological and Cellular Basis of Metabolic Bone Disease. The Williams & Wilkins Co., Baltimore.

2. Klein, D. C. and Raisz, L. G. 1970. Prostaglandins: stimulation of bone resorption in tissue culture. Endocrinology 86, 1436-1440.

3. Goodson, J. M., Dewhirst, F. E. and Brunetti, A. 1974. Prostaglandin E_2 levels and human periodontal disease. Prostaglandins 6, 81-85.

4. Raisz, L. G., Sandberg, A., Goodson, J. M., Simmons, H. A. and Mergenhagen, S. E. 1974. Complement-dependent stimulation of bone resorption mediated by prostaglandins. Science 185, 789-791.

5. Robinson, D. R. and Mcguire, M. B. 1975. Prostaglandins in the rheumatic diseases. An. N.Y. Acad. Sci. 256, 318-329.

6. Hausmann, E., Raisz, L. G. and Miller, W. A. 1970. Endotoxin: stimulation of bone resorption in tissue culture. Science 168, 862-864.

7. Hausmann,E., Luderitz, O., Knox, K., Weinfeld, N. 1975. Structural requirements for bone resorption by endotoxin and lipoteichoic acid. J. Dent. Res. 54 (Spec. Issue B), B94-99.

8. Horton, J. E., Raisz, L. G., Simmons, H. A., Oppenheim, J. J. and Mergenhagen, S. E. 1972. Bone resorbing activity in supernatant fluid from human cultured peripheral blood leukocytes. Science, 177, 793-795.

9. Horton, J. E., Oppenheim, J. J. and Mergenhagen, S. E. 1974. A role for cell-mediated immunity in the pathogenesis of periodontal disease. J. Periodont. 45, 351-360.

10. Pick, E. and Turk, J.L. 1972. The biological activities of soluble lymphocyte products. Clin. Exp. Immunol. 10, 1-23.

11. David, J. R. 1973. Lymphocyte mediators and cellular hypersensitivity. New Engl. J. Med. 288, 143-149.

12. Horton, J. E., Oppenheim, J. J., Mergenhagen, S. E. and Raisz, L. G. 1974. Macrophage-lymphocyte synergy in the production of osteoclast activating factor. J. Immunol. 113, 1278-1287.

13. Chen, P., Trummel, C., Horton, J. E., Baker, J. J. and Oppenheim, J. J. 1976. Production of osteoclast-activating factor by normal human peripheral blood rosetting and non-rosetting lymphocytes. Eur. J. Immunol. 6, 732-736.

14. Mundy, G. R., Raisz, L. G., Cooper, R. A., Schecter, G. P. and Salmon, S. E. 1974. Evidence for the secretion of an osteoclast stimulating factor in myeloma. New Engl. J. Med 291, 1041-1046.

15. Neiders, M. E., Horton, J. E., Kim, J. and Asofsky, R. 1978 Bone resorbing activity in supernatant fluids from established lymphoid tumor cell lines. J. Dent. Res. 57, (In press).

16. Mundy, G. R., Luben, R. A., Raisz, L. G., Oppenheim, J. J. and Buell, D. N. 1974. Bone-resorbing activity in supernatants from lymphoid cell lines. New Engl. J. Med. 290, 867-871.

17. Eisenstein, R., Sorgente, N., Soble, L. W., Miller, A., and Kuettner, K. E. 1973. The resistance of certain tissues to invasion: penetrability of explanted tissues by vascularized mesenchyme. Amer. J. Pathol. 73, 765-774.

18. Sorgente, N., Kuettner, K. E., Soble, L. W. and Eisenstein,R 1975. The resistance of certain tissues to invasion. II. Evidence for extractable factors in cartilage which inhibit invasion by vascularized mesenchyme. Lab. Invest. 32, 217-222.

19. Kuettner, K. E., Croxen, R. L., Eisenstein, R. and Sorgente, N. 1974. Proteinase inhibitory activity in connective tissue. Experientia 30, 595-597.

20. Sharkey, M., Veis, A. and Kuettner, K. 1973. Isolation and characterization of dental phosphoproteins. J. Dent. Res. 53 (Spec. Issue), (301), 134.

21. Kuettner, K. E., Harper, E. J. and Eisenstein, R. 1977. Protease inhibitors in cartilage. Arthr. & Rheum. 20, (Suppl.) S124-129.

22. Kuettner, K. E., Hiti, J., Eisenstein, R. and Harper, E. 1976. Collagenase inhibition by cationic proteins derived from cartilage and aorta. Biochem., Biophys., Res. Comm. 72, 40-46.

23. Kuettner, K. E., Soble, L., Croxen, R. L., Marczynska, B., Hiti, J. and Harper, E. 1977. Tumor cell collagenase and its inhibition by a cartilage-derived protease inhibitor. Science, 196, 653-654.

24. Eisenstein, R., Kuettner, K. E., Neopolitan, C., Soble, L. W. and Sorgente, N. 1975. The resistance of certain tissues to invasion. III. Cartilage extracts inhibit the growth of fibroblasts and endothelial cells in culture. Amer. J. Pathol. 81, 337-348.

25. Sakamoto, S., Sakamoto, M., Goldhaber, P. and Glimcher, M. J. 1975. Collagenase and bone resorption: isolation of collagenase from medium containing serum after stimulation of bone

resorption by addition of parathyroid hormone extract. Biochem., Biophys. Res. Comm. 63, 172-178.

26. Böyum, A. 1968. Isolation of mononuclear cells and granulocytes from human blood. Scand. J. Clin. Lab. Invest. 21, (Suppl. 97), 77-89.

27. Ostle, B., 1963. Statistics in research. Iowa State University Press, Ames, IA.

28. Sorgente, N., Kuettner, K. E. and Eisenstein, R. 1976. The isolation, purification and partial characterizaton of proteinase inhibitors from bovine cartilage and aorta. In, Protides of the Biological Fluids (Peeters, H., Ed.). Vol. 23, Pergamon Press, Oxford, pp. 227-230.

29. Raisz, L. G. and Niemann, I. 1969. Effects of phosphate, calcium, and magnesium on bone resorption and hormonal responses in tissue culture. Endocrinology 85, 446-456.

30. Rowe, D. J. and Hausmann, E. 1976. The alteration of osteoclast morphology by diphosphonates in bone culture. Calcif. Tiss. Res. 20, 53-60.

31. Raisz, L. G., Luben, R. A., Mundy, G. R., Horton, J. E. and Trummel, C. L. 1975. Effect of osteoclast activating factor from human leukocytes on bone metabolism. J. Clin. Invest. 56, 408-413.

32. Dudley, H. R. and Spiro, D. 1961. The fine structure of bone cells. J. Biophys., Biochem. Cytol. 11, 627-649.

33. Lucht, U. 1972. Osteoclasts and their relationship to bone as studied by electron microscopy. Z. Zellforsch. 135, 211-228.

34. Gothlin, G. and Ericsson, J.L.E. 1976. The osteoclast: Review of ultrastructure, origin, and structure-function relationship. Clin. Orthop. Rel. Res. 120, 201-231.

35. Cameron, D. A. 1968. The golgi apparatus in bone and cartilage cells. Clin. Orthop. Rel. Res. 58, 191-211.

36. Luben, R. A., Mundy, G. R., Trummel, C. L. and Raisz, L. G. 1974. Partial purification of osteoclast-activating factor from phytohemagglutinin-stimulated human leukocytes. J. Clin. Invest. 53, 1473-1480.

37. Raisz, L. G. 1970. Bone formation and resorption in tissue culture. Arch. Int. Med. 126, 887-890.

38. Vaes, G. 1971. A latent collagenase released by bone and skin explants in culture. Biochem. J. 123, 23-24P.

39. Sakamoto, S., Sakamoto, M., Goldhaber, P. and Glimcher, M. J. 1973. The effect of heparin on the amount of enzyme released in tissue culture and on the activity of the enzyme. Calcif. Tissue Res. 12, 247-258.

40. Sakamoto, S., Sakamoto, M., Goldhaber, P. and Glimcher, M. J. 1973. Isolation of tissue collagenase from homogenates of embryonic chick bones. Biochem. Biophys. Res. Comm. 53, 1102-1108.

41. Sakamoto, S., Sakamoto, M., Goldhaber, P. and Glimcher, M.J. 1975. Collagenase and resorption: isolation of collagenase from culture medium containing serum after stimulation of bone resorption by addition of parathyroid hormone extract. Biochem. Biophys. Res. Comm. 63, 172-178.

42. Dayer, J. M., Russell,R.G.G., and Krane, S. M. 1977. Collagenase production by rheumatoid synovial cells: stimulation by a human lymphocyte factor. Science 195, 181-183.

43. Horton, J. E., Wezeman, F. H. and Kuettner, K. E. 1978. Inhibition of in vitro bone resorption by a cartilage-derived anti-collagenase factor. Science, (In press).

44. Fritz, H., Tschesche, H., Greene, L. J. and Truscheit, E. 1974. Proteinase Inhibitors. Springer-Verlag, Berlin, Heidelberg, New York.

45. Bayer, A. G. Inhibitor of Proteinases. Trasylol. Brochure, 1977.

46. Kunitz, M. and Northrop, J. H. 1936. Isolation from beef pancreas of crystalline trypsinogen, trypsin, a trypsin-inhibitor, and an inhibitor-trypsin compound. J. Genl. Physiol. 19, 991-1007.

47. Harper, E., Hiti, J., Kuettner, K. E., and Goodman, M. 1976. Inhibition of collagenase activity by a proteinase inhibitor derived from cartilage. Fed. Proc. 35, (1961 Abs.), 1741.

48. Harris, Jr., E. D. and Krane, S. M. 1974. Collagenases. New Engl. J. Med. 291, 557-563, 605-609, 652-661.

49. Raisz, L. G., Wener, J. A., Trummel, C. L., Feinblatt, J. D. and Au, W.Y.W. 1971. Induction, inhibition and escape as phenomena of bone resorption. In, Calcium, Parathyroid Hormone and the Calcitonins. Proceedings of the Fourth Parathyroid Conference, Chapel Hill, N. C., March 15-19, 1971. Intl. Congress Series No. 243, Excerpta Media, Amsterdam, 446-453.

50. Holtrop, M. E. and King, G. J. 1977. The ultrastructure of the osteoclast and its functional implications. Clin. Orthop. Rel. Res. 123, 177-196.

51. Mears, D. C. 1971. Effects of parathyroid hormone and

thryrocalcitonin on the membrane potential of osteoclasts. Endocrinology 88, 1021-1028.

52. Kallio, D. M., Garant, P. R. and Minkin, C. 1972. Ultra-structural effects of calcitonin on osteoclasts in tissue culture. J. Ultrastruct. Res. 39, 205-216.

53. Lucht, U. 1973. Effects of calcitonin on osteoclasts in vivo: an ultrastructural and histochemical study. Z. Zellforsch. 145, 75-87.

54. Singer, F. R., Melvin, K.E.W. and Mills, B. G. 1976. Acute effects of calcitonin on osteoclasts in man. Clin. Endo-crinology, 5, Suppl. 333s-340s.

55. Mills, B. G., Haroutinian, A. M., Holst, P., Bordier, P. J. and Tun-Chot, S. 1972. Ultrastructural and cellular changes at the costochondral junction following in vitro treatment with calcitonin or calcium chloride in the rabbit. In, Endocrinology. Heineman Books, LTD., London, pp. 79-88.

56. Kuettner, K. E., Pauli, B. U. and Soble, L. 1978. Morpho-logical studies on the resistence of cartilage to invasion by osteosarcoma cells in vitro and in vivo. Cancer Res. 38 (In press).

57. Galasko, C.S.B. and Bennet, B. 1976. Relationship of bone destruction in skeletal metastases to osteoclast activation and prostaglandins. Nature 263, 508-510.

58. Sellers, A., Cartwright, E., Murphy, G. and Reynolds, J. J. 1977. An inhibitor of mammalian collagenases from fetal rabbit bone in culture. Biochem. Soc. Trans. 5, 227-229.

59. Hashimoti, K., Yamanishi, Y. and Dabbous, M. K. 1972. Electron microscopic observations of collagenolytic activity of basal cell epithelioma of the skin in vivo and in vitro. Cancel Res. 32, 2561-2567.

60. Hashimoto, K., Yamanishi, Y., Maeyens, E., Dabbous, M. K. and Kanzaki, T. 1973. Collagenolytic activities of squamous cell carcinoma of the skin. Cancer Res. 33, 2790-2801.

61. Heuson, J.-C., Pastells, J.-L., Legros, N., Heuson-Stiennon, J. and Leclerq, G. 1975. Estradiol-dependent collagenoly-tic enzyme activity in long-term organ culture of human breast cancer. Cancer Res. 35, 2039-2048.

62. Robertson, D. M. and Williams D. C. 1969. In vitro evi-dence of neutral collagenase activity in an invasive mammalian tumor. Nature 221, 259-260.

63. Yamanishi, Y., Dabbous, M. K. and Hashimoto, K. 1972. Effect of collagenolytic activity in basal cell epithelioma of the skin on reconstituted collagen and physical proper-

ties and kinetics of the crude enzyme. Cancer Res. 32, 2551-2560.

64. Rose, G. G. and Robertson, P. B. 1977. Collagenolysis by human gingival fibroblast cell lines. J. Dent. Res. 56, 416-424.

Discussion for Session III: The Role of Microbes, Mediators and Mononuclear Cells in Localized Bone Loss. Part A.

DR. RAISZ: Dr. Hausmann, two questions. One, have you seen whether indomethacin inhibits the effect?

DR. HAUSMANN: We have looked at the effect of indomethacin and it does not inhibit.

DR. RAISZ: And the other: on the DEAE cellulose chromatography, does it come out late, like highly acidic mucopolysaccarides would do? Or, does it come out closer to the beginning of an elution pattern?

DR. HAUSMANN: It comes off late. Let me say that we get the material, the marked enrichment, primarily from the avirulent strain, because we get a late peak in the virulent strain which we think represents this electronegative antigen that we see on immunoelectrophoresis. We do not get that peak on DEAE in the avirulent strains but we get a trailing-off spread, and it is within that area that we get the activity. It seems it is highly acidic.

DR. RAISZ: Do you know if it is sulfated?

DR. HAUSMANN: No.

DR. PECK: Is it neuraminidase degradable?

DR. HAUSMANN: We have not tried that.

DR. AVIOLI: Do you have any information concerning the in vivo effectiveness of this substance? What about animals? Can you infect certain species of animals with this material? Do they become hypercalcemic?

DR. HAUSMANN: Once we have a purified material, we will try to see if we can demonstrate an in vivo effect. We have not so far.

DR. TRUMMEL: Dr. Hausmann, is there any evidence that this is unique for Actinomyces viscosus, albeit is it associated with periodontal disease; is there any evidence that it is unique to this; or is it a phenomenon associated with bacteria growing in a medium?

DR. HAUSMANN: Since the only preparations that we have looked at are the three strains that I showed you, I can't answer beyond that.

DR. MUNDY: Dr. Stern, does br-A work on bone cells? Other than the hormonal effects, could it be working directly on the bone, independent of osteoclasts or other bone-resorbing cells?

DR. STERN: Do you mean an effect on release from dead bone? If that is what you are asking, it doesn't have any effect.

DR. MUNDY: What about the histology of the bones?

DR. STERN: There are large numbers of osteoclasts and not much cell proliferation.

DR. AVIOLI: Dr. Stern, I was interested in your results with the globulins, which you passed over casually. There are some specific species of globulins which bind calcium with the same affinity as albumin, or whatever is in crude albumin, suggesting that perhaps what you are looking at relates to the binding of calcium which is being released from your in vitro system. If that is the case, one could explain the results seen in the situations where you used substances or ingredients which blocked bone resorption.

Have you tried a variety of species of globulin to see if in fact IGG or IGA, etc. have more or less specificity in resorbing bone, or perhaps chelating calcium in your system?

DR. STERN: We haven't looked at the globulin effect. We thought that this might be similar to the complement-mediated bone resorption that has been described, or the bone resorption that has been studied by Fell and others.

We did look at calcium binding with the original albumin and it didn't seem to correlate with the amount of bone-resorbing activity. We haven't with the more purified fraction.

DR. MECHANIC: Dr. Stern, on your DEAE profile, you said that only one of the peaks had activity. That was peak two; is that correct?

DR. STERN: The residual albumin still had activity, the same thing I showed in the batch procedure, but only when we got up to high concentrations.

DR. MECHANIC: It is well-known that, using batch processes, you can never elute off all of the protein, no matter how much you try. Have you heated this protein in acid solution?

DR. STERN: No, we have not.

DR. MECHANIC: Could it be one of the gamma carboxyglutamiccontaining proteins, which would chelate calcium nicely from bone.

DR. STERN: We have not looked at acid stability. I assume that when you talk about chelation, you are talking about this as an initiating step.

DR. MECHANIC: Right.

DR. STERN: We don't think that this is just a binding phenomenon, because we do see a decrease in hydroxyproline in the TCA-insoluble extract from the bone, and we also see other characteristics that suggest it is resorption.

DR. MECHANIC: It could be an initiating step, because you have to demineralize bone before you get enzymatic digestion of it.

DR. RAISZ: Dr. Stern, does br-A induce? That is, does a short exposure produce prolonged resorption?

DR. STERN: We haven't looked at that.

DR. RAISZ: The indomethacin data are of great interest, but there seem to be definitely two components to it. We have found that in some experiments, when there is a lot of connective tissue on the bone, there is an indomethacin-inhibitable component of control resorption in the presence of albumin, which we assume is a major reason for our control resorption anyway.

I wonder if that could be an interaction between periosteal tissue and albumin, and whether you have tested albumin itself for indomethacin inhibitability, as well as the purified material.

DR. STERN: The answer to the second question is we had tested both. They were both on the graph.

DR. RAISZ: I am sorry. I meant the albumin that came off after the br-A was taken away.

DR. STERN: Oh. No; we hadn't tested that. I thought you meant the original material. To the other question, I would think that if part of this was something that was released from the connective tissue, we would have seen two phases, or we would have seen some effects, even with the parathyroid hormone-treated bones.

DR. RAISZ: We see it in some control cultures. I think when you get PTH in there you have so much resorption super-imposed on the control that you don't see it.

My idea would be that albumin somehow interacted with the periosteal tissue to make more prostaglandins, and that was one factor. There could be another factor in the albumin which caused resorption, because you have very substantial resorption up to 10^{-5} molar indomethacin.

DR. STERN: I think that may be difficult to dissociate.

DR. PECK: Dr. Stern, have you looked at serum extracts from patients with osteopetrosis on the one hand and Paget's disease on the other? It would be fascinating to see whether this resorptive material was present or not.

DR. STERN: We haven't looked at these diseases. However, we have also found this activity in human serum albumin.

DR. TEITELBAUM: Dr. Horton, does the inhibitory-factor inhibit other bone-resorbing agents?

DR. HORTON: Yes. We have also looked at PTH, as well as PGE-2, and the results are very similar.

DR. TEITELBAUM: 1-25?

DR. HORTON: We haven't looked at 1-25.

DR. RAISZ: Dr. Horton, what was the concentration of the material, and how does it relate to concentrations used for other inhibitors?

DR. HORTON: The concentration of the material in this series of experiments was 300 micrograms per mil. We have done dose-response concentrations with PTH, but not with OAF or PGE-2. We found that the inhibitory activity was lost around 40 to 50 micrograms of protein per mil.

DR. RAISZ: Do you have any idea whether cell function is maintained? You have mentioned the fact that osteoclasts are separated from the bone surface. Have you looked at any other cells in the tissue, or looked at DNA, or RNA, or protein synthesis in the tissue, or in the material?

DR. HORTON: With both light and electron microscopy, we find that when the AIF is removed from bones which were previously cultured with both OAF and AIF, and then subsequently cultured in OAF alone, the osteoclasts are reattached to the surface of the bone matrix. We are currently pursuing the other experiments to which you referred.

DR. MINKIN: Dr. Horton, I would be very much interested to know whether AIF had any effect on resorption from dead bones.

DR. HORTON: Are you asking about the exogenous addition, similar to what Dr. Mundy has done, with mononuclear cells on dead bones, or just on the dead bones themselves?

DR. MINKIN: On dead bones themselves. I noticed the percent release figure was very low for that first 48-hour period; lower than one might expect. One would be interested to know whether or not there was a great deal of proteolytic activity in these bones that was being inhibited by this material, which was a separate issue from any direct effect on cells.

DR. HORTON: We hadn't considered that experiment. Our first direction was to show that we didn't kill the bones nor the cells. Therefore, we designed the addition and removal experiments to show that the bones, i.e., the bone cells, in fact, recover.

DR. TASHJIAN: Dr. Horton, since AIF does inhibit parathyroid hormone-stimulated resorption as well as prostaglandin-stimulated resorption, have you looked at its ability to inhibit bone-specific enzymes released in the resorption process? In other words, have you looked at bone collagenase or lysozomal enzymes released from bone to know whether it has a differential effect on one of those two which might help all of us understand what is going on in resorption better?

DR. HORTON: No; we haven't. Those experiments are mandatory to be done, and we are attempting to pursue them very quickly.

DR. MATTHEWS: Since AIF is an extract of cartilage, and cartilage is resorbed when it mineralizes, then we must presume that the mineralization state may do something to the presence of this inhibitor. Since you are talking about mineralized bone resorption, can you equate these two?

DR. HORTON: If our hypothesis is correct that what we have indeed found is a local tissue enzyme regulator, then one would have to presume that there would be a regulator for AIF also, which may be involved with the process of mineralization.

DR. CANTERBURY: Dr. Stern, I am a little concerned because I don't understand this assay of yours for your factor which you have isolated from albumin which causes bone resorption.

If you pre-incubate this material in a high-calcium medium and then apply it to your cultures, do you still get resorption? Is it possible that this is just a binding phenomenon, that is, a chelating agent?

DR. STERN: The only answer I have is we haven't done that specific study. When we first began studying the albumins, we compared their calcium-binding capacity with their ability to cause resorption. There was no correlation. But we haven't done that with this partially-purified fraction.

DR. CANTERBURY: Dr. Hausmann, if you have looked at cell wall components from your bacteria, do you think this is some fraction from the cell wall?

DR. HAUSMANN: We looked at the cell wall after sonication, and it had no bone resorptive activity. However, I don't know if our factor is originally derived from the cell wall or not.

DR. STERN: May I ask a question back, since several people seem to be concerned about calcium binding. I wonder what the evidence is that an initial binding of calcium by a substance would be a trigger for bone resorption.

DR. RAISZ: I think we all would agree that there isn't any. You are right to bring it out in the open. One can reduce the medium calcium concentration by 50 percent, which is certainly more than any binding one could achieve with any amount of albumin one could get in there, and one can still differentiate resorption and control values which are rather similar to the ones we see now.

So, I don't see how anything could bind unless it did something to the membrane at the same time it bound; and I was going to ask you that question. Have you ever looked at this factor for its effect on bone cell calcium uptake? In other words, it might be a facilitator of the entry of calcium into the cell. I don't think you can bind out of the extracellular fluid, but it might work at the cell membrane. Have you looked at that?

DR. STERN: We have not looked at that.

DR. KUETTNER: Dr. Stern, do you have any idea about the molecular weight of your protein after you separated it through DEAE cellulose; and, how much of your total protein represents that particular fraction?

DR. STERN: We haven't put it back on Sephadex yet. The only thing we know is that the material is non-dialyzable. By dialyzing the material after preparation, we don't seem to lose any activity.

Now it could be some sort of aggregate, but then I would expect that when we dialyzed it, we would get some of the activity coming off just by sort of a mass action.

DR. KUETTNER: The second question was: how much of the total albumin does it represent?

DR. STERN: It varies between 3 and 10 percent. On the batch procedure which probably has more contamination, we get about 10 percent. On the column it is lower. So it is not a very potent substance at this point.

DR. KUETTNER: Dr. Hausmann, do you have any idea about the chemical composition of your carbohydrate? Do you know if it contains uronic acid, or hexosamines? You previously said that you do not know if it contains sulfate. Of course the story of cofactors, as Paul Goldhaber called it, of heparin, comes to mind. Heparin acts as a cofactor in bone resorption. I wonder if you have any idea of hexosamines, uronic acid, or any chemical data on your material?

DR. HAUSMANN: We have chemical data on the original material, but we haven't done any further analyses until we have a material of sufficient purity.

DR. AVIOLI: Dr. Stern, I have to disagree with Dr. Raisz a bit. He is going from an in vivo to an in vitro situation. In vivo, I would imagine he is absolutely correct. There is no precedent for a binding protein to affect calcium absorption from bone.

However, control resorption in this in vitro system is about 10 to 23 percent. If there are proteins in the bone of these rudiments which have an affinity for calcium and if your substance has an affinity for calcium which is greater than that in the bone rudiment, I can buy the fact that in vitro, in the system, there may be a very significant effect of a very powerful protein or calcium binder. I think Dr. Canterbury's suggestion of saturating it first, before you try it, may be appropriate.

DR. STERN: I can't speak to proteins. However, I can talk about other things that would bind calcium and demineralize, like EDTA or citrate. That is precisely what they do. They will demineralize the bone. But you don't see resorption; you don't see the cellular response, the effect on collagen, that you would see with something like this. A protein might be different, and there might be some more complex interaction like Dr. Raisz suggests.

DR. KLEIN: Dr. Stern, have you tried using guanadine 6-molar denaturation of your material to see whether, when you break the conformational aspects of your material, you lose all activity.

DR. STERN: We have not done that yet.

DR. PECK: I have a question for Dr. Stern and one for Dr. Horton. Dr. Stern, do you think that this is an albumin fraction, or do you think that this is a substance which just happens to be trapped in the albumin fraction?

DR. STERN: I don't know at this point. It is possible that it is a fragment that has different charge characteristics, and somehow it breaks off in a uniform manner. I don't know whether you would expect something like that to occur. I think more likely that it is one of the hundred thousand things that is bound to albumin.

DR. PECK: Dr. Horton, were there any morphological changes in any of the other cells of the bone treated with AIF; that is, osteoblasts, osteocytes, etc.?

DR. HORTON: Interestingly, that data is being examined right now. In bones which are treated with AIF alone, we are seeing a large increase in cellularity. That is all I could speak to at the moment.

DR. TEITELBAUM: Dr. Horton, do you have any data distinguishing the effects of AIF on a bone-resorbing agent, namely OAF or PTH, from a direct effect upon the cell? In other words, could you be looking at proteolysis of the bone-resorbing agent?

DR. HORTON: We do not expect this to be the case. The reason is that we find that AIF also inhibits control bone resorption, and that this control bone resorption is then restored when AIF is removed from these same cultures. This observation would indicate that the AIF inhibitor is working on the osteoclastic cell rather than affecting the bone resorbing stimulant.

DR. MILLER: Dr. Horton, the last few years, people, particularly Judah Folkman and his group at Harvard, have isolates from hyaline cartilage that have anti-angiogenesis properties. Is AIF related to these sorts of factors that they have reported? Are there similarities or are they dissimilar? What is the relationship between these?

DR. HORTON: I believe Dr. Kuettner should speak to that.

DR. KUETTNER: The material Judah Folkman isolated is probably identical to AIF. However, the system he is using is quite different. He is using it in the eye, and we have used it in the organ culture system.

The main component, probably, in AIF is the proteolytic enzyme-inhibitor. In Folkman's system, he places this proteolytic enzyme-inhibitor in a slow-release capsule. He probably could get the same effect if he implanted a piece of living cartilage between the tumor and the limbus of the eye. While these studies are indirect evidence, it appears as if the anti-angiogenesis factor and AIF may be the same material, or at least very similar.

DR. MUNDY: Dr. Horton, do you have any evidence that the osteoclasts stay healthy after they have been bathing in AIF? For example, if you took a bone away from AIF and then put it in with parathyroid hormone, which is one way of testing that, will the bone then resorb?

DR. HORTON: That is exactly what we have done with the same bone. The bone was cultured for 48 hours with PTH, or with OAF, or with PGE-2, concomitantly with AIF. It was then transferred into a second culture vessel for a subsequent 48 hours with only the bone-resorbing stimulant and without further addition of AIF. So it was done with the same bone.

Complement Dependent Bone Resorption.*
   *Dr. Sandberg was unable to present her paper during the
   conference due to illness.

Ann L. Sandberg, Lawrence G. Raisz, J. Max Goodson, Larry M. Wahl
and Stephen E. Mergenhagen.

Laboratory of Microbiology and Immunology, National Institute of
Dental Research, Bethesda, Md. 20014.
Department of Medicine, University of Connecticut Health Center,
Farmington, Connecticut, 06032.
Department of Pharmacology, Forsyth Dental Center, 140 The Fenway'
Boston, Massachusetts, 02115.

INTRODUCTION

Destruction of cartilage or bone may be due, in part, to
immunological activation of the complement (C) system (1-8).
Histologic examination of cartilage or bones and their adjacent
cellular components cultured in vitro in the presence of antibody
and C revealed marked degradation of these connective tissue
elements (1-6). These initial studies attributed this effect to
the enhanced release of lysosomal enzymes (3).

However, other factors, such as exogenous prostaglandin
(PGE) (9), have recently been demonstrated to be potent contri-
butors to the in vitro resorption of bone. An in vivo corollary
of this latter finding is the detection of high levels of PGE
in sites of inflammation associated with bone loss (10-12). The
in vitro synthesis and secretion of PG which resorbs bone have
been demonstrated in cultures of a mouse fibrosarcoma (13) and
synovial cells from patients with rheumatoid arthritis (14,15).

The present study focuses on the possibility that activation
of C may result in the enhancement of synthesis of prostaglandins
which may then mediate connective tissue destruction.

MATERIALS AND METHODS

Bone resorption. As previously described in detail (16), 19-
day fetal rat long bones (radii and ulnae) labeled in utero with
^{45}Ca were cultured in experimental or control media as described
in the table legends. The ^{45}Ca released into the media and that
remaining in the bones were determined. Resorption of bone is
expressed as the percentage of release of total ^{45}Ca initially
present in the bone or as the experimental to control ratio.
The data presented are representative of several experiments.

Prostaglandin E (PGE). Two radioimmunoassay procedures
were utilized to determine the release of PGE into the media.
The data in Table 1 and 4 were obtained by citric acid acidifi-
cation of the media and extraction with ethyl acetate. The
extracts were dried, dissolved in benzene-ethyl acetate (60:40)
and chromatographically purified by the method of Zusman et al.
(17). After conversion of the PGE to PGB by alkaline hydrolysis,

the samples were assayed with a commercial antibody to PGB_1 (Clinical Assays, Cambridge, Mass.) according to Jaffe and Behrman (18). These data are expressed in terms of PGE equivalents uncorrected for recovery (average recovery = 55%). The data in Table 5 were obtained by chloroform extraction of the acidified media and chromatographed as described above. The PGE content was determined by radioimmunoassay utilizing an anti-PGE_2 serum (Miles, Elkhart, Ind.).

Complement (C). Normal pooled rabbit serum served as the C source. When indicated, serum was heated at 56°C to destroy C activity. In specified experiements, 10 ml of rabbit C were absorbed twice for 10 min at 0°C with the pelleted washed cells from 3 adult rat spleens. Serum from rabbits genetically deficient in the sixth component of C (C6) was utilized in specified experiments. Functionally purified guinea pig C6 was obtained from Cordis Lab., Miami, Fla. Cultures containing C6 deficient serum plus C6 received an equal volume of each reagent.

Immunoglobulin preparations. Adult New Zealand White Rabbits were hyperimmunized with rat erythrocytes (2 x 10). The IgG fraction was obtained by DEAE cellulose chromatography (0.01 M phosphate, pH 8.0) of the 50% $(NH4)_2SO_4$ cut of the antiserum. $F(ab')_2$ fragments were obtained by peptic digestion of the IgG (19) and Sephadex G-150 column chromatography. The 19S and 7S fractions were prepared by Sephadex G-200 column chromatography.

Arachidonic acid was purchased from Sigma Chem.Co., St. Louis, Mo.

Indomethacin was obtained from Merck Sharp and Dohme Res. Lab., Rahway, N. J.

RESULTS

As shown in Table I, bone resorption, as determined by the release of ^{45}Ca, was significantly greater in cultures containing C (unheated serum) than in those which received heated serum. That this effect was attributable to C was verified by utilizing serum from rabbits genetically deficient in the sixth component of C (C6). ^{45}Ca release in cultures containing the C6 deficient serum alone was similar to that observed in those containing heat inactivated serum. However, bone resorbing activity could be restored to the C6 deficient serum by the addition of functionally purified guinea pig C6. Thus, the late acting C components, at least through C6, were required for this response.

The involvement of PG in this event was established by two criteria: addition of indomethacin to the cultures and radioimmunoassay of the culture media for PGE (Table 1). Indomethacin (1 x 10^{-5}M) inhibited the bone resorbing activity of the C6 deficient serum supplemented with C6. Radioimmunoassay revealed little PGE release into the media of bone cultures containing heated serum or C6 deficient serum. However, bones cultured

Table I

^{45}Ca and PGE Release by Bones Cultured in Rabbit Serum
and its Inhibition by Indomethacin[a]

Serum[b]	^{45}Ca Release (cpm/ml)	Experimental to Control Ratio[c]	Media PGE (ng/ml)
Heated	2280 ± 160		0.1 ± 0.1
Unheated	3390 ± 220^{d}	1.5	3.3 ± 0.4^{d}
C6 deficient	1990 ± 120	0.9	0.8 ± 0.5
C6 deficient + C6	2970 ± 190^{e}	1.5	4.0 ± 1.2^{e}
C6 deficient + C6 + indomethacin[f]	1760 ± 230	0.9	0.6 ± 0.5

[a] Bones were cultured for 6 days with a change of media on day 3.

[b] Cultures contained 50% rabbit serum.

[c] Heated serum served as the control for unheated serum and C6 deficient serum, and C6 deficient for C6 deficient + C6 and C6 deficient + C6 + indomethacin.

[d] Significantly different from heated normal serum, $p < 0.5$.

[e] Significantly different from C6 deficient serum, $p < 0.5$.

[f] Cultures contained a final concentration of 1×10^{-5}M indomethacin.

with unheated serum or C6 deficient serum supplemented with C6 released increased levels of PGE. In addition to its inhibition of bone resorption, indomethacin inhibited the production of PGE. Indomethacin does not inhibit bone resorption induced by exogenous PGE (7), demonstrating that the PGE was synthesized by the bone cultures.

Previous histologic studies suggested that C dependent destruction of cartilage was initiated by antibody to cell surface antigens (1-6). Studies were, therefore, carried out to determine the influence of immunoglobulin on ^{45}Ca and PGE release in bone cultures. Marked variability was observed in the concentrations of several pools of rabbit sera that induced in vitro bone resorption suggesting that the limiting factor might be antibody. The serum pool utilized for the studies in Tables II and III effectively resorbed bone at a final concentration of 10%. Absorption of this serum pool markedly decreased the ^{45}Ca release (Table II). Whereas 75% ^{45}Ca release occurred in the presence of untreated serum, only 34% ^{45}Ca was released in cultures containing absorbed serum in accord with the hypothesis that antibodies reactive with cell surface antigens initiated the destruction of bone. Additional evidence for the requirement of antibody derives from the finding that the resorbing activity could be restored to the absorbed C source by the addition of the 19S fraction of rabbit anti-rat erythrocyte (anti-rat RBC) serum. The 7S fraction of this antiserum was equally active as were the 19S and 7S fractions of anti-sonicated rat bone serum.

Since two pathways of C activation have been described (classical and alternative) it was of interest to examine which pathway was operative in this biological system. Although rabbit IgG activates the classical pathway, the biologic consequences of C activation by this immunoglobulin probably reflect some contribution of the alternative pathway. However, the F(ab')$_2$ fragments of rabbit IgG activate only the alternative pathway (20). As shown in Table III the IgG fraction of rabbit anti-rat erythrocyte antibody obtained by DEAE cellulose column chromatography was a potent inducer of C-dependent bone resorption. Of interest was the finding that the F(ab')$_2$ fragments of this IgG preparation were as active as the native immunoglobulin in initiating C dependent release of ^{45}Ca. Neither of the antibody preparations possessed any inherent bone resorbing properties since they did not induce the destruction of bone in the presence of heat inactivated serum. The pool of rabbit serum employed in these studies did not support ^{45}Ca at a final concentration of 10%.

Susceptibility to indomethacin inhibition and radioimmunoassay of the culture media for PGE further substantiated a role for PG in C dependent bone resorption initiated by antibody (Table IV). Addition of 7S anti-rat erythrocyte serum to an absorbed C source stimulated the release of ^{45}Ca from the bones and enhanced the levels of PGE in the culture media. Both effects were inhibited by indomethacin. Analagous results were obtained by the addition of 19S antibody.

Table II

Loss of Bone Resorbing Activity from Rabbit Serum by Absorption
with Rat Spleen Cells and Restoration by Antibody[a]

Serum[b]	% ^{45}Ca Release[c]
Heated serum	25.9 $\pm$ 1.1
Untreated serum	75.2 $\pm$ 3.1[d]
Absorbed serum	34.4 $\pm$ 3.2
Absorbed serum + 19S anti-rat RBC[e]	62.3 $\pm$ 1.3[d]

[a] Bones were cultured for 1 day without serum and then cultured under experimental or control conditions for 2 days.

[b] Cultures contained 10% rabbit serum.

[c] Mean $\pm$ S. E. of 3 cultures.

[d] Significantly different from heated serum, $p < .01$.

[e] Final concentration of antibody was 1%.

Table III

C-dependent Resorption of Bone Initiated by Rabbit Anti-rat
Erythrocyte IgG and F(ab')$_2$ Fragments[a]

Serum[b]	Antibody[c]	% ^{45}Ca Release[d]
Unheated		37.5 $\pm$ 4.6
Heated		37.0 $\pm$ 4.3
Unheated	IgG	60.6 $\pm$ 8.3[e]
Heated	IgG	34.4 $\pm$ 5.5
Unheated	F(ab')$_2$	71.7 $\pm$ 8.8[e]
Heated	F(ab')$_2$	30.4 $\pm$ 6.2

[a] Bones were cultures for 1 day without serum and then cultured under experimental or control conditions for 2 days.

[b] Cultures contained 10% rabbit serum.

[c] Final concentration of antibody was 1%.

[d] Mean $\pm$ S. E. for four bone cultures.

[e] Values differ significantly from control (heated serum), p < .05.

Table IV

Inhibition of Antibody-initiated C-dependent Resorption
of Bone and PGE Production by Indomethacin[a]

Antibody Addition to Absorbed Serum[b]	^{45}Ca Release Experimental to Control Ratio[c]	Media PGE ng/culture
None	1.00	2.4 ± 0.7
Indomethacin[d]	0.72 ± 0.04	0.4 ± 0.1
7S[e]	1.77 ± 0.12[f]	7.7 ± 3.1
7S + Indomethacin	1.14 ± 0.09	0.6 ± 0.1

[a] Bones were cultured for 1 day without serum and then cultured under experimental or control conditions for 2 days.

[b] Cultures contained 10% rabbit serum absorbed 2 times with rat spleen cells.

[c] Mean ± S. E. for four bone cultures

[d] Cultures contained a final concentration of 1×10^{-5}M indomethacin.

[e] Cultures contained 1% rabbit anti-rat erythrocyte 7S fraction.

[f] Significantly different from control, $p < .05$.

Since C is known to alter cell membranes, the possibility existed that it might enhance the cellular incorporation of the exogenously added PG precursor, arachidonic acid, into PGE. That this does in fact occur is demonstrated by the data in Table V. Minimal concentrations of PGE were detected in the media of bones cultured with C6 deficient serum and the 7S fraction of rabbit anti-rat erythrocyte serum in the presence or absence of arachidonic acid. The addition of C6 to the deficient serum enhanced PGE production in the absence of arachidonic acid (15.7 ng/ml). However, the addition of arachidonic acid to cultures containing C6 supplemented C6 deficient serum resulted in a dramatic increase in PGE production (158.3 ng/ml). ^{45}Ca release was slightly enhanced by the addition of arachidonic acid to cultures containing the deficient serum and C6. This minimal enhancement can be attributed to the high level of ^{45}Ca release in cultures which received C6 deficient serum plus C6. Additional studies utilizing limited C have demonstrated a marked enhancement of C dependent bone resorption by arachidonic acid correlating with enhanced PGE production.

DISCUSSION

These studies demonstrate that activation of C results in destruction of bone and that PG has a dominant role in this process. The release of ^{45}Ca from prelabeled bones in organ culture is initiated by antibodies reactive with cell surface antigens. Absorption of the C source with spleen cells or its dilution removed the activity and restoration of bone resorbing activity was achieved by the addition of immunoglobulins from sera of rabbits immunized with rat erythrocytes or sonicated rat bones. Utilization of $F(ab')_2$ fragments of IgG, which activate only the alternative C pathway, were as effective as native IgG in initiation of C dependent bone resorption indicating the possible importance of the alternative pathway in this biological function. The finding that some human antibodies reactive with cellular antigens activate the alternative pathway suggests a feasible in vivo correlate of these findings (21, 22).

This C dependent bone resorption was mediated by PG. Elevation of PGE levels was observed in cultures containing C and antibody and this increase as well as C dependent bone resorption were inhibited by indomethacin. These findings indicate that C activation at a cell surface results in bone destruction by enhancing PG production as well as by the previously described release of lysosomal enzymes (3).

Although the PG mediated mechanisms involved in C stimulated destruction of bone have not been completely delineated, several possibilities exist. The finding that C markedly enhances PG production and bone resorption in the presence of added arachidonic acid suggests one possible mechanism for this effect. C induced alterations of the cell membrane may allow greater accessibility of the PG precursor, arachidonic acid, to prostaglandin synthetase. In addition the demonstration of enhanced phospholipid metabolism in HeLa cells exposed to

Table V

C-dependent PGE Production and ^{45}Ca Release
by Bones Cultured in the Presence of Arachidonic Acid[a]

Serum[b]	% ^{45}Ca Release[c]	Media PGE ng/ml[d]
C6 Deficient	38.4 ± 3.0	0.3
C6 Deficient + C6	90.1 ± 4.1	15.7
C6 Deficient + Arachidonic Acid[e]	46.6 ± 6.8	1.1
C6 Deficient + C6 + Arachidonic Acid	95.4 ± 3.3	158.3

[a] Bones were cultured for 5 days with a change of media after 2 days.

[b] Cultures contained 20% serum and 0.1% 7S rabbit anti-rat erythrocyte serum fraction

[c] Means ± S.E. for 6 bone cultures.

[d] Mean of two samples each containing a pool of three cultures.

[e] Cultures contained a final concentration of 1×10^{-4}M arachidonic acid.

specific antibody and C suggests a mechanism for the intracellular accumulation of phospholipids which may provide a
source of the PG precursor (23). It has also been reported
that C releases phospolipids from cell membranes as well as
from liposomes (24-28). This may provide an additional source
of precursors for PG. Any or all of these C dependent effects
may contribute to the destruction of the structural elements
of connective tissue.

REFERENCES

1. Fell, H. B., and L. Weiss. 1965. The effect of antiserum, alone and with hydrocortisone, on foetal mouse bones in cultures. J. Exp. Med. 121:551.

2. Fell, H. B., R. R. A. Coombs, and J. T. Dingle. 1966. The breakdown of embryonic (chick) cartilage and bone cultivated in the presence of complement-sufficient antisera. I. Morphological changes, their reversibility and inhibition. Int. Arch. Allergy Appl. Immunol. 30:146.

3. Dingle, J. T., H. B. Fell, and R. R. A. Coombs, 1967. The breakdown of embryonic (chick) cartilage and bone cultivated in the presence of complement-sufficient antisera. 2. Biochemical changes and role of the lysosomal system. Int. Arch. Allergy Appl. Immunol. 31:283.

4. Lachmann, P. J., R. R. A. Coombs, H. B. Fell, and J. T. Dingle. 1969. The breakdown of embryonic (chick) cartilage and bone cultivated inthe presence of complement-sufficient antisera. 3. Immunologic analysis. Int. Arch. Allergy Appl. Immunol. 36:469.

5. Fell, H. B., and M. E. J. Barratt. 1973. The role of soft connective tissue in the breakdown of pig articular cartilage cultivated in the presence of complement-sufficient antiserum to pig erythrocytes. 1. Histological changes. Int. Arch. Allergy Appl. Immunol. 44:441.

6. Poole, A. R., M. E. J. Barratt, and H. B. Fell. 1973. The role of soft connective tissue in the breakdown of pig articular cartilage cultivated in the presence of complement-sufficient antiserum to pig erythrocytes. 2. Distribution of immunoglobulin G (IgG). Int. Arch. Allergy Appl. Immunol. 44:469.

7. Raisz, L. G., A. L. Sandberg, J. M. Goodson, H. A. Simmons and S. E. Mergenhagen. 1974. Complement-dependent stimulation of prostaglandin synthesis and bone resorption. Science 185:789.

8. Sandberg, A. L., L. G. Raisz, J. M. Goodson, H. A. Simmons and S. E. Mergenhagen. 1977. Initiation of bone resorption by the classical and alternative C pathways and its mediation by prostaglandins. J. Immunol. 119:1378.

9. Klein, D. C., and L. G. Raisz. 1970. Prostaglandins: Stimulation of bone resorption in tissue culture. Endocrinology 86:1436.

10. Robinson, H. J., Jr., and J. L. Granda. 1974. Prostaglandins in synovial inflammatory disease. Surg. Forum 25:476.

11. Goodson, M. J., F. E. Dewhirst, and A. Brunetti. 1974. Prostaglandin E_2 levels and human periodontal disease. Prostaglandins 6:81.

12. Harris, M., M. V. Jenkins, A. Bennett, and M. R. Wills. 1973. Prostaglandin production and bone resorption by dental cysts. Nature 245:213.

13. Tashjian, A. H., Jr., E. F. Voelkel, L. Levine, and P. Goldhaber. 1972. Evidence that the bone resorption-stimulating factor produced by mouse fibrosarcoma cells is prostaglandin E_2 (a new model for the hypercalcemia of cancer). J. Exp. Med. 136:1329.

14. Robinson, D. R., A. H. Tashjian, Jr., and L. Levine. 1975. Prostaglandin-stimulated bone resorption by rheumatoid synovia (A possible mechanism for bone destruction in rheumatoid arthritis). J. Clin. Inves. 56:1181.

15. Dayer, J. M., S. M. Krane, R. G. G. Russell, and D. R. Robinson. 1976. Production of collagenase and prostaglandins by isolated adherent rheumatoid synovial cells. Proc. Natl. Acad. Sci. 73:945.

16. Raisz, L. G., and I. Niemann. 1969. Effect of phosphate, calcium and magnesium on bone resorption and hormonal responses in tissue culture. Endocrinology 85:446.

17. Zusman, R. M., B. V. Caldwell, L. Speroff, and H. R. Behrman. 1972. Radioimmunoassay of the A prostaglandins. Prostaglandins 2:41.

18. Jaffe, B. M., and H. R. Behrman. 1974. Prostaglandins E, A, and F. In Methods of Hormone Radioimmunoassay. Edited by B. M. Jaffe and H. R. Behrman. Academic Press, New York. P. 19.

19. Nisonoff, A. 1964. Enzymatic digestion of rabbit gamma globulin and antibody and chromatography of digestion products. In Methods in Medical Research. Vol. 10. Edited by H. N. Eisen. Yearbook Medical Publishers, Chicago. P. 134.

20. Reid, K. B. M. 1971. Complement fixation by the $F(ab')_2$ fragment of pepsin-treated rabbit antibody. Immunology 20:649.

21. Ferrone, S., N. R. Cooper, M. A. Pellegrino, and R. A. Reisfeld. 1973. Activation of human complement by human lymphoid cells sensitized with histocompatibility alloantisera. Proc. Natl. Acad. Sci. 70:3665.

22. Perrin, L. H., B. S. Joseph, N. R. Cooper, and M. B. A. Oldstone. 1976. Mechanism of injury of virus-infected cells by antiviral antibody and complement: Participation of IgG, F(ab')$_2$ and the alternative complement pathway. J. Exp. Med. 143:1027.

23. Guttler, F. 1972. Phospholipid synthesis in HeLa cells exposed to immunoglobulin G and complement. Biochem. J. 128:953.

24. Wilson, L. A., and J. K. Spitznagel. 1968. Molecular and structural damage to Escherichia coli produced by antibody, complement and lysozyme systems. J. Bacteriol. 96:1339.

25. Wilson, L. A. and J. K. Spitznagel. 1971. Characteristics of complement-dependent release of phospholipid from Escherichia coli. Infect. Immun. 4:23.

26. Inoue, K., T. Kinoshita, Y. Akiyama, M. Okada, and T. Amano. 1976. Release of phospholipids from bacterial surface structure and liposomes by the action of complement. J. Immunol. 116:1737.

27. Giavedoni, E. B., and A. P. Dalmasso. 1976. The induction by complement of a change in KSCN-dissociable red cell membrane lipids. J. Immunol. 116:1163.

28. Shin, M. L., W. A. Pazrekas, A. S. Abramovitz and M. M. Mayer. 1977. On the mechanism of membrane damage by C; Exposure of hydrophobic sites on activated C proteins. J. Immunol. 119:1358.

Prostaglandins as Local Mediators of Bone Resorption.

Armen H. Tashjian, Jr.

Laboratory of Pharmacology, Harvard School of Dental Medicine, and Department of Pharmacology, Harvard Medical School, Boston, MA 02115

In concert with the theme of this Workshop, I shall summarize the results of studies on the local production of prostaglandins by bone and the resorption that follows.

The ability of exogenous PGE_1 to stimulate the resorption of bone in culture was first described by Klein and Raisz in 1970 (1). Subsequently, collaborative experiments from our laboratory and that of Lawrence Levine at Brandeis University have drawn attention to the role of PGE_2 produced by certain animal tumors in the pathogenesis of the hypercalcemia of malignant disease in these model systems (2-11).

In this summary I shall focus discussion on PGE_2 produced by bone in organ culture and on its role as a local mediator of bone resorption. There are several lines of evidence reported from different laboratories which indicate that bone can produce prostaglandins locally and respond to this endogenous stimulus for resorption (Table 1).

Against this background of information, we have performed two new sets of experiments which add further support to the conclusion that bone can synthesize PGE_2 and that locally produced PGE_2 can cause enhanced bone resorption. We have used two different pharmacologic approaches to stimulate PGE_2 synthesis in bone. First, we have used phorbol diesters and, secondly, the polypeptide toxin melittin.

The phorbol diesters are potent mitogens and tumor promoters which are isolated from croton oil (23-25). They have several actions which suggested that they might be interesting agents to examine for bone resorption-stimulating activity. These actions include decreased cylic AMP and increased cyclic GMP, enhanced phospholipid metabolism, release of lysosomal enzymes, and stimulation of prostaglandin synthesis in canine kidney cells by a mechanism that involves enhanced deacylation of cellular phospholipids, release of arachidonic acid and its conversion of PGE_2 and $PGF_2\alpha$ (26). Furthermore, some of the actions of the phorbol diesters are inhibited by glucocorticoid steroid hormones.

We have studied the action of several phorbol diesters

(1 Footnote see Page 176)

Table 1. Production of prostaglandins by bone and related tissues and the possible role of prostaglandins as local bone resorption-stimulating factors.

Experimental Observation	Reference
Prostaglandin production by dental cysts	12
Increased PGE_2 content of diseased human gingiva	13
Conditioned medium from cultures of gingival fragments stimulated bone resorption and that stimulation was inhibited by indomethacin	14
Complement-dependent stimulation of prostaglandin production by bone and bone resorption	15,16
Arachidonic acid stimulated bone resorption in organ culture and this process was inhibited by indomethacin	17
Phospholipase A_2 stimulated bone resorption in organ culture	18,19
Crude collagenase-induced bone resorption was inhibited by indomethacin	20
PGE_2 produced by synovial tissue and cells in culture and this prostaglandin stimulated bone resorption in culture	21,22
Conditioned medium from cultures of gingival fragments as well as arachidonic acid stimulated synthesis of PGE_2 in bone in culture *	unpublished data

* Drs. Goldhaber, Rabadjija and Tashjian, Harvard School of Dental Medicine, and Dr. Levine, Brandeis University.

on bone in organ culture using neonatal mouse calvaria in rotating Leighton tubes (2,6,9,21). Bone resorption was monitored by measuring the release of nonradioactive calcium (^{40}Ca) into the culture medium. Prostaglandins produced by the bones and released into the culture medium were measured by radioimmunoassay using an anti-PGE$_2$ which reacts with PGF$_2\alpha$ only 0.01%.

Phorbol Diesters

The potent phorbol diester in tumor promotion, 12-0-Tetradecanoylphorbol-13-acetate (TPA), was highly active in stimulating bone resorption. A maximum effect was observed with a concentration of TPA of about 50 ng/ml, and half-maximum stimulation was obtained at about 8 ng/ml in experiments of 48-hours duration. Analogs of TPA which are less active than TPA in tumor promotion were also less active in stimulating bone resorption; 4-0-methyl-TPA was a weak stimulator of bone resorption; and the unesterified parent alcohol, phorbol, had little or no activity.

Because TPA is known to affect cyclic AMP formation in certain tissues and because of the postulated role of cylic AMP in mediating the actions of certain bone resorption-stimulating agents, we measured cylic AMP in culture medium and in bones under a variety of conditions after treatment with TPA and found no statistically significant or reproducible change in cylic AMP. We, therefore, sought other possible mediators of bone resorption induced by TPA.

The effect of a supramaximal concentration of TPA, 100 ng/ml, on bone resorption was completely inhibited at 24, 48 and 72 hours when the culture medium contained indomethacin at concentrations as low as 5×10^{-8} M. We then performed experiments to examine bone resorption and prostaglandin production simultaneously. TPA, at a concentration of 100 ng/ml, stimulated bone resorption maximally by 48 hours and increased the concentration of PGE$_2$ in medium by 3- to 4-fold. The increase in PGE$_2$ production by bone was completely inhibited by indomethacin (5.6×10^{-7} M). Likewise, indomethacin prevented completely the enhanced release of bone calcium induced by TPA, while the inhibitor of fatty acid cyclooxygenase had no effect on bone resorption stimulated by exogenous PGE$_2$ (100 ng/ml). From these findings we conclude that TPA stimulates the production of PGE$_2$ by bone and that this endogenously produced prostaglandin then enchances bone resorption.

Melittin

I should now like to describe an entirely different means of stimulating PGE$_2$ synthesis in bone and subsequent bone resorption. Melittin is a 26-amino acid polypeptide isolated from bee venom (27). It has prominent surfactant properties due to its asymmetric arrangement of polar and nonpolar amino acid residues and is able to lyse cells and lysosomes. Other effects include histamine release from mast cells, stimulation of phospholipase A$_2$ activity in E. coli, and stimulation of phospholipase activity and prostaglandin biosynthesis by several cell lines in culture (28).

Melittin is a potent stimulator of bone resorption in organ culture. The dose-response curve was biphasic. Maximum stimulation of bone resorption, measured at 48 hours, occurred at a melittin concentration of about 25 ng/ml. Concentrations of 100 and 500 ng/ml were less active, and concentrations above 1 µg/ml were cytotoxic to bone cells. Melittin (25 ng/ml) stimulated the production of PGE_2 by bone about 2-fold. Indomethacin (5.6 x 10^{-7} M) prevented completely the increase in PGE_2 synthesis as well as the increase in bone resorption. Thus, like TPA, melittin stimulates PGE_2 synthesis in bone cells which, in turn, leads to enhanced bone resorption.

Conclusion

There is now abundant evidence that bone as a tissue can synthesize PGE_2, and that local synthesis of this prostaglandin leads to stimulation of local bone resorption. Using the two pharmacologic probes I have described, phorbol diesters and melittin, it should be possible in future experiments to examine the control of PGE_2 synthesis in bone, the local metabolism of endogenous PGE_2, as well as the mechanisms by which PGE_2 acts on bone cells to stimulate resorption.

Acknowledgment

The author wishes to thank his collaborators in these studies, Drs. Lawrence Levine and Joel L. Ivey, and Mr. Barry Delclos. The original investigations were supported in part by research grants from the National Institutes of Health (AM 10206 and DE 02849).

FOOTNOTES

1 Abbreviations used in this report are: prostaglandin E, PGE; prostaglandin E_2, PGE_2; prostaglandin $F_{2\alpha}$, $PGF_{2\alpha}$; and 12-0-tetradecanoylphorbol-13-acetate, TPA.

REFERENCES

1. Klein, D.C., and Raisz, L.G. 1970. Prostaglandins: stimulators of bone resorption in tissue culture. Endocrinology 86, 1436-40.

2. Tashjian, A.H., Jr., Voelkel, E.F., Levine, L, and Goldhaber, P. 1972. Evidence that the bone resorption-stimulating factor produced by mouse fibrosarcoma cells is prostaglandin E_2: A new model for the hypercalcemia of cancer. J. Exptl. Med., 136, 1329-43.

3. Levine, L., Hinkle, P.M., Voelkel, E.F., and Tashjian, A.H., Jr. 1972. Prostaglandin production by mouse fibrosarcoma cells in culture: Inhibition by indomethacin and aspirin. Biochem. Biophys. Res. Commun., 47, 888-96.

4. Tashjian, A.H., Jr., Voelkel, E.F., Goldhaber, P., and Levine, L. 1973. Successful treatment of hypercalcemia by indomethacin in mice bearing a prostaglandin-producing fibrosarcoma. Prostaglandins 3, 515-24.

5. Tashjian, A.H., Jr., Voelkel, E.F., Goldhaber, P., and Levine, L. 1974. Prostaglandins, calcium metabolism and cancer. Fed. Proc., 33, 81-6.

6. Voelkel, E.F., Tashjian, A.H., Jr., Franklin, R., Wasserman, E., and Levine, L. 1975. Hypercalcemia and tumor prostaglandins: The VX_2 carcinoma model in the rabbit. Metabolism 24, 973-86.

7. Franklin, R.B. and Tashjian, A.H., Jr. 1975. Intravenous infusion of prostaglandin E_2 raises plasma calcium concentration in the rat. Endocrinology 97, 240-43.

8. Tashjian, A.H., Jr., Voelkel, E.F., and Levine, L. 1977. Effects of hydrocortisone on the hypercalcemia and plasma levels of 13,14-dihydro-15-keto-prostaglandin E_2 in mice bearing the $HSDM_1$ fibrosarcoma. Biochem. Biophys. Res. Commun., 74, 199-207.

9. Tashjian, A.H., Jr., Tice, J.E., and Sides, K. 1977. Biological activities of prostaglandin analogs and metabolites on bone in organ culture. Nature 266, 645-47.

10. Tashjian, A.H., Jr., Voelkel, E.F., and Levine, L. 1977. Plasma concentrations of 13,14-dihydro-15-keto-prostaglandin E_2 in rabbits bearing the VX_2 carcinoma: Effects of hydrocortisone and indomethacin. Prostaglandins 14, 309-17.

11. Wolfe, H.J., Bitman, W.R., Voelkel, E.F., Griffiths, H.J. and Tashjian, A.H., Jr. In press. Morphometric, morphologic and radiologic evidence that the VX_2 carcinoma affects bone systemically in rabbits bearing localized tumor. Lab. Invest.

12. Harris, M., Jenkins, M.V., Bennett, A., and Wills, M.R. 1973. Prostaglandin production and bone resorption by dental cysts. Nature 245, 213-15.

13. Goodson, J.M., Dewhirst, F.E., and Brunetti, A. 1974. Prostaglandin E_2 levels and human periodontal disease. Prostaglandins 6, 81-85.

14. Goldhaber, P., Rabadjija, L., Beyer, W.R., and Kornhauser, A. 1973. Bone resorption in tissue culture and its relevance to periodontal disease. J. Am. Dent. Assoc., 87, 1027-33.

15. Raisz, L.G., Sandberg, A.L., Goodson, J.M., Simmons, H.A., and Mergenhagen, S.E. 1974. Complement-dependent stimulation of prostaglandin synthesis and bone resorption. Science 185, 789-91.

16. Sandberg, A.L., Raisz, L.G., Goodson, J.M., Simmons, H.A., and Mergenhagen, S.E. 1977. Initiation of bone resorption by the classical and alternative C pathways and its modulation by prostaglandins. J. Immunol., 119, 1378-81.

17. Rabadjija, L. and Goldhaber, P. 1974. Stimulation of bone resorption in tissue culture by arachidonic acid. J. Dent. Res., 53, 140, Abstr. No. 342.

18. Rabadjija, L. and Goldhaber, P. 1975. Stimulation of bone resorption in tissue culture by phospholipase A. J. Dent. Res., 54, 192, Abstr. No. 589.

19. Beyer, W., Rabadjija, L., and Goldhaber, P. 1976. Indomethacin inhibition of phospholipase A_2-stimulated bone resorption in tissue culture. J. Dent. Res., 55, B117, Abstr. No. 222.

20. Dowsett, M., Eastman, A.R., Easty, D.M., Easty, G.C., Powles, T.J., and Neville, A.M. 1976. Prostaglandin mediation of collagenase-induced bone resorption. Nature 263, 72-74.

21. Robinson, D.R., Tashjian, A.H., Jr., and Levine, L. 1975. Prostaglandin-stimulated bone resorption by rheumatoid synovia: A possible mechanism for bone destruction in rheumatoid arthritis. J. Clin. Invest., 56, 1181-88.

22. Dayer, J.-M., Krane, S.M., Russell, G.G., and Robinson, D.R. 1976. Production of collagenase and prostaglandins by isolated adherent rheumatoid synovial cells. Proc. Nat. Acad. Sci. USA 73, 945-49.

23. Boutwell, R.K. 1974. The function and mechanism of promoters of carcinogenesis. CRC Crit. Rev. Toxicol., 2, 419-43.

24. Sivak, A. 1977. Induction of cell division in Balb/c-3T3 cells by phorbol myristate acetate or bovine serum: Effects of inhibitors of cyclic AMP phosphodiesterase and

Na^+-K^+-ATPase. In Vitro 13, 337-43.

25. Mufson, R.A., Astrup, E.G., Simsiman, R.C., and Boutwell, R.K. 1977. Dissociation of increases in levels of 3': 5' - cyclic AMP and 3':5'-cyclic GMP from induction of ornithine decarboxylase by the tumor promoter 12-0-tetradecanoyl phorbol-13-acetate in mouse epidermis in vivo. Proc. Nat. Acad. Sci. USA 74, 657-61.

26. Levine, L. and Hassid, A. 1977. Effects of phorbol-12,13-diesters on prostaglandin production and phospholipase activity in canine kidney (MDCK) cells. Biochem. Biophys. Res. Commun., in press.

27. Habermann, E. 1972. Bee and wasp venoms. Science 177, 314-22.

28. Hassid, A. and Levine, L. In press. Stimulation of phospholipase activity and prostaglandin biosynthesis by melittin in cell culture and in vivo. Res. Commun. Chem. Pathol. Pharm.

Prostaglandin Regulated Macrophage Collagenase.

Larry M. Wahl, Charles E. Olsen, Sharon M. Wahl, Ann L. Sandberg
and Stephan E. Mergenhagen.

Laboratory of Microbiology and Immunology, National Institute of
Dental Research, Bethesda, Md. 20014.

INTRODUCTION

Elevated levels of prostaglandins (1,2) and collagenase
(3,4) are known to be associated with chronic inflammatory
lesions. Moreover a population of adherent cells isolated from
rheumatoid synovium has been shown to produce extremely high
levels of both prostaglandins and collagenase (5). These findings suggested that prostaglandins might have a regulatory role
in the production of collagenase in inflammatory lesions. Since
the macrophage is a predominant cell type found at an inflammatory site and since macrophages produce the enzyme collagenase
(6) it was of interest to determine whether prostaglandins regulate collagenase production by these cells. Macrophages
activated by endotoxin or lymphokines produce significant amounts
of collagenase (6,7). Macrophages have also been shown to produce prostaglandins (8-11). In recent studies we have
established that prostaglandins regulate the production of
collagenase by endotoxin stimulated macrophages (11) and here we
expand on those findings and also demonstrate that lymphokine
induced collagenase production is also prostaglandin dependent.

MATERIALS AND METHODS

Macrophages obtained from the oil-induced peritoneal exudate
of guinea pigs were cultured as previously described (6).
Activation of the macrophages in culture was achieved by exposure
of the cells to either endotoxin (lipopolysaccharide) from
Escherichia coli (055.B5 Difco Lab., Detroit, Mich.) or products from antigen stimulated lymphocytes obtained as previously
described (7). Prostaglandins E_1, E_2 and $F_{2\alpha}$ (PGE$_1$, PGE$_2$
and PGF$_{2\alpha}$) were a gift from John Pike (Upjohn Company, Kalamazoo,
Mich) and indomethacin was obtained from Merck, Sharp and
Dohme Research Lab., Rahway, N.J. Prostaglandins and indomethacin were dissolved in ethanol and added to medium with the
final concentration of ethanol never exceeding 0.1%. Media from
the macrophage cultures were harvested daily and frozen at -20°C
until assayed for collagenase or prostaglandins.

The culture media were assayed for collagenase activity on
[^{14}C] glycine labeled collagen fibrils as previously described
(6). Prostaglandin levels were determined by direct

radioimmunoassay or after extraction from the media and the prostaglandins separated according to the method of Auletta et al. (12). Anti-PGF$_{2\alpha}$ serum (Clincal Assays, Inc., Cambridge Mass.) or anti-PGE$_2$ serum (Miles, Elkhart, Ind.) were used in th radioimmunoassay. In all experiments the prostaglandin and collagenase data represent the mean value of duplicate samples.

RESULTS

The addition of 10^{-6}M PGE$_2$ to endotoxin-activated macrophag cultures significantly enhanced the production of collagenase (Table 1). However the addition of an equivalent amount of PGE$_2$ to macrophage cultures in the absence of endotoxin did not stimulate the production of collagenase. Addition of varying concentrations of prostaglandins to endotoxin treated cultures revealed that PGE$_1$ and PGE$_2$ enhanced collagenase production in an identical manner (Table 2) while PGF$_{2\alpha}$ had little effect (not shown). Prostaglandin enhancement of collagenase production was detected at 10^{-8}M with maximum stimulation between 10M^{-7} and 10^{-6}M. The increase in collagenase production with the addition of prostaglandins in various experiments ranged from 2 to 10 fold.

The simultaneous addition of indomethacin and endotoxin to macrophage cultures resulted in a significant inhibition of collagenase production (Table 3). While 10^{-5}M indomethacin was used for most of the experiments inhibition of both collagenase and prostaglandin could be demonstrated with concentrations as low as 10^{-8}M. However indomethacin was not effective in blocking collagenase if added 24 hrs after endotoxin.

Collagenase production could be restored in indomethacin blocked cultures by the additon of exogenous PGE$_1$ or PGE$_2$ but not PGF$_{2\alpha}$. The ability of varying concentrations of exogenous PGE$_2$ to overcome the inhibitor effect of indomethacin on endotoxin treated cultures is shown in Table 4. A concentration of 10^{-8}M PGE$_2$ increased the enzyme activity to a level comparable to that achieved with endotoxin in the absence of indomethacin. The peak production of collagenase was obtained with the addition of 10^{-7}M to 10^{-6}M PGE$_2$ while an inhibition of peak production occurred at 10^{-5}M PGE$_2$.

Radioimmunoassay for PGE$_2$ in the media of macrophage cultures exposed to endotoxin revealed that by 2-4 hrs after exposure to endotoxin a significant elevation in PGE$_2$ had occurred (Fig. 1). Maximal production of PGE$_2$ was reached within 14 hrs after the addition of endotoxin. A correlation between prostaglandin and collagenase production was observed when varying concentrations of endotoxin were added to macrophage cultures (Table 5). A small but significant increase in prostaglandin and collagenase production occurred with 0.01 µg/ml of endotoxin. A progressive increase in both was observed as the endotoxin concentration was increased. The peak production of prostaglandin and collagenase was seen at a concentration of 60 µg/ml of endotoxin. A higher concentration (100µg/ml) resulted in a decrease in both collagenase

TABLE 1

Effect of Prostaglandin E_2 on the Production of

Collagenase by Macrophages

Peritoneal Macrophages	Collagenase Activity (cpm)
Control	18
Control + PGE_2	13
Endotoxin	983
Endotoxin + PGE_2	1946

Culture Flasks (75 cm^2) contained 3 x 10^7 adherent macrophages in 10ml Dulbecco Modified Eagle's Media. Cultures received no PGE_2 or PGE_2 (10^{-6}M) alone or with endotoxin (30 μg/ml). The media were changed daily and the 48 hr media were dialyzed and lyophilized. The concentrated media from individual cultures were added to labeled reconstituted collagen fibers (3721 cpm/300 μg of substrate) and incubated for 7 hr. Collagenase activity was determined by the amount of label solubilized.

TABLE 2

Prostaglandin Concentration Effect on Macrophage

Collagenase Production

Stimulant	Collagenase Activity (cpm) Prostaglandin (conc.)				
	0	10^{-9}M	10^{-8}M	10^{-7}M	10^{-6}M
Endotoxin	894	---	---	---	---
Endotoxin + PGE_1	---	581	1486	1962	2054
Endotoxin + PGE_2	---	778	1424	1637	1972

The cells were plated and cultured as described in Table I. Endotoxin (30 μg/ml) was added to all cultures. Some of the cultures received varying concentrations of PGE_1 or PGE_2. The concentrated media products were incubated for 4 hr in the presence of labeled collagen fibers (2763 cpm/ 225 μg of substrate) to determine collagenase activity.

TABLE 3

Inhibitory Effect of Indomethacin on

Macrophage Collagenase Production

Time of Indomethacin Addition (hr)		Inhibition of Collagenase Activity (%)
0	24	
-	-	0
+	-	97
-	+	0
+	+	98

The cells were plated and cultured as described in Table I. Endotoxin (30 µg/ml) was added to all cultures on the first day of culture and indomethacin (10^{-5}M) was added as indicated at the onset of culture (0 hr) or 24 hr later.

TABLE 4

Prostaglandin E_2 Concentration Effect on the

Restoration of Collagenase in Indomethacin Treated

Macrophage Cultures

Additions	Collagenase Activity (cpm)
Control	45
Endotoxin	490
Endotoxin + Indomethacin	151
Endotoxin + Indomethacin + PGE_2	
10^{-9}M	161
10^{-8}M	614
10^{-7}M	1454
10^{-6}M	1557
10^{-5}M	1116

The cells were plated and cultured as described in Table I. The cultures were exposed to endotoxin (30 µg/ml), endotoxin and indomethacin (10^{-5}M) or endotoxin, indomethacin and varying concentrations of PGE_2. Collagenase activity was determined by incubating the concentrated media products with labeled collagen fibers (1847 cpm/150 µg of substrate) for 4 hr.

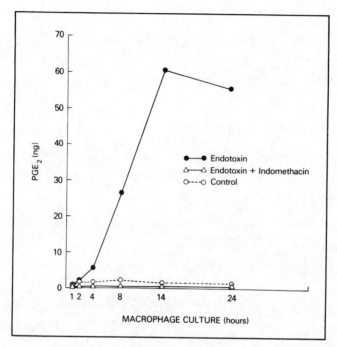

Figure 1.   Endotoxin stimulation of prostaglandin production by macropahges.   The cells were plated and cultured
as described in Table I.   Endotoxin (30 µg/ml) was added to
some of the cultures alone or in the presence of indomethacin
(10-5M).   Media was harvested at the indicated times and assayed
for PGE$_2$.

TABLE 5

Effect of Varying Concentrations of Endotoxin on Prostaglandin and

Collagenase Production by Macrophages

Peritoneal Macrophages	Prostaglandin E_2 (ng/5 x 10^7 cells)	Collagenase Activity (cpm)
Control	1.69	0
Endotoxin		
(µg/ml)		
0.01	3.78	452
0.1	9.10	1028
0.5	14.10	1199
1.0	25.20	1322
5.0	58.60	1599
10.0	97.20	2188
30.0	158.40	2340
60.0	186.60	2559
100.0	135.50	2099

The cultures contained 5 x 10^7 macrophages and were cultured as described in Table I. Prostaglandin determinations were made on the 24 hr media while the 48 hr media was concentrated and incubated with ^{14}C labeled collagen fibers (3766 cpm/ 300 µg of substrate) for 16 hr to determine the collagenase activity.

TABLE 6

Inhibition of Lymphokine Induced Macrophage

Collagenase Production by Indomethacin

Lymphocyte Supernatant	Macrophage Cultures	
	Prostaglandin E_2 (ng/5 x 10^7 cells)	Collagenase Activity (cpm)
None	4.35	0
DNP-OA	51.75	1513
DNP-OA + Indomethacin	2.30	194

The cultures contained 5 x 10^7 macrophages and were cultured as described in Table I. Supernatants (1:2 dilution) from lymphocytes exposed to the specific antigen, dinitrophenylated ovalbumin (DNP-OA), were added to some of the cultures in the presence or absence of indomethacin (10^{-5}M). The prostaglandin and collagenase determinations were made as described in Table VI. The collagenase assay was incubated for 20 hr and the substrate contained 3043 cpm/ 300 µg.

nd prostaglandin.

Supernatants from lymphocytes stimulated with the antigen o which they had been sensitized, dinitrophenylated ovalbumin DNP-OA), were added to macrophage cultures and the media from hese cultures assayed for collagenase activity and prostaglan-in levels. A significant increase in prostaglandins and ollagenase was observed (Table 6). Control supernatants from ultures of lymphocytes not exposed to antigen did not induce GE$_2$ or collagenase. The simultaneous addition of indomethacin nd supernatants from antigen-stimulated lymphocytes resulted n blockage of the production of PGE$_2$ (Table 6). Consequently, ollagenase, being prostaglandin dependent, was not significant-y elevated in these macrophage cultures (Table 6).

Discussion

Prostaglandins appear to have an essential role in the pro-uction of collagenase by macrophages. This conclusion is upported by the ability of PGE$_1$ or PGE$_2$ to enhance collagenase roduction in endotoxin stimulated cultures, the inhibition of nzyme activity by indomethacin, the restoration of collagenase ctivity in indomethacin blocked cultures by exogenous PGE$_2$ nd by the simultaneous elevation in the amount of PGE$_2$ nd collagenase produced by the macrophages in response to arying concentrations of endotoxin. Additionally, the con-entration of exogenous PGE$_2$ needed to restore collagenase ctivity in cultures blocked by indomethacin to the level ob-ained by endotoxin in the absence of indomethacin is nearly quivalent to the PGE$_2$ produced by the macrophages. Moreover, t appears that lymphokine induced macrophage activation which esults in collagenase production may operate through a mechanism omparable to endotoxin. Not only did the lymphokine trigger rostaglandin production by the macrophages but this elevation n prostaglandins was blocked by indomethacin which concurrently nhibited collagenase synthesis.

The results of these experiments suggest that following xposure to agents that activate macrophages there is a rapid and ignificant increase in PGE$_2$ production. Moreover the restora-ion of collagenase production in indomethacin-treated cultures y exogenous PGE$_2$ implies that the prostaglandins produced by the acrophage directly affect collagenase production. Activation f macrophages by endotoxin, lymphokines and presumably by other echanisms is required before prostaglandins can exert their ffect on the cell synthetic machinery involved in collagenase roduction since the addition of prostaglandins alone did not nduce the production of this enzyme. The mechanism by which rostaglandins regulate collagenase production is not known but ay involve a cyclic nucleotide dependent pathway. Several re-orts have indicated that macrophage function may be influenced y the changes in cyclic AMP levels brought about by prostaglandins 13,14,15) and we are currently investigating such a correlation n the regulation of collagenase activity. Thus it appears that roduction of prostaglandins by activated macrophages may serve as a regulatory mechanism in the induction of the enzyme colla-genase. This regulatory potential of prostaglandins, which are elevated in inflammatory lesions may have important implications in the inflammatory process.

ABBREVIATIONS

Prostaglandin E_1, E_2 and $F_{2\alpha}$ (PGE_1, PGE_2 and $PGF_{2\alpha}$)

Dinitrophyenlated ovalbumin (DNP-OA).

REFERENCES

1. Robinson, D.R. and McGuire, M.B. 1975. Prostaglandins in the Rheumatic Diseases. Ann. N.Y. Acad. Sci. 256, 318-329.

2. Goodson, J.M., Dewhirst, F.E. and Brunetti, A. 1974. Prostaglandin E_2 levels and human periodontal disease. Prostaglandins 6, 81-85.

3. Fullmer, H.M. and Gibson, W.A. 1966. Collagenolytic activity in gingivae of man. Nature 209, 728-729.

4. Krane, S.M. 1975. Collagenase production by human synovial tissues. Ann. N.Y. Acad. Sci. 25, 289-303.

5. Dayer, J-M., Krane, S.M. Russel, R.G.G. and Robinson, D.R. 1976. Production of collagenase and prostaglandins by isolated adherent rheumatoid synovial cells. Proc. Nat. Acad. Sci. USA 73, 945-949.

6. Wahl, L.M., Wahl, S.M., Mergenhagen, S.E. and Martin, G.R. 1974. Collagenase production by endotoxin-activated macrophages. Proc. Nat. Acad. Sci. USA, 71, 3598-3601.

7. Wahl, L.M., Wahl, S.M., Mergenhagen, S.E. and Martin, G.R. 1975. Collagenase production by lymphokine activated macrophages. Science, 187, 261-263.

8. Bray, M.A., Gordon, D. and Morely, J. 1975. Macrophages on intrauterine contraceptive devices produce prostaglandins. Nature, 257, 227-228.

9. Bray, M.A., Gordon, D. and Morely, J. 1976. Control of lymphokine secretion by prostaglandins. Nature, 262, 401-402.

10. Humes, J.L. Bonney, R.J., Pelus, L., Dahlgren, M.E., Sadowski, S.J., Kuehl, F.A. Jr. and Davies, P. 1977. Macrophages synthesize and release prostaglandins in response to inflammatory stimuli. Nature, 269, 149-150.

11. Wahl, L.M., Olsen, C.E., Sandberg, A.L. and Mergenhagen, S.E. 1977. Prostaglandin regulation of macrophage collagenase production. Proc. Nat. Acad. Sci. USA. 74, in press.

12. Auletta, F.J., Zusman, R.M. and Caldwell, B.V. 1974. Development and standardization of radioimmunoassays for prostaglandins E, F. and A. Clinical Chemistry 20. 1580-1587.

13. Koopman, W.J., Gillis, M.H. and David, J.R. 1973. Prevention of MIF activity by agents known to increase cellular cyclic AMP. J. Immunol. 110, 1609-1614.

14. Remold-O'Donnell, E. 1974. Stimulation and desensitization of macrophage adenylate cyclase by prostaglandins and catecholamines. J. Biol. Chem. 249, 3615-3621.

15. Gemsa, D., Steggemann, L., Menzel, J. and Till, G. 1975. Release of cyclic AMP from macrophages by stimulation with prostaglandins. J. Immunol. 114, 1422-1424.

Discussion for Session III: The Role of Microbes, Mediators
and Mononuclear Cells in Localized Bone Loss. Part B.

DR. PECK: Dr. Tashjian, did you see an effect of added
exogenous PGE's on cyclic AMP but not the endogenously-stimulated
PGE's? Was that a difference?

DR. TASHJIAN: Yes. I didn't show the numerical data.
Under experimental circumstances where PGE-2 exogenously added,
or PTH exogenously added, markedly, that is, 10-fold or 20-fold,
stimulates cyclic AMP accumulation, TPA had no effect at all.
Therefore, there were positive controls in all of those experiments in which we did not see either an increase or a decrease
in cyclic AMP with the phorbol diesters.

DR. PUZAS: Dr. Tashjian, have you tried additive effects
of phorbol and melittin and do you postulate that they work
through the same mechanism for increasing prostaglandin
synthesis?

DR. TASHJIAN: Well, I have shown that they both increase
prostaglandin synthesis.

DR. PUZAS: But is the effect additive, of maximal doses of
each of them?

DR. TASHJIAN: I have not actually done maximal doses of
both of those. I have done experiments with maximal doses of
exogenous prostaglandin, and either TPA or phorbol, and those
effects are not additive. You get the maximum effect from one,
and you get no further effect of the other. I have not done the
experiment in which one adds melittin and TPA together.

DR. WURTHIER: Dr. Tashjian, we have looked at prostaglandin
synthesis in the growth plate, and have also correlated this with
phospholipase-A activity. We find there a marked increase
in this level of activity as we approach the area of calcification.

This seems almost to be a paradox because of the fact that
in this area, where we know that calcification is just beginning,
we see this stimulation of prostaglandin synthesis. Would you
comment on the differences in the prostaglandin activity in these
two systems?

DR. TASHJIAN: It sounds very similar to the effect of PTH in stimulating resorption and formation. Have you measured locally, or can you measure locally, prostaglandin synthesis? Or are you referring primarily to measurements of phospholipase activity near the calcification front?

DR. WURTHIER: We are looking at both activities. Further, we have actually looked at the prostaglandin degradative enzymes. We found that the degradative enzymes are particularly prevalent in the proliferative zone; as one approaches the calcification area, then they give way and the dominant action seems to be the synthetase. As one goes toward the bone, you see again another spike of increase in the degradative enzyme.

DR. TASHJIAN: Yes. The comments I would make are as follows; and Dr. Raisz may want to comment additionally on it.

The one aspect that has intrigued me is the possible role of calcium as a trigger for stimulating the resorptive process. This is an indirect answer to your question in the following context.

We have looked at whether parathyroid hormone, prostaglandin E-2, or other agents that stimulate resorption, stimulate calcium uptake as an initial, very early event that precedes calcium release. We unfortunately have not been able, in a reproducible fashion, to demonstrate calcium uptake that precedes calcium release. Since others have, I presume that it is a problem for us, and not for them.

The question as to how prostaglandins might play a role in modulating formation I have not looked at at all, experimentally. Therefore, I have no data that are contrary to a dual role for prostaglandins and would be interested in Dr. Raisz's response.

DR. RAISZ: There is an important difference between cartilage and bone with respect to the one system we have studied both in, and that is complement-mediated destruction.

Complement-mediated destruction of cartilage, which was well demonstrated by Fell's group, is not prostaglandin-dependent, as far as we can make out; whereas complement-mediated bone resorption is prostaglandin-dependent. So I think the functions of prostaglandins must be quite different in the two systems.

If Dr. Sandberg were here, I know she would mention the fact that arachidonate increases prostaglandin synthesis in our culture systems. But interestingly, cortisol blocks all forms of prostaglandin-mediated bone resorption, including that where arachidonate is added to the culture system.

May I ask if you have looked at the glucocorticoid effect with these two compounds, or the arachidonate effect in their combination?

DR. TASHJIAN: The mechanism by which glucocorticoids

inhibit prostaglandin synthesis, I believe, is not entirely worked out at the molecular level. It is my understanding that the effect seems to focus on the phospholipase-phospholipid interaction, and is clearly not to be focused on the cyclo-oxygenase; so that one can dissect those two mechanisms at those loci, at least.

As far as phorbol and melittin are concerned, there is no inhibition of resorption by hydrocortisone or dexamethasone of those two compounds.

When one generates prostaglandin endogenously by melittin, there is an inhibition by the glucocorticoid. I have not looked at it in the case of phorbol. I think that the melittin is acting at the level of the substrate, the generation of arachodonic acid by deisolation of the phospholipids, presumably membrane phospholipids, and that probably is the area at which stabilization is taking place, by the glucocorticoid.

DR. RAISZ: Dr. Wahl, have you ever tried colchicine, which increases collagenase release, to see if it works with prosta-glandin?

DR. WAHL: Yes. We have tried several run-throughs with colchicine and we have seen elevated levels of both prostaglandin and collagenase. I must add, though, that while it is not always consistent, we do see them usually.

DR. WURTHIER: Dr. Wahl, in view of the recent discoveries of the thromboxines and the prostacyclines, have you by any chance tried to look at either of these, or the endoperoxides, PGG or PGH?

DR. WAHL: No; we have not. As you know, they are rapidly metablized. Further, as you have seen, the activation cycle seems to occur between two to 14 hours with PGE-2. One would anticipate that at least the thromboxines wouldn't be around that long, but that certainly doesn't mean that there is an indication that they wouldn't have a role at that early phase of activation.

DR. WURTHIER: I am sure they would never last more than just a few minutes; but they might actually turn something on during that transient period.

DR. WAHL: That is true.

DR. WURTHIER: It may very well be that they really don't have an effect but certainly in the platelet-mediated systems, they seem to be very powerful.

DR. BOCKMAN: Dr. Wahl, have you looked at unstimulated macrophages; that is to say, from peritoneal washings without the use of oil?

DR. WAHL: Yes. What we find in that case is that

unstimulated macrophages have higher basal levels of prostaglandins. However, we can activate comparable ratio increase in prostaglandins as we find with the oil, and get the collagenase production also with those cells.

But the wash-out cells seem to be a more mature cell, and to have elevated levels of background prostaglandins. They do not have collagenase production per se, without stimulation.

DR. BOCKMAN: We have looked at human and also mouse macrophages. The same thing appeared; in the human, they were peripheral monocytes. In the mouse, the unstimulated ones definitely produced more prostaglandin than the stimulated, just as you have found.

To comment to the prior discussion on endoperoxides: we have found using a different technique other than radioimmunoassay that I-2, that is to say prostacyclin, is produced by these cells.

DR. COHN: Dr. Wahl, do you have any idea what the molecular basis is for the increase in collagenase? Is this an increase in activity? Synthesis? And do you have any idea about the molecular link from the PGE; could it stimulate the activity?

DR. WAHL: That is a good point. There is considerable evidence in the literature now to suggest that prostaglandins elevate cyclic AMP. This is one thing that we are working on presently, and it appears that endotoxin will elevate cyclic AMP in these cultures.

This seems to be related to exogenous cyclic AMP added back that will also induce collagenase production. So it is most likely that we have a link here with the prostaglandins that are produced and the elevation in cyclic AMP. This is something we hope to publish shortly.

DR. KRANE: But Dr. Wahl, your data did not show that you could add back exogenous PGE-2 and produce any collagenase by yourselves in the absence of --?

DR. WAHL: That is correct and a very good point. We do get elevation of cyclic AMP there. There are obviously other events going on related to the increase in cyclic AMP.

DR. KRANE: Right. As we will show tomorrow. But you can't do that by the use of prostaglandin alone, so that you have to look at the prostaglandin as having some extra stimulating effect; some kind of modulating effect, rather than being the primary agent that changes your climate.

DR. SCHRAER: Dr. Tashjian, what is the effect of melittin on bone in vivo?

DR. TASHJIAN: It has never been looked at, as far as I know.

DR. BOCKMAN: Dr. Wahl, Dr. Webb has published that T cells produce prostaglandins. I wonder if in your lymphocyte supernates you looked, obviously before you tested them, for their prostaglandin levels.

DR. WAHL: Yes. We found very low levels. When the supernatants were added back to the macrophages in the presence of indomethacin, there was a very low basal level comparable to that found with the macrophages alone.

If we take out the adherent population in these preps, and then run experiments with mitogens on T cells, we remove most of the prostaglandin activity that we can induce in our supernatants. Albeit, there certainly is a small increase with T cells. Nonetheless, the macrophage, at least in our system, seems to be the prime producer of prostaglandin.

DR. PECK: Dr. Wahl, is there an increased elaboration of other enzymes in your system besides collagenase; that is, elastase, acid phosphatase, and so forth; and is the process inhibited by non-glucocorticoids, such as estrogens?

DR. WAHL: We have looked at elastase. Zena Werb has published some work with elastase, showing that there is a parallel increase in collagenase and elastase. We have seen this also. We have not measured directly in these cultures a relationship to prostaglandins. I would assume that both collagenase and elastase go up in this reponse to prostaglandins. Most of the true proteases in these cells tend to increase with stimulation.

DR. PECK: What about the steroids?

DR. WAHL: As you know, we have been looking. We have reported that progesterone, particularly, will inhibit these cells from producing collagenase. This seems to be more related to an inhibition within the cell, and we don't seem to block the prostaglandins per se. With dexamethasone, on the other hand, we block both very efficiently, down to 10^{-8} and 10^{-9} molar. But as has been brought out, dexamethasone has some initital problems, in that it may act on general protein synthesis. We know that it blocks protein synthesis in these cells, even at those concentrations, so the phospholipase may be blocked here as well as the collagenase.

So this steroid has some problems, at least with dividing between the two functions, based on protein synthesis.

DR. TASHJIAN: I just remembered one additional comment for Dr. Schraer. I know that melittin has been looked at in vivo in the rat and mouse. When given by intraperitoneal routes, it does produce up to at least a ten-fold increase in the circulating levels of 13, 14 dihydro-15-keto-PGE-2, which is the major circulating metabolite of E-2. In those experiments, unfortunately, no one thought to look at calcium levels. So, the experiment just doesn't have a result yet.

I also wanted to ask one of the previous questioners what the levels of PGI_2 synthesized by macrophages are?

DR. BOCKMAN: Very low. But that is hard to quantitate, and the identification of the substance that I am calling "I" is not complete.

DR. TASHJIAN: That is by mass spec?

DR. BOCKMAN: That is where we are failing, in the mass spec. But it is not any of the other classical prostaglandins, and it migrates where I_2 should be. Actually, we are measuring the stable metabolite, which is the 6-keto F_1 alpha.

DR. STERN: Dr. Tashjian, the group at Strangeways has shown that the resorption of cartilage produced by antiserum is enhanced or may even require the presence of loose connective tissue. Would you have any evidence that any of these agents which act through prostaglandin release might be releasing it from loose connective tissue? Does it make any difference, for example, how you dissect your calvaria?

DR. TASHJIAN: That is an interesting problem. After talking with Dr. Raisz on several occasions about the problems of basal resorption and especially at a time when we were suffering with high basal resorption, he mentioned to me that there was a correlation in the long bone system between the amount of connective tissue contamination and spontaneous resorption. So we have tried to examine that carefully by purposefully contaminating cultures with connective tissue; that is, doing a poor job at the section and then an ultra-meticulous job at the section.

With the calvaria from the mouse in our hands, there appears to be very little correlation between the amount of connective tissue contamination and spontaneous resorption. There is a very tight correlation between spontaneous resorption and prostaglandin E-2 in the medium; but I don't know where it is coming from.

DR. STERN: Not the connective tissue?

DR. TASHJIAN: It would seem not to be the case.

DR. WURTHIER: Dr. Tashjian, would you comment on the action of indomethacin? It appears that it is not at all clear just exactly what this drug does. I recently heard a report to the effect that its action may not be in the cyclo-oxygenase, but rather much earlier on, simply in the phospholipase A-2. I would be curious to know if anyone really has any hard data on the action of this drug.

DR. TASHJIAN: I have not worked myself on the mechanism of action of indomethacin. I would mention several relevant observations made by Levine, published in PNAS, who has been interested in the mechanism by which steroids inhibit prostaglandin synthesis.

And in experiments of the following design, if you pre-label cells in culture; now, these are not bone cells, but other sorts of cells that are able to synthesize prostaglandins; for example, dog kidney cells.

If you label the endogenous phospholipids with precursors so that they are, in fact, labeled and their endogenous arachidonic acid is also labeled, and then look for agents that stimulate the release of arachidonate, and also simultaneously measure the release of PGE synthesis, the effect of indomethacin on the release of arachidonate from pre-labeled endogenous phospholipids is not inhibited by indomethacin.

Now, that is a very specific cell system, and that release does depend on phospholipase activity. I do not know how one can generalize from that observation; but at least in that system, I would conclude that the effect of indomethacin, when it is inhibiting exogenous arachidonic acid's conversion, or endogenous conversion, to E-2, is not also affecting the phospholipase activation.

I have not seen the data which indicate that indomethacin inhibits phospholipase activity. I think from what has been said this afternoon, from the number of people who use indomethacin, one should always be concerned about the specificity of its action, and at the very least, measure for the product of the reaction, prostaglandin.

But, that in no way assures you that this is the only thing it is doing.

DR. WURTHIER: The reason that I really bring it up is the fact that the rate of synthesis of prostaglandins is so fast that anybody who has worked with them knows that you get a rapid burst of activity. It doesn't take very long; so that you almost might have a coupling effect. As soon as it is released, it gets coupled right to the synthetase system, and it would be very difficult to divorce one from the other.

DR. TASHJIAN: Just to emphasize the speed at which that reaction takes place, we have been interested in a tumor system that synthesizes prostaglandin very actively; the HSDM-1 fibrosarcoma system. In looking at the content of E-2 in those tumor cells in vivo, operating under circumstances where one can remove the tumor and have it in liquid nitrogen containing indomethacin in less than two seconds, we cannot demonstrate any inhibition of synthesis that occurs during the handling process. So, it is that fast.

DR. MILLER: I am trying to put this in some sort of anatomical perspective. Would either one of you care to speculate what bone cells in that particular microenvironment might be producing the prostaglandins in, say, a calvarial system?

DR. TASHJIAN: I can't tell you the answer to that. I would like to be able to. If there is another one of these workshops a year or so from now, more information should be available, because I think it is going to take a multifaceted approach.

One approach is going to be the sort of thing that Glenda Wong and Dave Cohn are doing; trying to separate the cells and get pure populations and then look at their responses. That will only be part of the story, because there are interactions between these cells and proliferative maturation phenomena which are not necessarily going to take place in isolated, pure populations. It will take others working with tissues in vitro, as well as animals in vivo, to find the answer to that kind of question.

I can visualize that it will be possible to do so by a variety of immuno-staining procedures, because it is now possible to localize prostaglandin at the cellular and probably subcellular level. It is not easy, because of their lipid solubility, but it can be done.

DR. MATTHEWS: I wonder whether any of the persons speaking to collagenase today could speak to where the collagenase is coming from. Is it lysosomal? If not, is it possible that cyclic AMP and/or prostaglandin might be affecting, or having its effect, by virtue of a lysosomal membrane effect, for example?

DR. WAHL: I know of no evidence that this is the case with lysosomal enzymes. There is some work in which prostaglandins have been added to polymorphonuclear leukocytes, and there was some stimulation; but with macrophages, I have no idea whether that is the case or if it has an effect on lysosomal membranes.

DR. RAISZ: Collagenase release is maintained, as Dr. Werb has shown and as we have also found in bone, in the presence of colchicine when lysosomal enzymes are markedly inhibited. In fact, collagenase release is increased; so I think any lysosomal activation of collagenase release seems unlikely.

DR. BOCKMAN: Dr. Raisz, I know you cut the ends off of your bones. Do you wash out the marrow?

DR. RAISZ: There isn't anything that you can recognize as marrow in a 19-day fetal long bone, as far as differentiated cells. I think they are all precursor cells.

DR. STERN: Dr. Tashjian, you were the first one in these talks who has brought up the subject of cyclic G, in saying that the phorbol esters do increase it. There is a great silence in the literature on the role of cyclic G in resorption. May I assume that means we all have negative data with everything we tried that might implicate it?

DR. TASHJIAN: I don't know whether the great silence is due to not finding any effect or problems with the assays. I certainly don't know of very many published results in this area. I would think that lack is methodologic, as much as it is anything else.

DR. RAISZ: Many of us have tried cyclic G analogs and cyclic G itself to stimulate bone resorption, all with consistently negative results. That certainly doesn't say what is going on inside the cell, but it is the kind of thing that happens and nobody ever publishes.

DR. TASHJIAN: How about the converse? How many people have actually measured changes in cyclic G in bone?

DR. RAISZ: Gideon Rodan has made such attempts, and he has measurements, but not changes.

DR. STERN: Dr. Jack Diamond at our institution has been measuring it in bone cells, in collaboration with us, after parathyroid hormone and after nitroprusside, which is a very potent stimulator of cyclic G in other cell systems. In a heterogeneous cell population, at a time when PTH causes a marked increase in cyclic A, we see no effects on cyclic G. Further, we have not found any effects with nitroprusside, which in other cell systems, causes like 13-fold increases.

He has been doing a lot of work with this in smooth muscle and has the capability of measuring it. But I wondered what other people's data were, and how it interacted with some of the other mediators.

DR. TASHJIAN: Is there a basal level of cyclic G, and is there a cyclic G synthetic system in your cells, but it is just not stimulatable?

DR. STERN: That is what it appears. It seems that there is a measurable basal level. I can't tell you at the moment what it is. However, it is certainly several orders of magnitude lower than the levels of cyclic A, but it doesn't seem to be stimulatable under the conditions that we have used.

DR. TASHJIAN: Dr. Wahl, in relation to the collagenase production and cyclic AMP, has the effect of cholera toxin been looked at in macrophages? There seems to be some uncertainty as to the role of cyclic AMP as a mediator of that effect.

DR. WAHL: We haven't yet looked at cholera toxin, but plan to. I might add that the addition of exogenous cyclic AMP only seems to enhance collagenase production in the macrophage population if they have been exposed prior to a stimulant, such as endotoxin. So there seems to be some common pathway between the initial stimulant to which the macrophage is exposed, and then also the sequence of prostaglandins and cyclic AMP.

DR. TASHJIAN: Do you know anything about prostaglandin binding before and after endotoxin?

DR. WAHL: We are looking at that at the present time.

DR. MECHANIC: I have noticed that there are a lot of stimulatory effects going on here; extra synthesis of prostaglandin, extra synthesis of collagenase. Could these possibly be primary responses of a cell which is sort of "sick"?

For instance, if you pneumonectomized one lung from a rabbit, and one day later look at the other lung, you will see a two- or three-fold increase in lysyloxidase. Also in the metaphasis of vitamin-D deficient chicks, you will see a two-fold increase in lysyloxidase, while the production of aldehydes are apparently normal or less than normal.

Apparently, the primary or compensatory response by "sick" tissue is to just blast off and synthesize something. There seems to be preliminary evidence for this. I wonder if there would be any comments on this from the audience or from the speakers.

DR. TASHJIAN: I would be interested in commenting on that. As far as prostaglandin synthesis is concerned, Dr. Mechanic, I think you have chosen a very penetrating shot, because an agonal gasp by most cells is prostaglandin synthesis. If you treat them with acetic acid, they will make prostaglandins; so dying cells do go through a burst of prostaglandin synthesis.

On the other hand, I don't think that most dying cells respond appropriately to exogenous hormonal signals, so I would separate and be concerned about dying cells responding to insults such as these or others from the outside; but when the response is appropriate, in a homeostatic sense, I would think that is unlikely to be the case.

DR. SAKAMOTO: Dr. Wahl, was the collagenase you found in macrophages all active collagenase, and no latent forms?

DR. WAHL: We have attempted some time ago to activate latent collagenase in these preps, and have been unsuccessful; that is, with trypsin in various concentrations from a time scale of 30 seconds up to about two to three hours.

This may be related to just a phenomenon of dialysis inactivation of latent enzyme. I don't know. There are others who have reported activation of latent enzyme in macrophage preparations; but we have been unsuccessful in doing so.

Secretion of Plasminogen Activator by Macrophages and
Polymorphonuclear Leukocytes.

Jean-Dominique Vassalli, Angela Granelli-Piperno, and E. Reich

The Rockefeller University, New York, New York   10021

Recent work has shown that many avian and mammalian cells -
both normal and neoplastic - can synthesize and secrete plasminogen activators. A partial list would include fibroblasts
(1-3), muscle cells (R. Miskin, T. Easton, and E. Reich, manuscript in preparation), epidermal cells (H. Green and E. Reich,
unpublished observations), synovial cells (4), ovarian granulosa
cells (5), Sertoli cells[1], trophoblast (6), parietal endoderm
(6), mammary epithelium (L. Ossowski and E. Reich, manuscript in
preparation), monocytes and macrophages (7,8), and polymorphonuclear leukocytes (PMNs) (9). Plasminogen is a catalytically
inactive zymogen that is present in body fluids at quite high
concentrations, and it is converted by plasminogen activator into
plasmin, a trypsin-like serine protease of broad specificity.
Secretion of activator allows cells to recruit the potential
proteolytic activity of the surrounding plasminogen, and thereby
to direct controlled proteolysis in their immediate environment.
Plasminogen activator is the only known catalyst of extracellular
proteolytic activity that is common to all of the cells listed
above, and since we have found that this enzyme functions in a
variety of biological contexts, its secretion may be a general
mechanism for performing localized and controlled extracellular
proteolysis.

A conspicuous property of plasminogen activator secretion is
the spectrum of regulatory phenomena associated with enzyme production. In some cells, such as trophoblast and parietal endoderm, synthesis appears to be regulated by endogenous synthetic
programming but, in the majority of cases, regulation is determined by hormonal mechanisms. For example, enzyme formation by
granulosa cells is maximal in vivo at the time of ovulation, and
can be induced in vitro by physiological concentrations of FSH
(10). Comparable hormonal responses have also been observed in
mammary epithelium (L. Ossowski and E. Reich, manuscript in preparation), and in Sertoli cells[1], and the evidence summarized
here points to the hormonal control of enzyme production in
macrophages and PMNs.

---

[1]Lacroix, M., Smith, F.E., and I.B. Fritz. Manuscript
submitted for publication.

Although we can only speculate on the possible functions of plasminogen activator in vivo, a growing and coherent body of evidence, assembled from the study of many normal and malignant cells, indicates that secretion of this enzyme is associated with cell migration and tissue remodelling. Some of the most persuasive of these results have been obtained with inflammatory cells, namely mouse peritoneal macrophages and human peripheral blood PMNs, and we describe here some of the evidence suggesting that plasminogen activator production by these cells is uniquely correlated with their participation in inflammatory responses; in particular we show that enzyme production is induced and stimulated by inflammatory substances, and inhibited by anti-inflammatory steroids.

1.   Macrophages Collected from Inflammatory Exudates Secrete Plasminogen Activator

Peritoneal macrophages obtained from mice that have been injected intraperitoneally with inflammatory substances such as thioglycollate medium, endotoxin, mineral oil, etc., produce plasminogen activator, whereas the resident peritoneal macrophages from unstimulated animals do not (7,8). Asbestos particles can also be used to induce such inflammatory exudates (11), and Figure 1 compares the fibrinolytic activity of resident peritoneal macrophages with that of cells obtained from mice injected with thioglycollate medium or with various amounts of asbestos particles: the rate of fibrinolysis by these cultures is a function of the amount of injected asbestos, and fibrinolysis is entirely due to secretion of plasminogen activator, since none is observed when plasminogen is omitted from the medium.

Among macrophage enzymes so far investigated, the correlations that link plasminogen activator secretion and responses to both inflammatory and anti-inflammatory stimuli (v. infra) appear to be unique, and they suggest that studies of the modulation of enzyme production may be useful for developing insights about the control of inflammtion. In contrast, secretion of lysozyme, or leakage of lysosomal hydrolases proceed at the same rate for "resident" as they do for "inflammatory" macrophages.

The plasminogen activator secreted by macrophages, like that from transformed mouse fibroblasts, is a DFP-sensitive serine protease with tryptic specificity (7). The secreted enzyme migrates in SDS-polyacrylamide gel electrophoresis in three bands, with apparent molecular weights of 48,000, 47,000 and 28,000 (Figure 2A); the relationship, if any between these three species is still unclear. In constrast, the enzyme present in the cell lysate migrates as a single band of apparent molecular weight 46,000 (Figure 2B), suggesting that it is synthesized by the cells as a single molecular weight species and subject to some post-synthetic modifications.

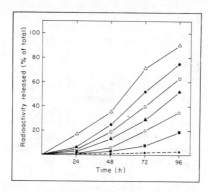

Fig. 1. Fibrinolysis by cultured peritoneal macrophages.
Peritoneal cells from asbestos, latex, PBS (2×10^6 cells
per well), and thioglycollate medium (8×10^5 cells per
well) -injected mice were plated on ^{125}I fibrin -coated
Linbro wells in Dulbecco's MEM containing 5% of heat-inactivated fetal bovine serum and 100 µg/ml soybean
trypsin inhibitor. The cultures were washed after 24hr,
and Dulbecco's MEM containing 5% of acid-treated, heat-
inactivated fetal bovine serum (AT HI FBS) (___) or 5%
of plasminogen-depleted AT HI FBS (----) was added; samples
were removed as indicated, and assayed for radioactivity
released into the medium. Cells were obtained from mice
injected with (Δ) thioglycollate medium; (●) 300µg,
(□)100µg, (▲) 10µg,(o) 1µg asbestos; (■) PBS or 500 µg
latex particles. Reproduced from (11).

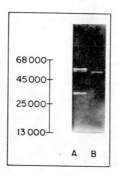

Fig. 2. Identification of plasminogen activator after
SDS-polyacrylamide gel electrophoresis of conditioned
medium and cell lysate from thioglycollate-induced
macrophages. Conditioned medium (lane A) and cell lysate
(lane B) were electrophoresed in an SDS-11% polyacrylamide
gel, and the gel processed for detection of plasminogen-
dependent fibrinolytic activity as described (9). The
figure is a photograph of the amido black-stained fibrin-
agar layer; the clear areas are due to lysis of fibrin
in the agar gel. No zones of lysis were observed if the
assay was performed in the absence of plasminogen.

2.   The Production of Macrophage Plasminogen Activator Can Be
Modulated in Vitro

a.   Inhibition by anti-inflammatory steroids, mitotic inhibitors, and cyclic AMP.   Glucocorticoids markedly inhibit the production of plasminogen activator by macrophages cultured from inflammatory exudates (12). Figure 3 shows both that this inhibition occurs at very low drug concentrations, and that the order of relative potencies strictly reflects the respective anti-inflammatory potencies in vivo. The effect of glucocorticoids on macrophages is rapid in onset (it is detectable within 90 minutes), reversible, and, like that in other systems influenced at low levels of glucocorticoids, also requires RNA synthesis; in addition, the macrophage response to glucocorticoids, appears to be quite selective since phagocytosis, lysozyme secretion, lysosomal hydrolase leakage, secretion of ^{3}H-DFP reactive enzymes, and overall rates of RNA and protein synthesis are not affected at hormone concentrations that inhibit plasminogen activator production by more than 90% (12). Since glucocorticoids administered in vivo produce a rapid decrease in circulating monocytes and prevent the migration of macrophages into inflammatory exudates, the results summarized here support the hypothesis that plasminogen activator secretion is correlated with the migration of these cells and with their involvement in inflammatory reactions; this also suggests that the anti-inflammatory effect of glucocorticoids may be mediated, at least in part, by a specific reduction of plasminogen activator secretion.

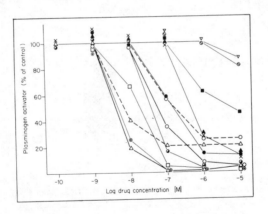

Fig. 3. Effect of steroid hormones and derivatives on plasminogen activator production by thioglycollate-induced macrophage cultures. Plasminogen activator in conditoned medium (___) and in cell lysates (---); the results are expressed as percentages of the activity present in control untreated cultures. (x) aldosterone; (•) cortexolone; (o) corticosterone; (▲) desoxycorticosterone; (△) dexamethasone; (◍) β-estradiol; (⊙) fluorocortisone; (◑) hydrocortisone; (□) prednisolone; (▪) progesterone; (▾) testosterone. Reproduced from (12).

In addition to the glucocorticoid hormones, other pharmacological agents also inhibit production of plasminogen activator (12): the mitotic inhibitors colchicine and vinblastine appear to inhibit preferentially the secretion process, whereas compounds related to cyclic AMP metabolism (dibutyryl cAMP, epinephrine, isoproterenol, prostaglandins E_1 and E_2, and cholera toxin) inhibit the production of active enzyme.

b. Induction by Concanavalin A and phorbol myristate acetate. Secretion of plasminogen activator by macrophages can be induced and stimulated in vitro by lectins such as Concanavalin A, and by the tumor promoter and inflammatory agent phorbol myristate acetate (PMA)(13). Table 1 shows that the majority of normal, resident macrophages can be induced to secrete plasminogen activator, and also that essentially all of the macrophages from thioglycollate-induced exudates can be stimulated to secrete the enzyme. By the manipulation of stimulatory (Con A, PMA) and inhibitory (glucocorticoids, cholera toxin) influences, enzyme production can be modulated continuously over a 200 fold range; in the same way the proportion of cells that secrete detectable levels of enzyme can be varied from 1 to 90% (13). These results demonstrate that production of plasminogen activator is a property of the macrophage population in general, and not only a subset of this population. In addition, since both Con A and PMA are potent inflammatory agents in vivo, their effect on plasminogen activator secretion in vitro supports the proposed correlation between enzyme secretion and the inflammatory response.

c. Induction by products of activated lymphoid cells. No information is as yet available about potential inducers of macrophage plasminogen activator in vivo. We have found that the conditioned medium from lectin-stimulated mouse lymphoid cells can both induce the synthesis of plasminogen activator by "resident" macrophages obtained from normal untreated mice, and it also stimulates enzyme production by macrophages obtained from thioglycollate-induced exudates (14). Figure 4 presents a dose curve showing the effect of such conditioned medium from Con A-stimulated mouse spleen cells on the proportion of normal macrophages secreting plasminogen activator: a majority of macrophages respond to high concentrations of lymphocyte conditioned medium, and a detectable effect is observed with a 100-fold dilution of this medium. These results suggest that macrophage plasminogen activator production may be regulated in part by lymphocytes, and they provide further evidence to link enzyme production with cell migration and inflammation.

Polymorphonuclear Leukocytes Secrete Plasminogen Activator

PMNs have many properties in common with monocytes and macrophages: both cell types are capable of digesting endocytosed materials, and both are migratory and are recruited to sites of inflammation by migration from the blood stream; in addition, the migration of both cell types in vivo is blocked by glucocorticoids.

TABLE I

Plasminogen Activator Production by Individual Macrophages

	Cells Surrounded by Lytic Zone (% of total)	
	5 hr	20 hr
"Normal" Macrophages:		
-	1	2
Con A	21	35
PMA	33	51
"Thioglycollate" Macrophages:		
-	36	52
Con A	51	68
PMA	70	89

Peritoneal cells (2 x 10⁴ from uninjected mice; 1 x 10⁴ from thioglycollate medium-injected mice) were plated in 60 mm tissue culture dishes in Dulbecco's medium supplemented with 10% HI FBS; Con A (10^{-7}M) or PMA (1.6 x 10^{-8}M) were added 8 hr later. After further incubation for 12 hr, the cultures were washed and overlayed with a casein-agar mixture containing 40 μg/ml purified human pl minogen, as well as Con A or PMA where required. Cultures were fixed and sta 5 and 20 hr later, and the proportion of individual cells surrounded by lytic zones was determined microscopically by scoring 400 cells from each culture. No lytic zones were ever observed after 20 hr in parallel cultures overlayed in the absence of plasminogen. (Modified from ref. 13).

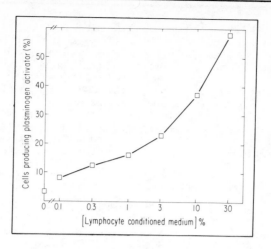

Fig. 4. Proportion of "normal" macrophages secreting plasminogen activator after incubation in presence of conditioned medium from cultures of stimulated spleen cells. The production of enzyme was assayed using a casein-agar overlay procedure that allows detection of secretion of enzyme by single cells. (see table 1) Reproduced from (13).

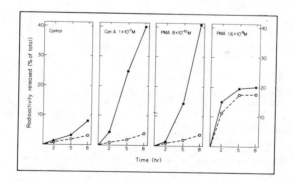

Fig. 5. Fibrinolysis by PMN's; effects of Con A and PMA. Purified PMN's (5 x 10^5) were plated in ^{125}I-fibrin coated wells of Linbro plates, in presence (o——o) or absence (o --- o) of plasminogen. Con A or PMA were present at the indicated concentrations during the whole period of fibrinolysis measurements. Reproduced from (9).

PMNs purified from human peripheral blood contain and secrete plasminogen activator (9). This secretion can be selectively stimulated by Con A and low concentrations of PMA without any increase in the release of plasminogen-independent proteases (Fig. 5). Plasminogen activator secretion is inhibited by low concentrations of glucocorticoids: Figure 6 shows a dose response curve for the effect of dexamethasone, and indicates that 50% inhibition of enzyme secretion is achieved at a steroid concentration of 10^{-9}M. Plasminogen activator secretion is also inhibited by cAMP and related compounds, and in addition appears to require RNA and protein synthesis since actinomycin D, cycloheximide and puromycin all strongly inhibit both the "spontaneous" secretion as well as that stimulated by Con A or low concentrations of PMA.

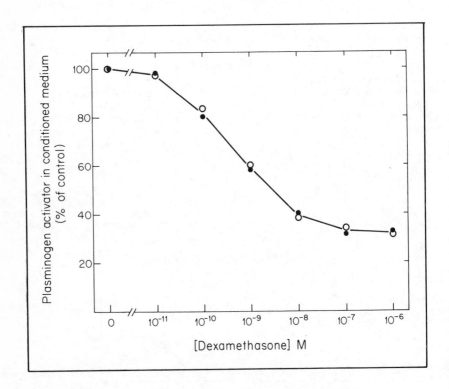

Fig. 6. Secretion of plasminogen activator by PMNs; effect of dexamethasone. Purified PMNs were cultured in Dulbecco's MEM supplemented with 1% of plasminogen-depleted acid-treated fetal bovine serum, in presence or absence of dexamethasone. After 2hr, some of the cultures received Con A (10^{-7}M), and the conditioned medium was collected and assayed 6hr later. The results are expressed as percentages of the plasminogen activator activity present in conditioned medium from dexamethasone -free cultures. Control: 0; Con A: ●. Reproduced from (9).

At high concentrations of PMA, PMNs release a plasminogen independent protease (Fig. 5), which has been clearly identified as elastase (9). This release of elastase is unaffected by glucocorticoids, by cAMP, or by inhibitors of RNA and protein synthesis, and it is associated with a marked decrease in cell viability. These differences between elastase release and plasminogen activator secretion, summarized in Table II, lead us to propose: (a) that elastase and other proteases of the azurophil granules are a static part of the enzymatic equipment of PMNs, and are destined to function inside the cell in conjunction with endocytosis; (b) that, in contrast, plasminogen activator synthesis and secretion form part of the response of PMNs to extracellular stimuli and mediators, the normal function of this enzyme being expressed in the local microenvironment after secretion by PMNs.

TABLE II

Plasminogen Activator Production by PMNs	Release of Elastase by PMNs
Repressed by glucocorticoids	Unaffected by glucocorticoids
Repressed by cAMP	Unaffected by cAMP
Requires RNA and protein synthesis	Does not require RNA and protein synthesis
Stimulated by Con A	Unaffected by Con A
Stimulated by low concentration of PMA	Elicited by high concentration of PMA
No loss of cell viability accompanies secretion.	Associated with loss of cell viability

CONCLUSION

The secretion of plasminogen activator by macrophages and PMNs is sensitive to both stimulatory and inhibitory influences, and the wide range of cellular responses to this variety of effectors suggests that enzyme production in vivo reflects the interplay of these antagonistic modulating stimuli. The response to glucocorticoids is the most impressive of these effects and, since these hormones are active at concentrations within the physiological range, it can be proposed that, in vivo, enzyme production by macrophages and PMNs is constantly subject to some degree of tonic inhibition. On the other hand, the substantial synthesis of plasminogen activator that accompanies inflammatory reactions indicates that this tonic inhibition can be overcome, presumably through the action of stimulatory effectors; likewise, the anti-inflammatory effects of higher glucocorticoid concentrations can be regarded as an opposed pharmacological perturbation of this basic balance.

In addition to the glucocorticoids, the effects of cAMP-related compounds suggest the existence of other inhibitory mechanisms, and it would not be surprising if multiple stimulatory effectors are ultimately discovered. For the time being the only candidate for such a function is an activity found in the secretion products of activated lymphoid cells, but the stimulatory actions of asbestos and thioglycollate medium might well be expected to be mediated by pathways independent of lymphocytes.

The potential role of plasminogen activator and/or plasmin in inflammation cannot be deduced with confidence at this time. The association of these enzymes with tissue remodelling in other systems might imply their involvement in digesting some supportive structures of blood vessels, thereby allowing the migration of inflammatory cells between the various body compartments. Other possibilities include fibrin removal from sites of inflammation, and whatever consequences might ensue from the proposed (15) interactions between the fibrinolytic system and other circulating enzyme cascades.

Despite present uncertainties, the observation that plasminogen activator production by macrophages and PMNs is responsive to a spectrum of modulating stimuli suggests some significant role for this enzyme in the cellular control of inflammatory reactions; this also emphasizes the potential usefulness of the enzyme as a tool for the study of the physiological and pharmacological control of inflammation.

References

1. Unkeless, J. C., Tobia, A., Ossowski, L., Quigley, J. P., Rifkin, D. B., and E. Reich, (1973). An enzymatic function associated with transformation of fibroblasts by oncogenic viruses. I. Chick embryo fibroblast cultures transformed by avian RNA tumor viruses. J. Exp. Med. 137, 85-111.

2. Ossowski, L., Unkeless, J. C., Tobia, A., Quigley, J. P., Rifkin, D. B., and E. Reich, (1973). An enzymatic function associated with transformation of fibroblasts by oncogenic viruses. II. Mammalian fibroblast cultures transformed by DNA and RNA tumor viruses. J. Exp. Med. 137, 112-126.

3. Rohrlich, S T., and D. B. Rifkin, (1977). Patterns of plasminogen activator production in cultured normal embryonic cells. J. Cell. Biol. 75, 31-42.

4. Werb, Z., Mainardi, C.L., Vater, C. A., and E. D. Harris, (1977). Endogenous activation of latent collagenase by rheumatoid synovial cells; evidence for a role of plasmino- gen activator. N.E.J.M. 296, 1017-1023.

5. Beers, W. H., Strickland, S., and E. Reich, (1975). Ovarian Plasminogen Activator: relationship to ovulation and hormo- nal regulation. Cell 6, 387-394.

6. Strickland, S., Reich, E., and M. I. Sherman, (1976). Plas- minogen Activator in early embryogenesis: enzyme production by trophoblast and parietal endoderm. Cell 9, 231-240.

7. Unkeless, J., Gordon, S., and E. Reich(1974). Secretion of plasminogen activator by stimulated macrophages. J. Exp. Med., 139, 834-850.

8. Gordon, S., Unkeless, J., and Z. A. Cohn, (1974). Induction of macrophage plasminogen activator by endotoxin stimulation and phagocytosis; evidence for a 2 stage process. J. Exp. Med., 140, 995-1010.

9. Granelli-Piperno, A., Vassalli, J.-D., and E. Reich (1977). Secretion of plasminogen activator by human polymorphonu- clear leukocytes. Modulation by glucocorticoids and other effectors. J. Exp. Med., in press.

10. Strickland, S., and W. H. Beers, (1976). Studies on the role of plasminogen activator in ovulation. In Vitro re- sponse of granulosa cells to gonadotropins, cyclic nucleo- tides, and prostaglandins. J. Biol. Chem. 251, 5964-5702.

11. Hamilton, J., Vassalli, J.-D., and E. Reich (1976). Macro- phage plasimogen activator: induction by asbestos is blocked by anti-inflammatory steroids. J. Exp. Med. 144: 1689-1694.

12. Vassalli, J.-D., Hamilton, J., and E. Reich, (1976). Mac- rophage plasminogen activator: modulation of enzyme pro- duction by anti-inflammatory steroids, mitotic inhibitors, and cyclic nucleotides. Cell 8: 271-281.

13. Vassalli, J.-D., Hamilton, J., and E. Reich, (1977). Mac- rophage plasminogen activator: induction by Concanavalin A and Phorbol Myristate Acetate. Cell 11: 695-705.

14. Vassalli, J.-D., and E. Reich, (1977). Macrophage plasmi- nogen activator: Induction by products of activated lymphoid cells. J. Exp. Med. 145, 429-437.

15. Ratnoff, O. D. (1969). Some relationships among hemostasis, fibrinolytic phenomena, immunity, and the inflammatory re- sponse. Adv. Immunol. 10, 145-227.

ACKNOWLEDGEMENTS

J-D.V. is a postdoctoral fellow of the Arthritis Foundation, and A.G-P. is a postdoctoral fellow of the National Institutes of Health, USPHS. This work was supported in part by grants from the National Institutes of Health (CA-08290) and the American Cancer Society, Inc. (ACS PDT 1H).

Pathways for the Modulation of Macrophage Collagenase Activity.

Zena Werb

Laboratory of Radiobiology, University of California, San Francisco, CA 94143

Introduction

It is well documented that vertebrate collagenases catalyze the major step in collagen breakdown (1). Specific collagenases are secreted by a number of cell types in vivo. Of particular interest is the secretion of collagenase by macrophages (2-6). Although macrophages (2) produce rather small quantities of this enzyme compared to fibroblasts[1] (7) they may play an important role in initiating the extracellular degradation of collagen in bone and in sites of chronic inflammation. Moreover, because phagocytosis and macrophage activation induce the secretion of collagenase by mononuclear phagocytes, the localized regulation of collagenase production is possible.

Macrophage collagenases are able to attack the triple helix of the three distinct collagens found in the interstitial structures of tissues--type I, type II, and type III (2,4)--and thus could contribute to the breakdown of the extracellular matrix of bone, cartilage, and blood vessels.

Recent data support the concept that most collagenases are secreted in a latent or precursor form (4,5,8-14). Although the nature of this latent form has not been established, evidence for both an enzyme-inhibitor complex (8,11) and a proenzyme (9,13,14) exists.

In addition to latent collagenase, macrophages secrete at least two enzymes capable of activating the latent form and at least two inhibitors of collagenase activity. In this report I describe the pathways regulating the expression of macrophage collagenase activity.

Factors Influencing the Rates of Collagen Breakdown by Macrophages

The extracellular activity of collagenase is the net result of secretion from the cells, activation of the latent form of the enzyme, and clearance of the active molecules by proteinase inhibitors (Fig. 1). In macrophages these processes are intimately interrelated. Macrophages secrete collagenase, potential activating enzymes (plasminogen activator [15] and neutral

(Footnotes see Page 225)

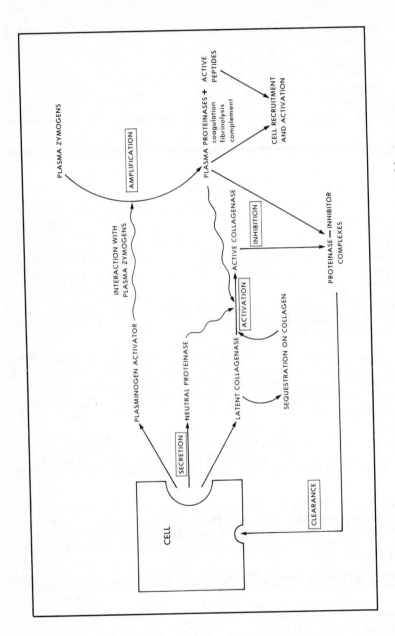

Fig. 1. Extracellular expression of macrophage collagenase activity.

proteinase [3,5]), and inhibitory molecules (α_2-macroglobulin [21]).

The rate of collagen degradation by macrophages is enhanced by increased production of collagenase after phagocytosis and by interaction with activated lymphocytes (Table I). As tissue inhibitors are saturated more collagenase is activated, and additional monocytes can be recruited through the chemotactic activity of fragments of collagen and complement components.

Collagen degradation by macrophages is retarded by local concentrations of glucocorticoids that inhibit secretion of the collagenolytic enzymes (Table II). Inhibitors of collagenase produced locally, from interstitial fluid or from cartilage, also slow the rate of collagen breakdown.

Activation of Latent Forms of Macrophage Collagenase

The rate-limiting step in the regulation of macrophage collagenase activity is likely to be the rate of activation of latent forms of the enzyme (Table III). It has been suggested that collagenase is secreted along with its endogenous activator (5,10). The collagenases secreted by thioglycollate-elicited mouse peritoneal macrophages (2), by BCG-induced rabbit alveolar macrophages (4), and by WEHI-3, a cell line with macrophage properties including lysozyme (27) and collagenase secretion (manuscript in preparation), were largely latent (Table IV). Collagenase is generally secreted in parallel with other neutral proteinases from macrophages, some of which may be endogenous activators (5,10) (Fig. 2). Plasminogen activator appears to be secreted by stimulated macrophages coordinately with collagenase. The secretion of both enzymes is increased in response to phago-cytosis (2,15), and anti-inflammatory steroids inhibit the secretion of both enzymes[2,3] (20,28). However, these enzymes may have independent regulatory mechanisms; e.g., colchicine inhibits synthesis of plasminogen activator (20) while markedly stimulating collagenase secretion (3).

Four distinct pathways for the enzymatic activation of macrophage collagenase are possible in vivo (Table III). Because trypsin activates most of the latent forms of collagenase in vitro (4,9,10) it is possible that collagenase is activated by trypsin-like serine proteinases occurring in interstitial fluid.

Lysosomal cathepsin B, an enzyme that could be present extracellularly in sites of inflammation and bone resorption, has been shown to activate bone collagenase (14). Although cathepsin B has an acid pH optimum, sufficiently low pH values can be achieved in these locations; thus, this enzyme could have some physiological or pathological role in activating latent collagenase.

A neutral proteinase secreted by macrophages may play a role in activating collagenase (4). The presence of this enzyme correlates with "auto-activation" of collagenase preparations during concentration and storage. However, this enzyme has not been shown to act in culture, and despite its presence in most of

(Footnotes See Page 225)

Table I

Factors Enhancing the Rate of Collagen Degradation by Macrophages

Factor	References
Increased secretion of macrophage collagenase after phagocytosis	2
Increased secretion of collagenase in response to lymphokines and macrophage "activation"	2,6,15
Activation of macrophage collagenase by macrophage neutral proteinases or plasmin	5,10,12
Saturation of tissue inhibitors of collagenase	2,9,10,16
Increased recruitment of macrophages by chemotaxis to collagen peptides and complement fragments	17
Greater susceptibility to degradation of collagen types I and III in soluble or uncrosslinked forms	3,4,18
Sequestration of latent collagenases on collagen fibers, followed by activation	10,12
Increased temperature in inflamed sites	18,19
Possible collagenase secretion by fibroblasts induced by macrophage proteinases	29[1]

Table II

Factors Retarding the Rate of Collagen Degradation by Macrophages

Factor	References
Inhibition of secretion of collagenase, neutral proteinase and plasminogen activator by glucocorticoids	10,20,28
Inhibition of macrophage recruitment by glucocorticoids	20,28
Greater resistance to degradation of crosslinked mature collagens and cartilage collagen (type II)	4,18
Secretion of α_2-macroglobulin by macrophages and clearance of saturated α_2-macroglobulin complexes	21,22
Increased tissue collagenase inhibitors	11,23
Cartilage collagenase inhibitors	24,25
Decreased activation of latent forms of collagenase	3
Slower degradation of mineralized tissues	26

Table III

Activation of Latent Forms of Macrophage Collagenase

Activating Stimulus	References
Trypsin	4,9,13
Plasmin, other plasma proteinases	10,14
Endogenous neutral proteinase	3,5
Lysosomal cathepsin B	14
Plasminogen plus plasminogen activator	10
Nonenzymatic activation (organomercurials, NaI, NaSCN)	2,7,8,11,23
"Autoactivation" by dialysis and concentration	2,3,4,6,14

Table IV

Activation of Macrophage Collagenase by Proteinases

Macrophage Collagenase	Collagenase Activation[*]			
	"Spontaneously" Active (%)	Trypsin, 10 µg/ml (%)	Plasmin, 1 µg/ml (%)	Plasminogen, 1 µg/ml (%)
Mouse thioglycollate-elicited macrophages	2	100	121	0
WEHI-3 macrophages	6	100	94	4
BCG-induced rabbit alveolar macrophages	7	100	106	10

[*]Approximately 0.05 U of latent collagenase was used in each assay. Activation was at 25°C for 30 min with added proteinases, followed by addition of soybean trypsin inhibitor (40 µg/ml) and assay on reconstituted collagen fibrils. Activation by trypsin was considered to be 100%.

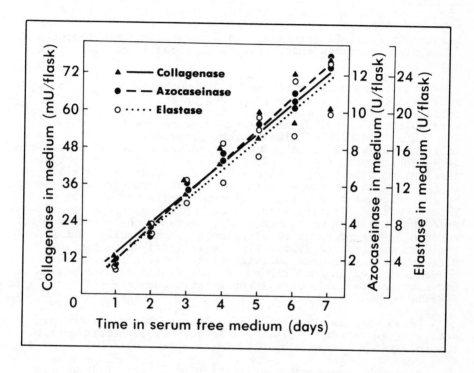

Fig. 2.   Parallel secretion of collagenase, elastase, and non-
specific neutral proteinase (azocaseinase) by
thioglycollate-elicited mouse macrophages. Macrophages
(1.4 x 10[6]/flask) were cultured in Dulbecco's modified
Eagle's medium plus 0.2% lactalbumin hydrolysate (DME-
LH). Every 24 h the conditioned medium was decanted and
fresh DME-LH was added to each culture. Cumulative
enzyme activities are shown. Assays were made as described previously[3](2,3).

the preparations the collagenases are still latent immediately after decanting the medium from the cells.

The fourth enzymatic pathway for activation of macrophage collagenase utilizes macrophage plasminogen activator and plasminogen to generate plasmin (10). Plasmin was an efficient activator of collagenases found in the serum-free culture fluid of macrophages, whereas its zymogen, plasminogen, did not activate collagenase under these conditions (Fig. 3: Table IV). Kallikrein (14), Cl-esterase, and activated Hageman factor are other plasma enzymes that, potentially, could activate collagenase.

Conditions under which viable macrophages degrade collagen were examined by plating macrophages on gels of radioactive collagen. Little collagen breakdown occurred when macrophages were cultured on collagen in serum-free medium (Fig. 4,; Table V). After addition of plasminogen, progressive lysis of the collagen film took place. Degradation was inhibited by addition of α_1-antitrypsin (an inhibitor of plasmin but not of collagenase) along with the plasminogen. The degradation of collagen in this system correlated with collagenase activity demonstrated by conventional assays with collagen fibrils and by viscometry. Thioglycollate-elicited macrophages, which secrete more collagenase than resident macrophages (2), degraded their collagen substratum in the presence of plasminogen more readily than did resident macrophages (Table V). It is intriguing that the plasminogen-independent collagenase-activating systems that can be demonstrated in conditioned culture fluids of macrophages did not cause appreciable activation in this complete collagenolytic system.

Dexamethasone inhibition of collagenase and plasminogen activator secretion[2],[3] (20,28) also prevented the degradation of the collagen substratum by the macrophages (Table V).

Although nonenzymatic activation of latent collagenases or dissociation of collagenase-inhibitor complexes can be achieved in reaction mixtures (Table III), these effects do not take place in the presence of cells. However, locally synthesized inhibitors of collagenase may play a role in controlling local activity of collagenase (11,23-25).

A General Scheme for Modulation of Macrophage Collagenase Activity (Fig. 5).

Macrophages synthesize latent collagenase, plasminogen activator, and (in the case of human monocytes) α_2-macroglobulin. Once secreted the latent collagenase can bind to collagen fibrils. The inactive collagenase escapes trapping by α_2-macroglobulin, but active enzyme is bound and inhibited (9, 10, 16) and the proteinase-inhibitor complexes are cleared (22) by macrophages. Latent collagenase may remain bound to collagen indefinitely if it escapes initial activation by plasmin generated by the macrophage plasminogen activator. Later, other

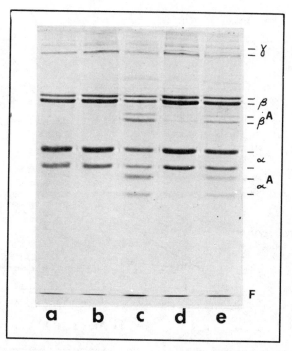

Fig. 3. Plasmin activation of macrophage collagenase. Conditioned culture medium from WEHI-3 macrophages was incubated with collagen in solution at 25°C, and then the reaction mixtures were examined by SDS-polyacrylamide gel electrophoresis (2,7,18): (a) control collagen incubated with DME-LH alone; collagen incubated with (b) WEHI-3 medium; (c) WEHI-3 medium activated with 2.3 μg of bovine plasmin/ml for 30 min at 25°C, followed by addition of 40 μg of soybean trypsin inhibitor/ml (10); (d) activated WEHI-3 medium plus 10 mM EDTA (an inhibitor of collagenase activity added after activation); (e) activated WEHI-3 medium plus 1 mM phenylmethylsulfonyl fluoride (an inhibitor of plasmin activity added after activation). (β,α) intact collagen subunits; (βA,αA) 3/4-length cleavage fragments produced by the action of specific collagenase. The 1/4-length fragments (αB) migrated with the buffer front in gels (c) and (e).

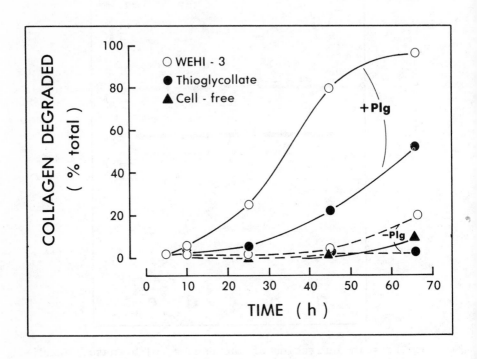

Fig. 4. Plasminogen-dependent degradation of collagen by macrophages. WEHI-3 macrophages (2 x 10^5) (o) and
thioglycollate-elicited mouse peritoneal macrophages
(5 x 10^5) (•) were cultured on ^{3}H-collagen films
(10). At time 0, the cells were plated in DME-LH
(---) or DME-LH containing 50 nM bovine plasminogen
(—). Aliquots were removed at the times indicated.
Collagen degradation is expressed as a percentage of
the total available radioactivity in the wells, as
described previously (10). Each point represents the
mean of 3 determinations. Cell-free wells containing
plasminogen (▲) released very little radioactivity.

Table V

Collagen Degradation by Macrophages and Its Inhibition by Dexamethasone

Mouse Macrophages	Dexamethasone (nM)	Collagen Degraded per 24 h[*]		
		Control (%)	Plasminogen (%)	Plasminogen + α_1AT (%)
Resident peritoneal	0	0	2	0
	100	0	0	0
Thioglycollate-elicited	0	0	18	0
	100	0	3	0
WEHI-3	0	5	38	0
Cell-free control	0	0	2	0

[*]Cells (1×10^6) were plated on 200 µg of ^{3}H-collagen gel (10) in Dulbecco's modified Eagle's medium (DME) + 10% fetal calf serum. After 24 h, cultures were placed in DME plus lactalbumin hydrolysate (0.2%) with or without dexamethasone, and bovine plasminogen (50 nM) was added as indicated. Addition of plasmin (urokinase + plasminogen) to cell-free wells for 24 h resulted in the release of 4% of the available radioactivity. α_1-Antitrypsin (α_1AT) was added to the wells at 100 µg/ml.

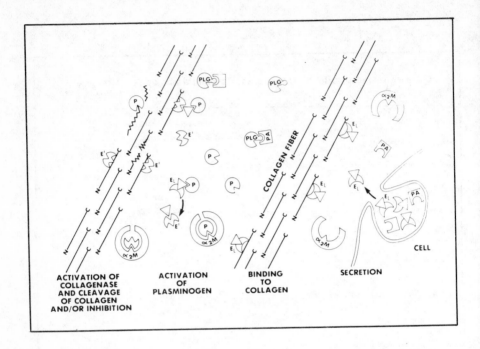

Fig. 5. General scheme for secretion, activation, and clearance of macrophage collagenase. Macrophages secrete collagenase in a latent form (E_L), as well as plasminogen activator (PA) and, possibly, α_2-macroglobulin (α_2M). E_L and PA cannot bind to α_2M and thus are protected from being cleared. E_L may bind to its substrate, collagen fibers, but is unable to cleave collagen. If plasminogen (Plg) is present, PA converts this zymogen to plasmin (P). The active plasmin may be inactivated by binding to α_2M. Once the α_2M is saturated locally, plasmin can activate E_L, generating active collagenase (E'). E' may be cleared by α_2M, but, once all the inhibitors are saturated, collagen breakdown commences with production of specific collagen fragments. At physiological temperatures these fragments melt to gelatin, which is susceptible to degradation by many proteinases, including plasmin.

activating proteinases, perhaps those produced by newly recruited macrophages and vascular endothelium, may activate the collagenolytic system. The combined effects of these proteolytic enzymes on interstitial macromolecules and on connective tissue cells (29)[1] could mediate connective tissue remodelling.

Summary

The extracellular expression of macrophage collagenase activity is the net result of secretion of collagenase by the macrophages, activation of the latent form of the enzyme by endogenous or exogenous enzymes, and clearance of the active collagenase by proteinase inhibitors. Interrelationships between proteinase inhibitors and the collagenase, plasminogen activator, and neutral proteinases secreted by the macrophages were examined by cultivation of macrophages in the presence of reconstituted collagen fibrils.

Acknowledgments

I thank Ingrid Vander Heiden, Judy Power, and Jennie Chin for excellent technical assistance, Dr. Peter Ralph for the gift of the WEHI-3 line, and Dr. E.D. Harris, Jr. and Dr. Saimon Gordon for stimulating discussions about many aspects of this work. This investigation was supported by the U. S. Department of Energy.

Footnotes

[1] Werb, Z., and Aggeler, J. 1977. Proteases induce secretion of collagenase and plasminogen activator by fibroblasts. In press P.N.S.

[2] Werb, Z., Foley, R., and Munck, A. 1977. Interaction of glucocorticoids with macrophages. Identification of glucocorticoid receptors in monocytes and macrophages. In press J. Exp. Med.

[3] Werb, Z. 1977. Biochemical effects of glucocorticoids on macrophages in culture. Specific inhibition of elastase, collagenase, and plasminogen activator secretion and effects on other metabolic parameters. In press J. Exp. Med.

References

1. Harris, E.D., Jr., and Krane, S.M. 1974. Collagenases. New Engl. J. Med., 291, 557-563, 605-609, 652-661.

2. Werb, Z., and Gordon, S. 1975. Secretion of a specific collagenase by stimulated macrophages. J. Exp. Med., 142, 346-360.

3. Gordon, S., and Werb, Z. 1976. Secretion of macrophage neutral proteinase is enhanced by colchicine. Proc. Natl. Acad. Sci. USA, 73, 872-876.

4. Horwitz, A.L., and Crystal, R.G. 1976. Collagenase from rabbit pulmonary alveolar macrophages. Biochem. Biophys. Res. Commun., 69, 296-303.

5. Horwitz, A.L., Kelman, J.A., and Crystal, R.G. 1976. Activation of alveolar macrophage collagenase by a neutral protease secreted by the same cell. Nature, 264, 772-774.

6. Wahl, L.M., Wahl, S.M., Mergenhagen, S.E., and Martin, G.R. 1975. Collagenase production by lymphokine-activated macrophages. Science, 187, 261-263.

7. Werb, Z., and Reynolds, J.J. 1974. Stimulation by endocytosis of the secretion of collagenase and neutral proteinase from rabbit synovial fibroblasts. J. Exp. Med., 140, 1482-1497.

8. Nagai, Y. 1973. Vertebrate collagenase:further characterization and the significance of its latent form in vivo. Mol. Cell. Biochem., 1, 137-145.

9. Birkedal-Hansen, H., Cobb, C.M., Taylor, R.E., and Fullmer, H.M. 1976. Synthesis and release of procollagenase by cultured fibroblasts. J. Biol. Chem. 251, 3162-3168.

10. Werb, Z., Mainardi, C.L., Vater, C.A., and Harris, E.D., Jr. 1977. Endogenous activation of latent collagenase by rheumatoid synovial cells. Evidence for a role of plasminogen activator. New Engl. J. Med., 296, 1017-1023.

11. Sellers, A., Cartwright, E., Murphy, G., and Reynolds, J.J. 1977. Evidence that latent collagenases are enzyme-inhibitor complexes. Biochem. J., 163, 303-307.

12. Woessner, J.F., Jr. 1977. A latent form of collagenase in the involuting rat uterus and its activation by a serine proteinase. Biochem. J., 161, 535-542.

13. Vaes, G. 1972. The release of collagenase as an inactive proenzyme by bone explants in culture. Biochem. J., 126, 275-289.

14. Eeckhout, Y., and Vaes, G. 1977. Further studies on the

activation of procollagenase, the latent precursor of bone collagenase. Effects of lysosomal cathepsin B, plasmin, and kallikrein, and spontaneous activation. Biochem. J., 166, 21-31.

15. Gordon, S., Unkeless, J.C., and Cohn, Z.A. 1974. Induction of macrophage plasminogen activator by endotoxin stimulation and phagocytosis. Evidence for a two-stage process. J. Exp. Med., 140, 995-1010.

16. Werb, Z., Burleigh, M.C., Barrett, A.J., and Starkey, P.M. 1974. The interaction of α_2-macroglobulin with proteinases. Binding and inhibition of mammalian collagenases and other neutral proteinases. Biochem. J., 139, 359-368.

17. Postelthwaite, A.E., and Kang, A.H. 1976. Collagen- and collagen peptide-induced chemotaxis of human blood monocytes. J. Exp. Med., 143, 1299-1307.

18. Burleigh, M.C, Werb, Z., and Reynolds, J.J. 1977. Evidence that species specificity and rate of collagen degradation are properties of collagen, not collagenase. Biochim. Biophys. Acta, 494, 198-208.

19. Harris, E.D., Jr. and McCroskery, P.A. 1974. The influence of temperature and fibril stability on degradation of cartilage collagen by rheumatoid synovial collagenase. New Engl. J. Med., 290, 1-6.

20. Vassalli, J.-D., Hamilton, J., and Reich, E. 1976. Macrophage plasminogen activator: modulation of enzyme production by anti-inflammatory steroids, mitotic inhibitors, and cyclic nucleotides. Cell, 8, 271-281.

21. Hovi, T., Mosher, D., and Vaheri, A. 1977. Cultured human monocytes synthesize and secrete α_2-macroglobulin. J. Exp. Med., 145, 1580-1589.

22. Debanne, M.T., Bell, R., and Dolovich, J. 1975. Uptake of proteinase- α_2-macroglobulin complexes by macrophages. Biochim. Biophys. Acta, 411, 295-304.

23. Murphy, G., Cartwright, E.C., Sellers, A., and Reynolds, J.J. 1977. The detection and characterization of collagenase inhibitors from rabbit tissues in culture. Biochim. Biophys. Acta, 483, 493-498.

24. Kuettner, K.E., Soble, L., Croxen, R.L., Marczynska, B., Hiti, J., and Harper, E. 1977. Tumor cell collagenase and its inhibition by a cartilage-derived protease inhibitor. Science, 196, 653-654.

25. Ehrlich, M.G., Mankin, H.J., Jones, H., Wright, R., Crispen, C., and Vigliani, G. 1977. Collagenase and collagenase inhibitors in osteoarthritic and normal human

cartilage. J. Clin. Invest., 59, 226-233.

26. Evanson, J.M., Jeffrey, J.J., and Krane, S.M. 1968. Studies on collagenase from rheumatoid synovium in tissue culture. J. Clin. Invest., 47, 2639-2651.

27. Ralph, P., Moore, M.A.S., and Nilsson, K. 1976. Lysozyme synthesis in established human and murine histocytic lymphoma cell lines. J. Exp. Med., 143, 1528-1533.

28. Werb, Z. 1977. Glucocorticoid receptors and glucocorticoid sensitivity of macrophages. J. Cell. Biol., 75, 191a.

29. Power, J.A., and Werb, Z. 1977. Protease stimulation of collagenase and plasminogen activator secretion by fibro-blasts. J. Cell. Biol., 75, 412a.

Non-Bone Cell Mediated Bone Resorption.

Gregory R. Mundy, Gabriel Eilon, Arnold J. Altman, Jesus H. Dominguez

Departments of Medicine and Pediatrics, University of Connecticut Health Center, Farmington, Connecticut 06032

Bone is a living tissue which is constantly being remodeled by the coupled processes of bone resorption and bone formation. Bone is comprised of an acellular mineralized matrix. The organic matrix consists mostly of collagen (about 95%), but also contains non-collagen glycoproteins and other acidic proteins. The mineral phase of bone is interspersed within the collagen molecules of the matrix in the form of poorly crystalline calcium hydroxyapatite and amorphous calcium phosphate. The resorption of bone is a complex process which involves release of bone mineral, removal of glycoproteins and breakdown of the collagenous bone matrix. The factors responsible for mineral release, the sequence of events in the resorption process and the respective roles of lysosomal enzymes and bone collagenases are largely unknown.

The giant multinucleated osteoclast is the major cell responsible for bone resorption. The osteoclast responds to the known humoral stimulators of bone resorption such as parathyroid hormone (1), prostaglandins-E (2), 1,25-dihydroxycholecalciferol (3), thyroxine (4) and osteoclast activating factor (5) to resorb bone. Osteoclast activity is inhibited by calcitonin (transiently) (6), phosphate (7) and corticosteroids (8) (although the response to corticosteroids depends on the stimulus). The mechanisms by which stimulated osteoclasts resorb bone are still not clear. The activity of osteoclasts in organ culture correlates closely with the release of lysosomal enzymes by the bones (9). Cultured bones release lysosomal enzymes when stimulated by humoral mediators of bone resorption and this lysosomal enzyme release is decreased by inhibitors of bone resorption. There is a less perfect correlation between bone resorption and collagenase release. Collagenase is released also by bones stimulated to resorb. However, colchicine, which is a powerful inhibitor of bone resorption and lysosomal enzyme release by bones, causes increased collagenase release (9). Thus collagenase production alone cannot account for the degradation of the bone matrix by osteoclasts. It has not been possible as yet to separate lysosomal enzyme release from the resorption process.

The role of the osteocyte in bone resorption is even less clear. It is probable that osteocytes can both resorb (10) and

229

form bone (11) under certain circumstances. Osteocytic bone
resorption has only been measured by changes in the osteocyte
lacunar size. However, these effects on lacunar size are difficult to interpret because relative increases in lacunar size due
to decreased bone formation could be misinterpreted as increased
resorption effects. Osteocyte lacunae appear to enlarge in
hyperparathyroidism (12) and after vitamin D treatment (13).
Although the exact role of osteocytic bone resorption is unknown,
it is likely that osteocytic bone resorption is much less important than osteoclastic bone resorption (13).

In order to identify cells which are capable of resorbing
bone, we devised a dead bone model in which we took live fetal
rat long bone shafts which were labeled previously with ^{45}Ca
or ^{3}H-proline and killed the endogenous bone cells. We then
cultured different cells on the acellular mineralized matrices
and assessed the direct effects of these cells on bone by measuring the release of ^{45}Ca from the bones into the media. The
cells which were assessed for effects on dead bones were isolated
rat calvarial cells, human monocytes and human breast cancer
cells.

Resorption of Bone by Isolated Calvarial Cells

During the past few years, much interest has been shown in
studying factors which influence bone metabolism using cultures
of isoalted bone cells (14-16). The bone cells are usually
obtained from fetal rat or newborn mouse calvaria by enzyme
digestion. These cultured bone cell preparations respond to
both parathyroid hormone and calcitonin with increased intracellular generation of cyclic AMP (15). However, at no time
during culture do these isolated bone cells differentiate
morphologically to recognizable mature cells although it is
apparent that there may be some cells in the heterogeneous population which respond preferentially to parathyroid hormone and
some which respond preferentially to calcitonin (16).

Our starting hypothesis was that isolated cells may require
culture with their tissue of origin to differentiate fully both
functionally and morphologically. Both in vivo and in organ
culture, bone cells grow in the bone micro-environment. In
order to determine if the bony environment is necessary for the
morphological differentiation of cultured bone cells, we cultured fetal bone cells on endosteal bone surfaces. Long bones
obtained from the 21-day fetal rat radius, ulna and tibia were
split vertically with the endosteal surfaces of the split bone
halves turned upwards. The bone halves were exposed to ultraviolet light to kill all of the endogenous bone cells and leave
an acellular calcified bone matrix. Fetal rat calvarial cells
obtained without enzyme digestion were layered across the bone
surfaces for periods up to 21 days.

When cultured away from bone surfaces on a plastic petri
dish, these calvarial cells assumed the appearances of fibroblasts and were usually mononuclear, although occasionally
binucleate cells were seen. These cells remained viable in

culture for a period of 4 to 5 weeks and although during this time they divided and rapidly became confluent, at no time did they look like recognizable mature bone cells. However, when the same cells were cultured on dead bone surfaces, the histological appearances were markedly different. Under these circumstances the cells differentiated into a heterogeneous population of bone cells which were interwoven with the calcified matrix. Different types of cells were present in this population including plump polygonal cells with perinuclear haloes (possibly representing Golgi apparatus) and having the histologic features of osteoblasts, other cells which looked like fibroblasts and some giant multinucleated cells which looked like osteoclasts. These cells were apparent after a period of 10 days of culture of the calvarial cells on the killed bone surfaces.

Some of these cells which were growing on the endosteal bone surfaces were examined histologically by smearing the endosteal bone surfaces across a microscope slide and staining with Wright's stain. Under these circumstances clearly discernible giant multinucleated cells were seen. Some of these cells were located in lacunae and contained foamy vacuolated cytoplasm as well as multiple nuclei.

At the same time that these giant multinucleated cells were appearing in the calvarial cell population, the killed bones were resorbing. This was demonstrated by using bones which had been previously labeled with ^{45}Ca or ^3H-proline. The incorporation of the label was performed by injecting a pregnant rat subcutaneously on the 18th day of gestation with ^{45}Ca or ^3H-proline which were incorporated into bone mineral or bone matrix respectively. The following day, the fetal rat long bones were explanted and cultured with the bone cells. At the 10th day of culture the release of the labeled isotopes was increased from those bones which were cultured with the calvarial cells compared with paired control bones. In parallel experiments we cultured live bones with bone cells and found that mineral was also released from these bones. This effect was apparently not due to the generation of prostaglandins by the cultured cells because co-culture with indomethacin at $10^{-5}M$ had no discernible effect on ^{45}Ca release.

Peptide hormones which stimulate or inhibit bone resorption did not effect mineral release from dead bones. Bovine parathyroid hormone and osteoclast activating factor did not further enhance mineral release by the cultured bone cells on killed bone nor did calcitonin substantially inhibit it. Failure of hormone responsiveness may be due to the calvarial cells being maximally activated by the cultured conditions and not responding further to a stimulus to bone resorption or may be due to the degradation of the peptide hormones by proteases released from the dead bones. However, mineral release from the killed bones by the cultured cells was substantially inhibited by cortisol $10^{-6}M$ and colchicine $10^{-7}M$. Both of these agents have been shown to inhibit the release of lysosomal enzymes (17) which are probably responsible for normal osteoclast-mediated bone resorption (9, 18).

Resorption of Bone Monocytes

Isolated calvarial cells are not the only exogenous cells which will release ^{45}Ca from killed bones. We have found in other studies that normal human monocytes as well as their supernatants are also capable of causing mineral release and matrix resorption from dead bones (19).

Circulating human monocytes were obtained from platelet-pheresis donations at the American Red Cross in Farmington, Connecticut. The leukocyte rich buffy coats were separated from neutrophils by Ficoll-Hypaque density sedimentation. The monocytes were separated from the lymphocytes by adherence to plastic petri dishes. Monocytes were then cultured on dead bones at a concentration of 1 to 2 by 10^6 cells per ml. The period of culture was for 10 days. During this period of time it was found that monocytes and their supernatants caused ^{45}Ca release which had been previously incorporated into killed fetal rat long bones. Again the bones were killed by exposure to ultraviolet light overnight. Matrix resorption was also verified by using some killed bones which were previously labeled with ^{3}H-proline. Bone was resorbed both when cells were added directly to bone surfaces or when supernatants taken from monocyte cultures were applied to the bone (Table 1). The effects of the monocytes on bone were not modified by hormones which normally regulate osteo-clastic bone resorption. Parathyroid hormone, vitamin D and calcitonin had no effect on monocyte-mediated bone resorption. On the other hand, cortisol 10^{-6}M and colchicine 10^{-7}M inhibited these effects. Although the mechanism for this inhibition is not known, it may be related to the effects of these agents on the release of lysosomal enzymes. It is thought that normal osteo-clastic bone resorption may be mediated by lysosomal enzymes (9, 18) and it may be that inhibition of lysosomal enzyme re-lease by cortisol or colchicine would inhibit the monocyte-mediated resorptive response.

The significance of the effects of monocytes on bone resorp-tion is unknown. However, there is a lot of circumstantial evidence which indicates that monocytes may be precursors for the major bone resorbing cell, the multinucleated osteoclast. The experiments recorded here indicate that monocytes themselves have the intracellular machinery necessary for the direct resorption of bone. Monocyte-related bone resorption may also be important in some pathologic situations. Monocytes are often found adjacent to bone resorbing margins in patients with meta-static tumor deposits in bone and chronic inflammatory diseases associated with bone resorption such as periodontal disease and rheumatoid arthritis. These experiments indicate that monocytes in these situations may not be mere innocent bystanders but may take an active part themselves in bone destruction.

Monocyte Chemotaxis by Resorbed Bone

The frequent appearance of monocytes near bone resorbing margins raises the possibility that bone or bone products may be

Table 1

Relationship of position of cultured bones relative to mononuclear
cells and bone mineral release. Cells were cultured for 5 days
(Experiment 1) and 8 days (Experiments 2 and 3) at 2×10^6 cells/ml
in 0.5 ml of media in plastic Linbro dishes. The culture medium
was BGJ supplemented with 10% heat-inactivated fetal calf serum.
Values are expressed as percent increases ± S.E.M. in medium ^{45}Ca
from killed bones cultured with mononuclear cells compared with
paired bones cultured without mononuclear cells.

Position of killed bones	Percent increase in ^{45}Ca release
Experiment 1	
Suspended on screens	24 ± 7*
Floating in medium	20 ± 5*
Adherent to dish floor	24 ± 2*
Experiment 2	
Suspended on screens	26 ± 7*
Adherent to dish floor	18 ± 8*
Experiment 3	
Cell free supernatant media	31 ± 6*

*Significantly greater than zero, $p < 0.05$.

chemotactic for monocytes. To test this hypothesis we cultured circulating human monocytes with the conditioned media taken from resorbed bone. Nineteen day fetal rat long bones were cultured for 48 to 120 hours in BGJ medium. Some bones were cultured with PTH 400 ng/ml which stimulates bone resorption. Conditioned media from resorbing bone was added to the lower compartment of Boyden chambers and monocytes were placed in the upper compartment. The migration of cells into the filter separating the compartments after four hours incubation was quantitated. It was found that media taken from resorbed bones contained factors which produced a two-fold increase in monocyte chemotaxis compared with media taken from unresorbed bones.

Chemotaxis was demonstrated in other experiments by culturing monocytes under an agarose layer in petri dishes with bones placed in adjoining wells. In some dishes PTH was added to the cell suspension. The linear distance monocytes moved towards resorbing bones over an 18-hour period was measured and found to be 30% greater in dishes containing PTH. Thus, resorbing bone produces factors which cause unidirectional monocyte movement.

Direct Resorption of Bone by Human Breast Cancer Cells

Advanced breast cancer is frequently associated with hypercalcemia (20). To examine the mechanisms responsible for hypercalcemia in breast cancer, we assayed the supernatant media of a stable cultured human breast cancer cell line for the presence of bone resorbing activity. This cell line, called MCF-7, is a stable epithelial tumor cell line which was derived from a malignant pleural effusion of a patient with advanced breast cancer (21). The assay for bone resorbing activity we have used is based on the release of previously incorporated ^{45}Ca from fetal rat long bones in organ culture.

The supernatant media from MCF-7 were tested for their effects on the release of ^{45}Ca and breakdown of bone matrix. We found that MCF-7 caused ^{45}Ca release from live bones (22). We also found that MCF-7 caused the release of isotope from bones previously labeled with ^{3}H-proline. Resorption of bone occurred whether the bone was alive or the bone had been previously killed by exposure overnight to ultraviolet light. Thus resorption of the dead bone indicates that the bone resorption occurred independent of endogenous bone cells or osteoclasts and was due to a direct effect of the breast cancer cells themselves on bone.

To investigate further the cellular mechanism of bone resorption in breast cancer, we examined live bones cultured with MCF-7 supernatants histologically and compared these bones cultured with other stimulators of bone resorption such as prostaglandins. The bones cultured with prostaglandins showed intense osteoclastic bone resorption whereas those which were cultured with the breast cancer cells and were resorbing as measured by ^{45}Ca release showed little evidence of increased osteoclast number or activity.

To confirm that endogenous bone cells such as osteoclasts are not required for breast cancer cells to resorb bone, live bones were treated with drugs which inhibit osteoclast activity. Two of these inhibitory agents are phosphate (3 mM) and cortisol (10^{-6}). Phosphate and cortisol were added to PGE-stimulated live bones and bone resorption was totally inhibited. On the other hand, when supernatant media from the MCF-7 cultures were added to live bones in the presence of cortisol and phosphate in the same concentration there was no inhibitory effect of these agents on the bone resorbing activity present in the MCF-7 supernatants.

Thus there may be two mechanisms for the bone destruction which occurs in patients with malignant disease. Firstly, bone destruction may be bone cell or osteoclast mediated and this is the mechanism of bone breakdown which occurs in patients with myeloma (23) and in patients with solid tumors who develop ectopic hormone syndromes. However, these studies also suggest that there may be another mechanism for bone breakdown which is important particularly in breast cancer. In this situation, the breast cancer cells themselves have the intracellular machinery necessary to directly resorb bone independent of osteoclasts. The actual mechanism by which breast cancer cells breakdown bone awaits further study.

REFERENCES

1. Raisz, L.G. 1965. Bone resorption in tissue culture.
    Factors influencing response to parathyroid hormone. J. Clin.
    Invest., 43;103-116.

2. Klein, D.C. and L.G. Raisz 1970. Prostaglandins: Stimula-
    tion of bone resorption in tissue culture. Endocrinology
    85:1436-1440.

3. Raisz, L.G., C.L. Trummel, M.F. Holick and H.F. DeLuca 1972.
    1,25-dihydroxycholecalciferol, a potent stimulator of bone
    resorption in tissue cultures. Science 175:768-769.

4. Mundy, G.R., J.L. Shapiro, J.G. Bandelin, E.M. Canalis,
    L.G. Raisz 1976. Direct stimulation of bone resorption by
    thyroid hormones. J. Clin. Invest. 58:529-534.

5. Horton, J.E., L.G. Raisz, H.A. Simmons, J.J. Oppenheim and
    S.E. Merhenhagen 1972. Bone resorbing activity in super-
    natant fluid from cultured human peripheral blood leukocytes.
    Science 177:793-795.

6. Raisz, L.G. and I. Niemann 1967. Early effects of para-
    thyroid hormone and thyrocalcitonin on bone in organ culture.
    Nature 214:486-487.

7. Raisz, L.G. and I. Niemann 1969. Effect of phosphate,
    calcium and magnesium on bone resorption and hormonal
    responses in tissue culture. Endocrinology 85:446-452.

8. Raisz, L.G., C.L. Trummel, J.A. Wener and H.A. Simmons 1972.
    Effect of glucocorticoid on bone resorption in tissue
    culture. Endocrinology 90:961-967.

9. Eilon, G. and L.G. Raisz 1977. Comparison of effects of
    stimulators and inhibitors of resorption on the release of
    lysosomal enzymes and radioactive calcium from fetal bone in
    organ culture. Endocrinology (in press).

10. Jande, S.S. and L.F. Bélanger 1973. The life cycle of osteo-
    cyte. Clinical Orthopedics 94:281-305.

11. Baylink, D.J. and J.E. Wergedal 1972. Bone formation by
    osteocytes in: Cellular Mechanisms for Calcium Transfer in
    Homeostasis, edited by Jean Nichols Jr. and R.A. Wasserman,
    New York Academic Press, pages 257-289.

12. Bélanger, L.F. 1965. Osteolysis: An outlook on its mech-
    anism and causation in: The Parathyroid Glands, edited by
    P.J. Gaillard, R.V. Talmage and A.M. Budy, University of
    Chicago Press, pages 137-143.

13. Liu, C.C., D.J. Baylink, J.E. Wergedal. 1974. Vitamin D-
    enhanced osteoclastic bone resorption at vascular channels.
    Endocrinology 95:1011-1018.

14. Peck, W.A., S.J. Birge Jr. and S.A. Fedak 1964. Bone Cells: Biochemical and biological studies after enzymatic isolation. Science 146:1476-1477.

15. Rodan, S.B. and G.A. Rodan 1974. The effect of parathyroid hormone and thyrocalcitonin on the accumulation of cyclic adenosine 3', 5'-monophosphate in freshly isolated bone cells. J. Biol. Chem. 249:3068-3074.

16. Wong, G. and D.V. Cohn 1975. Target cells in bone for parathormone and calcitonin are different: Enrichment for each cell type by sequential digestion of mouse calvaria and selected adhesion to polymeric surfaces. Proc. Nat. Acad. Science USA 72:3167-3171.

17. Wiener, E. and Y. Marmary 1969. The in vitro effect of hydrocortisone on cultures of peritoneal monocytes. Lab. Invest 21:505-510.

18. Vaes, G. 1969. Lysosomes in the cellular physiology of bone resorption in: Lysosomes in Biology and Pathology, edited by J.T. Dingle and H.G. Fell, North Holland, London, page 217-253.

19. Mundy, G.R. and G. Eilon 1977. Direct resorption of bone by cultured human breast cancer cells. Clinical Research 25:410A.

20. Galasko, C.S.B. and J.I. Burn 1971. Hypercalcemia in patients with advanced mammary carcinoma. British Medical Journal 3:573-577.

21. Soule, H.D., J. Vasquez, A. Long, S. Albert and M. Brennan 1973. A human cell line from a pleural effusion derived from a breast carcinoma. Journal of the National Cancer Institute 51:1409-1416.

22. Mundy, G.R., A.J. Altman, M.D. Gondek and J.G. Bandelin 1977. Direct resorption of bone by human monocytes. Science: 196:1109-1111.

23. Mundy, G.R., L.G. Raisz, R.A. Cooper, G.P. Schechter and S.E. Salmon 1974. Evidence for the secretion of an osteoclast stimulating factor in myeloma. New England Journal of Medicine 291:1041-1046.

Discussion for Session III: The Role of Microbes, Mediators and Mononuclear Cells in Localized Bone Loss. Part C.

DR. WURTHIER: Dr. Vassali, what is PMA?

DR. VASSALI: PMA is phorbol myristate acetate. It is a very potent inflammatory agent.

DR. TASHJIAN: Dr. Mundy, in the breast cancer tumor cell resorption system, do you believe that actual physical contact of the tumor cells with the bone is required in order for resorption to be mediated? Or can you culture breast cancer cells independently of bone, harvest the conditioned medium from those cultures, and show dissolution of bone by some product of the tumor cell?

DR. MUNDY: I can't give you a complete answer to that yet. I am sure that we can take media from these MCF-7 cultures and cause calcium-45 release from bones, but I am not sure whether we can cause matrix breakdown.

DR. TASHJIAN: My other question concerns specificity of the migration of monocytes. How about conditioned media from other kinds of active cultures? In other words, something other than bone that also could attract macrophages? Is this a general property of metabolically-active tissues, or is it special to bone?

DR. MUNDY: I don't know; we haven't tested anything else. However, the fact that we are getting this sort of correlation between the resorbing bone, that is different from live bone which is resorbing less, suggests that it is something produced by resorbing bone.

The other question, is this effect specific for monocytes? We have taken purified neutrophils in separate experiments and found that this factor in the resorbed bone media isn't chemo-tactic for neutrophils, which makes it different from those other two standard chemotactic factors I mentioned.

DR. COHEN: Dr. Mundy, two questions. The first: what time interval is involved in the Boyden assay system? Secondly, is there any evidence for selectivity among cells in the monocyte population? That is, does every cell appear to react, or are some cells more sensitive than others?

DR. MUNDY: The time is four hours. That is one of the reasons I wanted to use the other technique, because it is a much longer incubation period. The incubation period we are operating now is the standard way of measuring monocyte chemotaxis.

The other part of your question, can we define different populations of monocytes? We see monocytes come through, but I don't know if we are selecting out a subpopulation.

DR. COHN: Dr. Mundy, I was trying to decide from your data whether you think that this chemotactic factor has to be produced during the active metabolic process of bone resorption; or whether during the process of bone resorption, a pre-existing factor is uncovered and perhaps released into solution?

I am thinking of the work of Reddi and Huggins and Urist, that there is a factor unassociated with the cellular elements of bone, that apparently affects bone formation; and, in this case, would be resorption.

DR. MUNDY: It is an interesting question, and there are likely possibilities from other systems. One is, that this could be a fragment or a product of matrix resorption; and I think one of Werb's slides covered monocyte chemotaxis by collagen peptides. This is a possibility, since these collagen peptides and other forms of collagen are chemotactic for mono-cytes. All I know at the moment is that the material we have is non-dialyzable.

DR. COHN: Are platelets required for this chemotactic process? We all know that platelets release a variety of factors, some of which could participate in the activation process.

DR. MUNDY: From my data I couldn't say that we weren't, but I would suspect based on Minkin's data that they aren't.

DR. PECK: Dr. Mundy, if you partially demineralize bone, and then incubate it with medium, will you release a chemotactic factor?

DR. MUNDY: We haven't done that.

DR. HORTON: Dr. Mundy, you showed that CLL lymphocytes, as well as nonadherent rat spleen cells, caused a 4 percent and 11 percent increase in mineralization. I wonder if you interpret this as an enhancement of mineralization, or accretion of calcium? May something be elaborated by these cells to cause that?

DR. MUNDY: I interpret that as negative data, because the standard errors were such that there was no difference in those particular cells between dead bones treated with cells and the corresponding control bones.

DR. MINKIN: I might add a few comments. We were aware of the work that had been done on collagen peptides, and the possibility that they were chemotactic, at least for human peripheral blood monocytes.

In thioglycollate-elicited mouse cells that we have used for our experiments, purified mouse type I collagen is not chemotactic at concentrations up to the point where it jelled in the lower compartment of the chemotactic chamber.

Alpha-1 chains purified from carboxymethyl cellulose columns from calf skin were not chemotactic, and we have yet to test degraded collagen preparations with either pepsin or collagenase, although based on observations available in the literature, we doubt that we will see chemotactic activity.

In response to the comment that Dr. Cohn made, we have tested material from Urist. By either crushing the material and putting it in the chemotactic chamber, or letting it soak in the chemotactic medium for periods of time to allow substances to diffuse out, we haven't found chemotaxis.

One more comment to perhaps clarify the issue that Dr. Tashjian raised: we have been able to show that calcitonin-treated bones don't have the amount of chemotactic activity that either control bones or bones that have been stimulated to resorb have. So, there may be more than a specific relation to a metabolically-active tissue on the basis of these observations.

DR. KUETTNER: A question to Dr. Vassali, and also to Dr. Werb. Are there any cells which do not secrete plasminogen activator? And to Dr. Werb: are there certain particular connective tissue cells which do not have the potential to secrete collagenase?

DR. VASSALI: The normal resident macrophages do not secrete any plasminogen activator; normal primary cultures of mouse, chicken, and other fibroblasts secrete only very low levels of enzyme. There is at least one cell type where we have looked at some aspects of regulation, and we haven't found any activator. This is the lymphocyte, either resting peripheral blood lymphocytes or after stimulation.

DR. KUETTNER: How about chondrocytes? Can you stimulate chondrocytes, or have you tried with chondrocytes at all?

DR. VASSALI: We have not looked.

DR. WERB: I don't believe that chondrocytes have been tested for collagenase, but lymphocytes don't make collagenase. Fibroblasts make only when they are activated; they don't under other conditions.

DR. PARFITT: I have two questions, the first addressed to Dr. Mundy, and the second perhaps to all members of the panel.

The first question is: you demonstrated that the chemical mediator of resorption was not a critical factor in determining whether or not chemotaxis occurred, but I believe all the agents you used normally operate via the osteoclast. Have you demonstrated chemotaxis with non-osteoclast-mediated resorption?

In other words, you demonstrated that you could induce resorption with monocytes. Do these, then, act chemotactically for further monocytes in the second kind of system that you studied?

DR. MUNDY: I don't know. That is an interesting question, and it would be worth pursuing.

DR. PARFITT: The second question concerns the mechanisms of localization of resorption in the normal skeleton. For all of the local mechanisms being studied, there is an obvious reason why resorption occurs in one part of the skeleton rather than another, e.g., there is a breast cancer cell or a myeloma cell.

But with normal bone turnover, where resorption is occuring only on a small part of the surface, and not somewhere else, there is no such obvious reason why a particular surface of the bone is resorbing at one moment, rather than some other portion of the surface.

Do any of the speakers have any ideas as to what might determine this localization in normal bone, as opposed to around the pathologic foreign type of cell?

DR. MUNDY: We know very little about the regulation of why cells move around in bone. They are interesting questions, but I suspect answers are quite a way down the line yet.

DR. SHAPIRO: A comment and two questions. The comment is that a monocyte chemotactic factor has been isolated from dental plaque, which may link up the initiation of peridontal disease with monocytic resorption. One question is: Dr. Mundy, are PMN's in your system osteoclastic? Secondly, would you speculate on the relationship between chemotactic factors and OAF?

DR. MUNDY: Apparently PMN's are not osteoclastic. Since they are full of lysosomal enzymes, they probably could resorb bone if you got enough of them together; but we haven't been able to demonstrate it in the numbers we have used. My bias would be that they are probably not very important in the bone resorption process.

To the speculation between osteoclast activating factor and monocyte chemotaxis: I am not sure what the effects are of these agents, and whether there are real differences between these agents on osteoclast precursor cells. That is clearly a very interesting question.

DR. SHAPIRO: Are you worried by the fact that you don't see ruffled borders on monocytes which are resorbing bone?

DR. MUNDY: It would worry me if I was trying to call them "osteoclasts," but I am not doing that. I see a ruffled border as a specialized area of the cell membrane which, in some way, makes it easier for the osteoclast to resorb mineralized tissue that is lying underneath. It seems reasonable if the monocyte is really a precursor of the osteoclast, that monocytes should have similar intracellular machinery to resorb bone. It may not have all the specialized features, because that may require further differentiation. In vitro it appears that monocytes are much less effective bone resorbers than osteoclasts. We are certainly not suggesting they are as good as osteoclasts. So it doesn't really worry me that there is not a ruffled border.

DR. KAHN: A question to Dr. Werb. There has been a fair amount of discussion during the course of this meeting about collagenase. I wonder about the evidence that really relates collagenase activity to the removal of resorption of mineralized matrices.

Could one consider that perhaps the organic component, collagen, is removed by other kinds of proteases?

DR. WERB: There is no direct evidence that the osteoclast makes collagenase that removes the collagen at this point. All the evidence for collagenase in bone is somewhat indirect. That is, you put a little bone into culture, and you can measure collagenase in the medium. That is essentially it.

DR. KAHN: Is it possible, theoretically?

DR. WERB: Collagenase is an enzyme that produces the first clip in collagen at neutral pH; but there are lysosomal hydrolases, particularly cathepsin B, which could nibble away at collagen and eventually do it in. For that matter, a combination of the neutrophil proteases can nibble away at it and do it in too.

DR. TEITELBAUM: Dr. Mundy, I would like to underscore what Dr. Parfitt said about tumor-mediated bone resorption relating to osteoclast activation. If one looks at bone taken from lesions of patients with breast cancer, one invariably sees osteoclasts. This would suggest that indeed, if non-osteoclastic bone resorption did occur, it probably does in some way relate to releasing chemotactic agents, which in turn are responsible for attracting osteoclasts to the bone.

DR. MUNDY: I would like to see the documentation for that. I have looked at breast cancer, and I can't see it. Of course, I realize not finding osteoclasts doesn't mean anything, and there are a few case reports where one occasionally sees osteoclasts; but they seem to be far outnumbered by the other cells.

There is one other point I would like to make about breast cancer. It is incredibly rare to get hypercalcemia with widespread bone destruction. Most patients who get hypercalcemia in breast cancer have lots of bone metastases. The situation is uncommon in breast cancer where you get a patient with hyper- calcemia with just a tumor, and no obvious bone metastases. And that has really pointed me in this direction.

What I am looking at are the tumor cells, the cultured, cloned, established human breast cancer cell line and I am trying to look at how those cells break down bone.

In the whole animal, there may be other mechanisms invoked by the presence of a tumor which could stimulate osteoclasts and cause resorption, which would be another process involved, as well.

DR. TEITELBAUM: Yes. The point doesn't obviate what you said; except that if, indeed, there are osteoclasts, and I am convinced there are; there are osteoclasts involved in the resorption of bone in breast cancer. The monocyte-related, or the non-osteoclast-related resorption may be a stimulus to the activation of the osteoclasts. In other words, the non-tumor resorption occurs first.

DR. MUNDY: That is one theory. Okay.

DR. HEERSCHE: Dr. Mundy, is monocyte-stimulated, or breast cell stimulated, resorption inhibited by calcitonin?

DR. MUNDY: The data are negative, but that doesn't mean it is not. In the ways that we have tried to inhibit it, we haven't been able, because calcitonin is a drug which has a transient effect in our system on inhibiting bone resorption.

DR. HEERSCHE: Yes, but you could have some corticosteroids to overcome that escape, as you have shown, right?

DR. MUNDY: If we have high enough doses of corticosteroids, we can block the effect; and that may be due to an effect on lysosomal enzymes.

DR. HEERSCHE: Okay. The reason I ask the question is because I think if we combine this information with Dr. Parfitt's remark and with Dr. Minkin's observation, then you have an opportunity of testing whether or not resorbing bone, which is not osteoclastic resorption, is indeed inducing chemotaxis. So it would be a neat experiment.

DR. MUNDY: Yes.

DR. BOCKMAN: In regard to what Dr. Teitelbaum just said, there was a paper in Nature last year which used the Walker 256 carcinosarcoma, derived originally from a mouse mammary line. They did what you can't do in a patient, because by the time you find a patient with breast cancer and bone disease, the lytic disease has been going on for a while; but by following the sequence of events from the introduction of the tumor into the bone of the animal, they first saw resorption by osteoclasts, then tumor replacement, and then what was obviously tumor resorption, suggesting that this was the natural sequence of events in that model tumor system.

The second thing is that I have a slide, but I won't try to show it, that clearly demonstrates, in the human, mononuclear cell bone resorption. It is a case, on which Dr. Mundy collaborated, of hypercalcemia in immunoblastic lymphadenopathy.

DR. MUNDY: Yes. I read those papers in Nature, but I didn't think it was very new that that particular tumor caused osteoclast stimulation. I thought that had been demonstrated quite well, only if by Dr. Tashjian, and I wasn't really convinced about the data, one way or the other, which showed that the tumor cells themselves were directly resorbing bone. I wouldn't want to use that data to support what I am saying, or have it used that way.

DR. MARKS: I would like to mention a brief clinical anecdote that I think bears on this question of how breast disease is associated with hypercalcemia.

A few years ago, we participated in the evaluation of an adolescent girl who had persistant hypercalcemia over several years, with calciums in the 12 to 13 range. She underwent several attempts at parathyroidectomy, which were unsuccessful, and ultimately came to a rather unusual treatment for her hypercalcemia. She had developed massive adolescent hyperplasia of both breasts during the previous several years, and underwent cosmetic surgery with deliberate removal of both of her breasts. Immediately after the operation, she actually became hypocalcemic. She had no breast cells in any of her lymph nodes, and over five years has not had any recurrence of her hypercalcemia.

I think this is a rather bizarre case that illustrates a humoral mechanism whereby breast disease can be associated with hypercalcemia.

DR. GOLDHABER: Dr. Mundy, I would like to caution you and the whole conference that this may not be an adequate model for studying bone resorption.

DR. MUNDY: If we have a model where we show positive effects, and you are saying it is not an adequate model, then I think you have to explain why you think it isn't.

DR. GOLDHABER: I think you are not showing resorption of bone, but are showing resorption of a devitalized tissue which is not the usual problem in bone physiology. I think we may be dealing with two different problems when we look at that model.

The other point I would make is the question of resorption of bone by tumors. Many years ago, we tested a whole series of tumors, human tumors, and found slight effects in stimulating resorption, depending upon the amount of tissue that was around. We did test breast carcinoma, and were a little disappointed to find that they were not very good bone-resorbing stimulators.

Now, the HSDM-1 tumor that Dr. Tashjian mentioned in his talk did show that when you put a fragment of that tumor on the bone, you got tremendous resorption around the fragment, even at distant places. At that time, we went through the same process of reasoning as you are now in trying to find out whether this was the tumor cells or some mediator coming off the tumor cells. Until you do what Dr. Tashjian suggested; that is, look at either conditioned medium or extracts of the tumor, you will not really have the answer as to whether or not this is direct action of a tumor cell, or some factor coming off the cell.

DR. MUNDY: There are some points I think need to be made here. We are putting these MCF-7 cells with live bones, as well as with the dead bone models, and we have something happening in both the live as well as dead bones.

The effect that we are seeing in live bones doesn't appear to depend on osteoclast activity; and I have further evidence for this which wasn't shown because of the time.

Now, it may be that the dead bone model isn't the right model. However, we are able to demonstrate that when we put the tumor cells in with dead bone, we cause, by some means, the mineral to be released and the matrix to be broken down, as measured by release of tritiated hydroxyproline from the matrix. So there is something happening in that dead bone which is akin to what happens in the live bone.

Clearly, the breakdown of the matrix must be an enzymatic process. Presumably, that process is through the release, rather than by phagocytosis, of enzymes from the tumor cell.

Now, it may require something that is very local. It may need, for example, an acid environment, right at the cell membrane; I don't know. And it may be very difficult to show that with supernatant media taken from the bone. We have still to test that to find out, one way or the other. But negative results wouldn't mean that it is not an important observation.

DR. GOLDHABER: If you use a devitalized bone assay system, then you would not be able to do the experiment, because in the system that we are talking about with vital bone, when you take the tumor extract, or the factors coming off bone, which seem to be prostaglandins, that in itself will not have any effect on a piece of dead bone. So that you have to use vital bone to study the tumor effect.

DR. MUNDY: But clearly, Dr. Goldhaber, what you are looking at is a humoral mediator which is working indirectly in that system by stimulating osteoclasts.

DR. GOLDHABER: That is correct.

DR. MUNDY: We are not dealing with that in this system,

apparently; and all the data says we are not.

DR. KUETTNER: I would like to enter this discussion between Dr. Mundy and Dr. Goldhaber because I think we have to be very cautious. The discussion may be true with metastatic bone diseases; but if you are talking about an osteogenic sarcoma, or osteosarcoma, we have evidence that I will show in the paper after the coffee break, that these tumor cells directly will resorb bone where there is no osteoclastic activity involved.

In metastases, it may be a different story; so whenever one talks of "tumor cells", it should be specified whether these are metastatic tumor lines or not.

DR. WURTHIER: I believe there is a point that is important to bring out in these discussions. It is that the removal of both living and devitalized bone is important biologically. In bone fractures, clearly in the area of the injury, there is devital bone which must be removed; so this model is important. I think we should keep this in mind so that we don't think that if we are not looking at a living bone system, it doesn't have any biological relevance.

SESSION IV

DISORDERS OF BONE ASSOCIATED WITH
INFLAMMATION AND NEOPLASIA

Resistance of Cartilage to Normal and Neoplastic Invasion.

Klaus E. Kuettner* and Bendicht U. Pauli[+]

Departments of Biochemistry*, Orthopedics* and Pathology[+],
Rush Medical College (*[+]) and Rush College of Health Sciences(*),
Rush Presbyterian St. Luke's Medical Center, Chicago, IL 60612

INTRODUCTION

The penetration of a tissue by cells from another tissue is characteristic of various physiological and pathological processes. Examples of physiologic invasion are the sperm migration through the cervical mucus, the penetration of the zona pellucida of the ovum, neovascularization of tissues during embryogenesis, and vascular penetration of calcified cartilage in the epiphyseal growth plate. Pathologic invasion is most obviously displayed by the infiltration of tumor cells into adjacent tissues (1). Invasion, both physiologic and pathologic, has been defined as the passing, interpenetration or infiltration of a cell into adjacent tissues. Though simple, this definition recognizes the complexity of the interaction between the invader and the host tissue.

This interaction is classically displayed in the neovascularization of tissues during embryogenesis. For most tissues, neovascularization is necessary to provide nutrients and to eliminate waste products. However, there are several tissues such as cartilage, cornea, dentin and epithelia, which do not normally vascularize. These tissues receive nutrients and eliminate waste products by diffusion. The cause for selective vascularization of tissues may well be related to tissue specific "anti-invasive" factors, which may express themselves as a physical barrier to the advancing endothelium or as a system translated into the specific inhibition to the penetration by endothelial cells.

This report discusses the possible role of anti-invasive factors for determining the natural resistance of postnatal mammalian hyaline cartilage to blood vessel and tumor invasion. The mechanisms for this tissue's anti-invasive system may provide insight for other invasion, both physiologic and pathologic.

I.   Studies on Cartilage Vascularization

A.   Experimental Approach:

Mammalian hyaline cartilage lacks an intrinsic capillary blood supply. Vessels are only present in the cartilage nutrient

canals (2). At the growth plate, vascular loops penetrate to
the area of the last hypertrophic chondrocyte and its calcified
matrix (3). This resistance of cartilage to vascular penetration was studied by grafting hyaline cartilage and other
mammalian tissues onto the chick embyro chorioallantoic membrane
(CAM) (Fig. 1) by methods previously described (4-6). Direct
observations of the tissue grafts during the incubation period
were made through a window in the egg shell. After completion
of an experiment, each graft was histologically examined. Re-
vascularization of explants depended on the type of grafted
tissue. Vascularized tissues were readily penetrated by the
vessels of the CAM (Fig. 2). In contrast, tissues devoid of an
intrinsic capillary blood supply such as hyaline cartilage and
cornea were closely surrounded but never penetrated by the
vessels of the CAM (4). (Figs. 2 and 3). Accordingly, in
grafted rib costochondral junctions the hyaline cartilage, although it was eventually completely covered by a pannus of
vascularized mesenchyme, was never penetrated. Only the vascularized parts of the explant, such as bone and calcified
cartilage of the growth plate were penetrated by the blood
vessels of the CAM (Figs. 2 and 4). At the growth plate,
vessels reached to the area of the last hypertrophic chondrocyte and its calcified matrix, but were stopped by the uncalcified columnar cartilage (Fig. 5). This inhibition of the
vascular mesenchyme did not appear to be directly controlled
by the activity of chondrocytes since it persisted after the
cells of the explant were devitalized by freezing and thawing(4).

Experiments were designed to study the relationship between these biological properties and diffusible or extractable
substances of cartilage which might prevent invasion. Normal
and physically or chemically altered cartilage explants were
placed on Millipore membranes and grafted onto the CAM. It
was noted that bare filters were covered by arcades of blood
vessels. However, when cartilage explants were placed on the
filters, the vascular proliferation was markedly diminished (6),
suggesting that a diffusible factor inhibited blood vessel proliferation. This inhibitory effect on vascular proliferation
was also evident when Millipore membranes carrying cartilage
powder were transplanted onto the CAM. Blood vessels and connective tissue elements which normally would cover the Millipore
membrane were unable to approach or penetrate the cartilage
powder pellet. These observations were consistent with those
described by Folkman and his collaborators (7,8) who showed that
cartilage placed between a tumor and a potential vascular source
in the anterior chamber of the rabbit eye inhibited the proliferation of limbus vessels that otherwise were stimulated by
the tumor transplant. Isolated chondrocytes as well as cartilage
extracts injected intradermally can also inhibit the angiogenesis induced by lymphocytes in vivo during local graft versus
host reactions (9). From this inhibition of the vascular response, it can be concluded that cartilage contains factors
which influence blood vessel proliferation. Therefore, hyaline
cartilage segments were mildly extracted with various molarities
of guanidinium hydrochloride (1M, 2M, 4M GuHCl), washed with

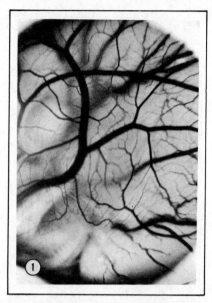

Fig. 1:   Normal chorioallantoic membrane (CAM) of a 7 day old chick embryo as photographed through a window in the egg shell. (x6)

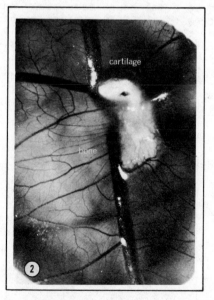

Fig. 2:   Human rib costochondral junction was grafted onto the CAM of a 7 day old chick embryo. One week after explantation, the bone is penetrated by a dense capillary network, whereas the cartilage resists vascular invasion. (x6).

Fig. 3-5: Human rib costochondral junctions were grafted onto the CAM of a 7 day old embryo, incubated for 7 days at 37°C, and then processed for light microscopic examination.

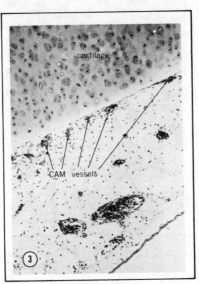

Fig. 3: The cartilage, although completely surrounded by blood capillaries of the CAM (typically characterized by nucleated chick red cells), resists vascular invasion. (H&E, x150)

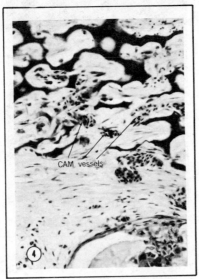

Fig. 4: The bone is densely penetrated by vascular mesenchyme. (H&E, x370)

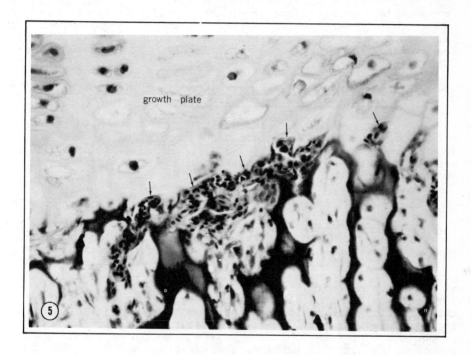

Fig. 5:   At the growth plate, CAM vessels reach to the area of
the last hypertrophic chondrocyte and its calcified
matrix but were stopped by the uncalcified columnar
cartilage (arrows).   (H&E, x510)

physiologic saline and then explanted onto the CAM (5). These devitalized, extracted explants had no inhibitory effect on the proliferation of CAM blood vessels. Explants were covered with a dense vascularized mesenchyme and were invaded by numerous capillary branches (Fig. 6). It was also noted that the proliferative response by the vascularized mesenchyme of the CAM was more extensive on and near extracted than unextracted tissues (Figs. 2 and 6). This suggests that the factor(s) in the cartilage causing this inhibitory response is, in part, diffusible and extractable. Chemical assays of the cartilage after extraction showed that 1M GuHCl extracted only 7% of the tissue uronic acid (an indicator for proteoglycans) and virtually no collagen (5). The extracts, however, contained a spectrum of lower molecular weight proteins (10-12).

B. The Effect of Cartilage Extracts on the Growth of Endothelial Cells in Culture.

In vitro studies on neovascularization have shown that this biologic process is determined by proliferation and invasion of endothelial cells (13,14). Therefore we studied the effect of cartilage extracts on the growth of isolated aortic endothelial cells in culture (15-17).

At a concentration of 500 µg/ml, material derived from a 1M GuHCl extract of bovine hyaline cartilage inhibited the growth of bovine endothelial cells completely. At lower concentrations, the growth curve was dose responsive,showing some activity at concentrations of less than 100 µg/ml. In contrast, the growth of bovine skin fibroblasts in culture was not affected and human foreskin and bovine fetal fibroblasts were inhibited only at very high concentrations of the cartilage extracts. Cartilage proteoglycans as subunits or as aggregates even in high concentrations did not affect the growth of endothelial cells in vitro significantly. Evidence that the biologically active compound was of relatively low molecular weight was obtained by preparing ultrafiltrates of the cartilage extract. The filtrate which contained substances of molecular weight of 50,000 daltons or above had no effect on the growth of endothelial cells in doses as high as 500 µg/ml. The lower molecular weight substances, however, were more potent than the crude cartilage extract showing a dose-dependent activity with some growth inhibition even at concentrations of less than 5 µg/ml (15).

Correlation between morphologic observations and analytic data on the crude cartilage extract permit the following conclusion. The "rejection" of blood vessels by the cartilage does not seem to be due to the physical arrangement of its matrix molecules but rather to diffusible compounds synthesized and released by chondrocytes. The increased susceptibility to invasion of the tissue extracted with relatively low molarities of GuHCl indicates that its resistance to invasion is not entirely due to proteoglycans or to any particular packing array of proteoglycans into the collagenous meshwork of the matrix. The hypothesis on which our experiments was based implies that

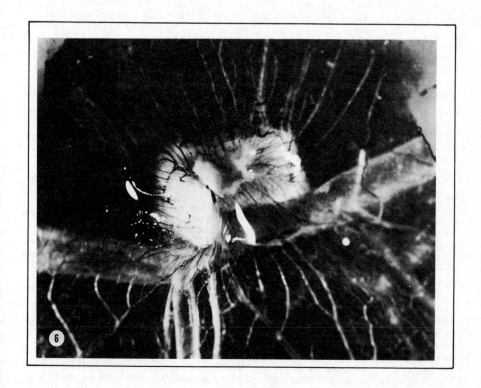

Fig. 6:   Hyaline human rib cartilage was extracted with 1M
guanidinium hydrochloride and grafted onto the CAM
of a 7 day old chick embryo. At day 14, the extracted
cartilage was covered with a dense vascularized
mesenchyme and invaded by numerous capillary branches.
(x15)

for endothelial cells to penetrate a tissue like cartilage, they must not only degrade the extracellular matrix in order to penetrate it, but that this process is also accompanied by a proliferative activity of the cells involved.

C. Isolation and Identification of a Protease Inhibitor From Cartilage.

The ingrowth of endothelial cells into tissues may be caused by the release of proteolytic enzymes (18) which are able to degrade the connective tissue matrix proteins (collagen, proteoglycans, etc.) to provide space for their proliferation. Since cartilage shows specific resistance to endothelial cell penetration, both in vivo and in vitro, and since a cartilage extract can inhibit the proliferation of these cells, we postulated that the extractable anti-invasion factor derived from cartilage may well be related to proteolytic enzyme inhibitors. This concept was supported by our observation that specific protease inhibitors such as soybean trypsin inhibitor suppresses the growth of endothelial cells in vitro, but to a lesser extent than the cartilage extracts (15).

Several connective tissues were surveyed for the presense of proteinase inhibitors. For that purpose, slices of connective tissue such as cartilage were submerged in agar containing denatured fibrinogen as substrate for proteolytic enzymes. Trypsin and chymotrypsin were then placed in wells surrounding the explants (19). Due to radial diffusion of these enzymes, the substrate was digested except in areas on the side of the tissue explants. Here proteolysis was inhibited, indicating that trypsin or chymotrypsin inhibitors were diffusing from the tissue (Chart 1). The greatest anti-protease activity was found in poorly vascularized, bradytrophic connective tissues such as cartilage and blood vessel walls (20). There was also some inhibitor activity in dentin (20,21). Recent unpublished experiments show that the protease inhibitory activities are not present in serum and are synthesized by chondrocytes in culture. In an electrophoretic field, the inhibitor activity migrates as a single band with a net positive charge (20). In addition, a trypsin inhibitor was isolated from cartilage and partially characterized by a series of chromatogrophic steps, including affinity chromatography on insoluble trypsin (19,22). The inhibitor is a cationic protein showing a single band on SDS-polyacrylamide electrophoresis with a molecular weight of less than 13,000 daltons. Further chemical characterization of this molecule is currently in progress. Cartilage also contains activity which inhibits α-chymotrypsin, and which has not yet been isolated (22). Work is currently in progress to test whether or not the purified protease inhibitors can inhibit endothelial cell proliferation or if other specific molecules present in cartilage are involved.

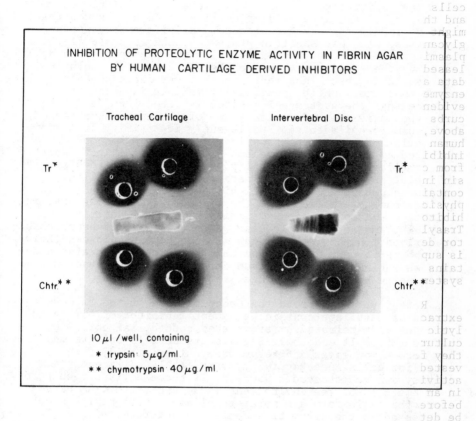

INHIBITION OF PROTEOLYTIC ENZYME ACTIVITY IN FIBRIN AGAR
BY HUMAN CARTILAGE DERIVED INHIBITORS

Tracheal Cartilage   Intervertebral Disc

Tr.*   Tr.*

Chtr.**   Chtr.**

10 μl /well, containing

* trypsin: 5 μg/ml

** chymotrypsin 40 μg/ml

Chart 1: Human tracheal and intervertebral disc cartilage
slices are shown submerged in agar containing denatured fibrinogen. Twenty-four hours later, trypsin (5
μg/ml) and chymotrypsin (40 μg/ml) were placed into
wells surrounding the tissues and the Petri dish was
incubated in a wet chamber at 37°C for 17 hours. The
areas of clearance due to the proteolytic activity
appear dark because the photograph was taken against a
dark background. Note a significant inhibition of
the proteolytic enzyme activities on the side of the
explant, where the freely diffusing enzyme does not
form a circular ring of clearance due to an inhibitor
diffusing from the tissue.

D. Identification of the Cartilage-Derived Trypsin
    Inhibitor as a Collagenase Inhibitor.

In the previous section, we postulated that endothelial
cells may be invasive because they secrete proteolytic enzymes
and thereby erode extracellular matrices. Among enzymes that
might be involved in such a process are collagenase, proteo-
glycanases, and less specific proteases such as those of the
plasminogen-plasmin system, kallikrein or other proteases released by these cells. Although there are no such biological
data available that might indicate that cartilage contains
enzyme inhibitors which specifically inhibit invasion, there is
evidence that the protease inhibitor isolated from cartilage
curbs the activities of at least one of the enzymes mentioned
above, namely collagenase. Collagenolytic activity from normal
human skin and human hypertrophic scar tissue was found to be
inhibited by the purified protease (trypsin) inhibitor isolated
from cartilage, but only slightly by Trasylol^R and soybean trypsin inhibitor (23,24). These data suggest that cartilage
contains a potent collagenase inhibitor which differs in its
physical characteristics from the serum derived collagenase inhibitor, α_2-macroglobulin and in its biological activity from
Trasylol^R, another low molecular weight cationic trypsin inhibitor derived from bovine tissues. The concept of biospecificity
is supported by our observation that human cartilage also contains an inhibitor which acts on human skin collagenase in a
system using human skin collagen as a substrate (24).

Recently, we observed that the fraction of the 1M GuHCl
extract of cartilage contains a potent inhibitor of collagenolytic activity released by stimulated endothelial cells in
culture (25). If endothelial cells are kept in culture until
they form a monolayer and serum-free culture medium is harvested for collagenase activity, very little collagenolytic
activity can be detected. However, if these cells are cultured
in an elevated oxygen environment (40%) and the medium harvested
before the cells form a monolayer, collagenolytic acvitity can
be detected in the serum-free medium. Therefore, we hypothesize
that endothelial cells in culture have to be in an "active
proliferative and migrating" state in order to secrete or synthesize collagenase activity.

In addition, we reported recently that the same cartilage
material which inhibits the endothelial cell proliferation as
well as their secreted collagenolytic activity was found to
reversibly block bone resorption induced in vitro (26). Morphologic examination revealed that this factor modulates osteoclastic activities. Since active osteoclasts share with
endothelial cells the characteristic of bone matrix collagen
degradation, such bone cells could also be interpreted as being
"invasive". We therefore have tentatively named the above mentioned collagenase inhibitor enriched substance(s) isolated from
cartilage "anti-invasion factor" (AIF) (27).

II. Studies on Tumor Invasion

A. Inhibition of Tumor Cell Collagenase by the Cartilage Derived Protease (trypsin) Inhibitor.

Invasive tumor cells share the following growth characteristic with normal proliferating endothelial cells: both cells have to "digest" their way into the tissue they penetrate. Since the cartilages of the epiphyseal growth plate and articular surfaces seem to inhibit the "invasiveness" of primary bone tumors such as osteosarcomas as well as of bony metastases in vivo (28,29), we decided to use two human tumor cell lines to test their ability to elaborate collagenase into tissue culture media. For the experiments we used a well-defined human osteosarcoma (TE-85) (30) cell line and a human breast carcinoma cell line (ALAB) (31) derived from a lung metastasis. Based on the experiments described in the proceding sections, the two tumor cell lines were cultured in the presence of 10% fetal calf serum under conditions recently described (32). After the cells reached confluence (usually 5 days), the cell layers were rinsed thoroughly in serum-free Dulbecco-Eagles medium (serum contains the strong collagenase inhibitor, α_2-macroglobulin) and then cultivated at 37^0 in Dulbecco-Eagles's medium in the absence of serum, according to the method described by Werb and Burleigh (33). The media of 2 and 4 day old cultures were pooled processed and assayed for collagenase activity. The presence of small amounts of collagenase activity indicated that the enzyme was secreted or released by these cells into the media. Stimulated by the observation that heparin acts on a co-factor in experimentally-induced bone resorption in organ culture (34,35, 36), possibly by enhancing bone collagenolytic activity, we added heparin (50 U/ml) to the serum-free media of confluent cultures of tumor cells. Two interesting phenomena were observed: first, the tumor cell morphology was well preserved and the tumor cells did not detach from the culture dishes and could be maintained in serum-free media for up to 25 days. Second, collagenase activity in the media of heparin-stimulated cultures was significantly increased over control values. As recently reported (32), this collagenolytic activity harvested from the osteosarcoma and mammary carcinoma cell cultures was substantially inhibited by the cartilage-derived collagenase inhibitor (19). As indicated by polyacrylamide gel electrophoresis, the mammary carcinoma cells produced a large spectrum of reaction products from the collagen, probably due to the presence of other proteases within the media which further degraded the normal fragments TC^A and TC^B derived from collagenase digesion of collagen. The collagen breakdown could be totally inhibited by prior incubation of the media with the cartilage collagenase inhibitor, indicating that the first collagenolytic step in the collagen breakdown is inhibited (32).

B. Inhibition of Collagenolytic Activity Derived From Primary Human Mammary Carcinomas In Vitro.

The growth of human breast tumors is frequently dependent upon hormones, i.e., estrogens (37). In the following experiments, the estrogen effect on explants of primary mammary carcinomas was studied and the results compared with the effect of heparin as described in the previous paragraph. Mammary carcinoma explants (1 mm^3 tissue) were prepared from 20 patients who underwent diagnostic biopsy or mastectomy. The explants were placed into 35 mm^2 Falcon plastic Petri dishes and medium added in a ratio of 50 mg tumor/ml medium. Explants were then incubated for 17 hours at 37°. In some experiments, explants were co-incubated with human hyaline rib cartilage (100 mg/ml medium) which was obtained during surgical correction of Pectus Excavatum deformity. Incubation media were prepared as follows: a) Control - Standard RPMI-1640 Tissue Culture Medium, b) Heparin medium - Standard Medium + Heparin (50 U/ml), c) Estradiol medium - Standard Medium + 17 β-estradiol (10 ng/ml). Following incubation, the specimens were centrifuged and the media processed and analyzed for collagenolytic activity. In explants from 14 of the 20 patients, heparin stimulation showed the greatest collagenolytic activity. Three explants showed greatest activity when stimulated by estradiol and 3 explants showed no discernible difference in activity when stimulated by heparin, estradiol or in control media (38). Co-incubation of the tumor with cartilage slices showed total inhibition of the collagenolytic activity in the media and contributed to a better morphologic preservation of the explants Incubation of the tumor media with AIF isolated from human rib cartilage also showed a marked decrease in collagenolytic activity which appeared to be dose related.

Random morphologic examination of tumors for the presence of mast cells showed that tumors which were diagnosed as scirrhous carcinoma contained mast cells in, or close to, the collagen network surrounding the tumor. Numerous mast cells were found in the proximity of tumor cell nests. A partial degranulation was indicative of the release of heparin. These preliminary data indicate that heparin potentiated collagenolytic activity of most of these tumors.

C. Morphologic Studies on the Resistance of Cartilage to Tumor Cell Invasion.

a) In vivo observations on an osteogenic sarcoma:

In general, solid tumors expand or invade along paths of least resistance through pre-existing tissue clefts and spaces and destroy normal tissue as they grow. Dense tissues like the walls of arteries resist destruction for a time and provide an effective barrier to the spread of tumors. Therefore, tumor growth is not entirely unconfined, and is subject to important checks and restraints (1).

In bone neoplasms, the most common primary malignant tumor is the osteosarcoma (28,29). The five year survival rate for patients with this malignancy is poor. Osteosarcomas arise in the metaphyseal ends of the shafts of long bones, particularly the lower end of the femur, the upper end of the tibia, and the upper end of the humerus. Occasionally, the neoplasm arises in the middle portion of the shaft of a long bone. The disease is seen most frequently in children and young adults, where about 75% occur in patients between 10 and 25 years of age. Males are affected about twice as often as females. Primary osteosarcoma usually replaces the metaphyseal cancellous tissues before it destroys the cortex. The unossified endochondral cartilage is rarely invaded by osteosarcoma and remains intact until quite late in the disease (28). If the endochondral growth plate is fused or locally violated, the tumor grows through the ossified nucleus of the epiphysis up to the articular cartilage which usually restrains the neoplastic process (28). This phenomenon was also seen in bony metastases derived from other primary tumors (e.g., breast and prostate).

Detailed histological examinations were recently pursued in an osteogenic sarcoma arising in the distal metaphysis of the femur of a 10 year old girl (39). The tumor had a diameter of 10 cm and filled the marrow cavity in the metaphyseal region. The cortex was laterally eroded and the tumor invaded the epiphyseal bone, but did not invade the articular cartilage. Specimens from the metaphyseal bone, growth plate, epiphyseal bone, and the interface between the epiphysis and articular cartilage were obtained during surgery (amputation). They were immediately fixed with 10% phosphate buffered formalin and routinely processed for light microscopic examination. It was found that the residual cortical and metaphyseal cancellous bone was embedded in tumor masses showing surface irregularities and numerous lacunae in bone spicules with closely attached tumor cells. This can be interpreted as morphologic evidence for direct bone erosion by the tumor cells in the absence of osteoclasts (Fig. 7). The epiphyseal cartilage, however, had resisted the invasion by the tumor cells, except for a central area of the growth plate which was penetrated by the tumor leading to the invasion of the entire distal epiphyseal bone (Fig. 8). This extension of the tumor from the metaphysis to the epiphysis was probably through pre-existing connective tissue canals and promoted by microfractures and associated hematoma. At the interface of the epiphyseal bone and the articular cartilage, the tumor cells closely followed the outline of the articular cartilage spreading as far as the vascular loops extended to the area of the calcified cartilage matrix (Fig. 9). The articular cartilage therefore appeared to represent a barrier to further tumor spread.

   b) The resistance of human cartilage to osteosarcoma cell invasion in vitro.

These in vivo observations indicate that tumor cells will only occupy spaces in the cartilage where blood vessels are

Fig. 7-9: Osteogenic sarcoma arising in the distal metaphysis of the femur of a 10 year old girl.

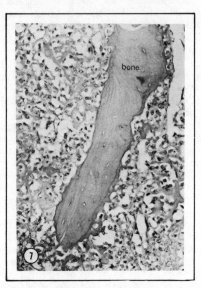

Fig. 7:   Bone spicule in the metaphysis is tightly surrounded by osteosarcoma cells. The irregularities in the bone surface suggest bone resorptive activity mediated by tumor cells. Osteoclasts are absent. (H&E, x160)

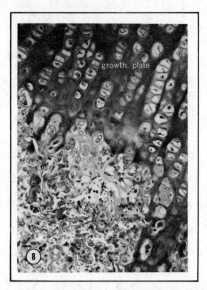

Fig. 8:   The columnar cartilage of the growth plate resists invasion by both blood vessels and tumor cell. (H&E, x160)

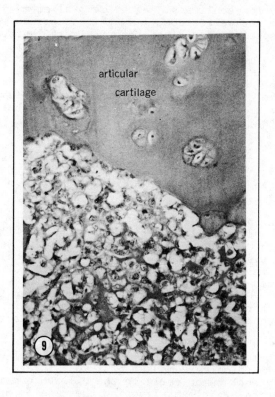

ig. 9:   Articular cartilage acts as a barrier for further tumor
          spread.   (H&E, x200)

found. This suggests that the mechanisms by which cartilage resists endothelial cell invasion may be similar in tumor cell invasion. Therefore, we co-cultured interfaces of human cartilage-bone explants and human osteosarcoma cells in a specially designed organ-cell-culture system. Light microscopy techniques were used to evaluate the results (29).

Human rib growth plates from the costochondral junctions of children aged 11 to 13 years were obtained at the time of therapeutic surgery for scoliosis. After removal of muscle, fascia, perichondrium, and periosteum, 1 mm thick segments were prepared so that each specimen contained both the cartilaginous growth plate and bone. All specimens containing bone were briefly trypsinized and mildly agitated to remove marrow and endothelial cells and then immediately cultured. The cartilage-bone-explants were placed onto Millipore membranes which served as a growth surface for the explants. These membranes were elevated on Falcon stainless steel grids 2 to 3 mm above the bottom of the culture dish and the medium was added until the fluid level wetted the membrane to sustain viability of the tissues. The explants were cultured for an initial period of 2 to 3 days during which the growth and viability of the tissue was monitored microscopically. The RPMI-1640 medium supplemented with 50 µg/ml gentamycin and 5 µg/ml amphotericin-B, 25mM HEPES and 10% fetal calf serum was used (39).

After the initial culture of the explants for 2 to 3 days, 2×10^4 osteosarcoma cells (TE-85, the human cell line described above) or primary human foreskin fibroblasts were seeded onto the explanted tissues. In control cultures both cell types were cultured in the absence of explants. After 3, 7, or 10 days of combined organ-cell culture the explants were processed for histology. Millipore membranes were processed for light microscopy either immediately after the removal of the explants from the membrane or in some cases after the cells were cultured further for different time intervals.

Osteosarcoma cells cultured in the absence of explants formed multiple colonies composed of 1 to 5 layers of spindle-shaped or polygonal tumor cells on the Millipore membranes. During the entire experimental period these cells appeared healthy. Human foreskin fibroblasts formed a confluent contact-inhibited monolayer of the Millipore membranes. At all times, cartilage explants showed viability as indicated by the morphology of the chondrocytes, the preservation of shape and size of the tissue and the stainability of its matrix. Similarly, the mesenchyme of the cartilage canals was well preserved. In contrast to cartilage, bone did not survive for long periods of time in organ cultures. At the end of the 10 day culture period some necrosis of osteocytes was indicated by the appearance of empty spaces in the bone matrix. Therefore the experiments were generally terminated after 1 week or 10 days of culture.

Fibroblasts cultured in the presence of rib explants covered the entire cartilage top surface with a coherent monolayer. At the lateral surfaces they intermingled with and became morphologically indistinguishable from outgrowing cartilage derived mesenchymal cells (39). In the bone cavity, fibroblasts formed strands between the bone spicules mostly without adhering to them, leaving surfaces of the bone spicules smooth.

When explants were cultured in the presence of osteosarcoma cells, the surface of the cartilage was generally devoid of tumor cells. The few osteosarcoma cell colonies observed consisted of 1 to 2 layers of less than 10 tumor cells. They were restricted to roughened cartilage surfaces which were due to the preparation of the tissue prior to explantation. Tumor cells or their cytoplasmic processes did not penetrate into the cartilaginous matrix. However, tumor cells or tumor nests were frequently observed within the nutrient cartilage canals which represent connective tissue invaginations containing blood vessels (39). At the growth plate, tumor cells reached only as far into the cartilage as the vascular loops extended to the area of the last hypertrophic chondrocyte and its calcified matrix (Fig. 10). These observations were the same as those in the biopsy specimen from the human osteosarcoma (Fig. 8).

In contrast to the cartilage, the bone explants, however, contained multiple osteosarcoma cell clusters. Tumor cells surrounded the bone spicules in a tight girdle of several cell layers and followed the contours of the bone surface (Fig. 11). Bone spicules surrounded by multiple cell layers or embedded in tumor cell clusters had rough and irregular surfaces similar to those observed in osteosarcoma specimens. This suggests that active erosion of the bone by osteosarcoma cells was occurring. No osteoclasts were observed in these explants nor in the numerous biopsies.

Osteosarcoma cells cultured in the presence of cartilage explants grew in multiple layers on the Millipore membrane, but failed to overgrow the mesenchymal cell outgrowth from cartilage. There was no evidence of mixing or interdigitating of the two cell types. In contrast, control fibroblasts growing on the membrane adjacent to the explants intermingled with and became morphologically indistinguishable from the outgrowing cartilaginous cells. After immediate removal of explants, areas on the membrane previously occupied by the cartilage explants were practically devoid of osteosarcoma cells (Fig. 12). At the border of these areas of "no growth", cells grew together to lower densities and several osteosarcoma cells appeared necrotic. In contrast, areas where bone explants had been cultured, cells grew beneath the explants, although their density was somewhat less than that outside the explant.

In some experiments, osteosarcoma cells were cultured after the explant was removed. Areas where the cartilage explants were originally positioned on the Millipore membrane resisted overgrowth with tumor cells for approximately 5 days. In contrast, human foreskin fibroblasts immmediately overgrew these areas and covered them with a continous monolayer. In some experiments, where osteosarcoma cells were cultured in the

Figs. 10 & 11: Human osteosarcoma cells (TE-85) were cultured
                in the presence of human rib costochondral junctions.

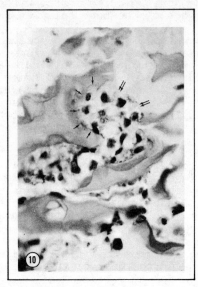

Fig. 10: Calcified cartilage of the growth plate and bone are
          both eroded by tumor cell clusters (single arrow).
          Uncalcified cartilage resists tumor invasion (double
          arrow). (H&E, x 450)

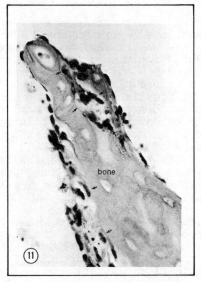

Fig. 11: Osteosarcoma cells are in intimate contact with a
          bone spicule. Surface irregularities and a deep
          invagination (arrows) suggest bone resorption by
          tumor cells. Osteoclasts are absent. (H&E, x380)

presence of cartilage explanted directly onto the stainless
steel grids, the bottom of the Petri dish directly underneath
the cartilage explant was found to be devoid of osteosarcoma
cells. Upon removal of the cartilage explant, this zone of "no
growth" was overgrown within 5 days (39). No such effect was
observed beneath bone explants or if human foreskin fibroblasts
were cultured in the presence of either cartilage or bone.

These morphological data provide evidence that bone spicules
from both explants and biopsies of osteogenic sarcoma were eroded by osteosarcoma cells, whereas cartilage was able to resist
the invasion by osteosarcoma cells. Osteosarcoma cells infil-
trated the cartilage matrix only to areas which were originally
occupied by vascularized mesenchyme (capillary loops at the
growth plate (40); nutrient cartilage canals (2)). Inhibition
of tumor cell growth underneath the explant and on the bottom
of the Petri dish and the delayed outgrowth into membrane areas
previously occupied by cartilage explants suggest that the cartilage explants release substances which inhibit growth and
proliferation of the tumor cells. These observations lead to
the possible conclusion that the inability of tumor cells to
penetrate cartilage is not due to a physical barrier provided
by the tissue matrix against the invading cells but rather to
molecular anti-invasion factor(s) (AIF) which prohibits the degradative process of invasion. Whether or not this anti-tumor-
invasion factor is identical to the extractable material (AIF)
from cartilage which inhibits endothelial cell proliferation
and osteoclastic function is currently under investigation.

c) Experimental alterations of cartilage and tumor cells
    to "induce" cartilage invasion.

In previous studies we have shown that chemically altered
hyaline cartilage loses its resistance to invasion by endothelial
cells (5). This phenomenon was explained by the extraction of
the anti-invasive factor (AIF) from the cartilage which was
found to inhibit collagenolytic activity secreted by endothelial
cells. The release of this enzyme activity was enhanced when
endothelial cells were stimulated with heparin in vitro (25).
Therefore, we stimulated tumor cells with heparin and co-cultured them with altered hyaline cartilage explants from human ribs.
The cartilage explants were extracted with 1M GuHCl as described.
Normal (living) or extracted (devitalized) explants were cultured in a) medium (RPMI-1640) supplemented with 10% fetal calf
serum (FCS), b) serum-free medium, c) medium supplemented
with 10% FCS and 50 U heparin/ml, and d) the serum free medium
supplemented with 50 U heparin/ml. After the initial culture
period of 2 days, human foreskin fibroblasts, osteosarcoma
cells (TE-85) or metastatic mammary carcinoma cells (ALAB) were
added to some organ cultures and cultured for an additional 5
days. Other cultures where no cells were added served as control.

Histologic examination of control and extracted explants
indicated that the various media combinations had no significant
effects on their morphology. In control (living) explants, the

cartilage appeared well preserved; in the extracted explants (devitalized), a peripheral rim of decreased stainability, surface irregularities and increased numbers of necrotic chrondrocytes were observed. In the presence of osteosarcoma cells or mammary carcinoma cells, control explants were covered with numerous often confluent tumor cell clusters only when the culture medium was supplemented with heparin (Fig. 13). They contained only few clusters of tumor cells when heparin was absent. No evidence of invasion was detected in either case. Similar effects were observed when the explants were devitalized by sequential freezing and thawing prior to explantation. These data thus are similar to those obtained with devitalized cartilage on the CAM (4). Increased tumor cell densities, however, were observed when the normal control explants were replaced by extracted cartilage (Fig. 14). Here, especially in the presence of heparin, tumor cells clearly invaded the loosened peripheral tissue of the extracted explants. This effect was most pronounced when both heparin and serum were present in the medium (Fig. 15).

Our observations indicate that heparin may stimulate tumor cells to yield an increased attachment to cartilage, a tissue which otherwise inhibited the attachment of these cells. In addition, mildly extracted cartilage from which only small amounts of proteoglycans but the majority of the low molecular weight proteins (AIF) including the protease inhibitor have been removed (19) and which became devitalized in the process also became more susceptible to invasion by heparin stimulated tumor cells. It is likely, therefore, that heparin stimulates tumor cells to secrete enough collagenase to exhaust the inhibitory system present in the living tissue. In extracted cartilage we assume that both the absence of the protease inhibitor and the inability of the cells to re-synthesize it as well as the heparin stimulated collagenase release are responsible for increased susceptibility of the tissue matrix to tumor invasion.

CONCLUSIONS

In this report we propose that the naturally occurring resistance of cartilage to both physiologic invasion (vascular penetration) and pathologic invasion (tumor invasion) is, at least in part, due to a protease-collagenase inhibitor which seems to be a component of cartilage matrix. This collagenase inhibitor is of low molecular weight, synthesized and secreted by chondrocytes, and has been proven in vitro to be a part of a system that effectively restricts invasion by both endothelial and tumor cells. In this system of relative resistance to invasion, selective growth inhibition of invasive cells by a cartilage-derived anti-invasion factor (AIF) may well play an important role. The observation that potentially invasive cells can be stimulated by heparin to release collagenase and therefore become invasive may also be physiologically important. With respect to the invasive mechanism(s), our results lead to new emphasis upon the physiologic role of the mast cell in these processes.

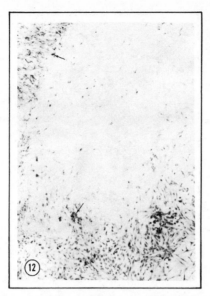

Fig. 12: Millipore membrane area previously occupied by a
          cartilage explant for 10 days is devoid of osteosar-
          coma cells. At the border to the area of "no growth",
          tumor cells grow together to different densities,
          whereby few osteosarcoma cells appear necrotic
          (arrow). (H&E, x60)

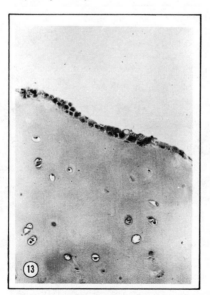

Fig. 13: In the presence of heparin, a normal cartilage ex-
          plant is covered with a confluent sheet of ALAB
          metastatic mammary carcinoma cells. (H&E, x145)

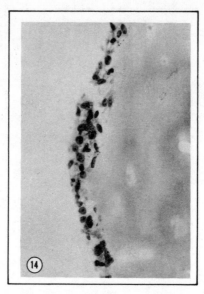

Fig. 14:   In the absence of heparin, numerous osteosarcoma
cells are piling on a roughened surface of a 1M
guanidinium hydrochloride extracted cartilage.   There
is no clear evidence of tumor cell invasion.   (H&E,
x240)

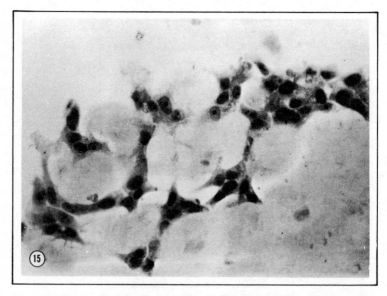

Fig. 15:   In the presence of heparin, ALAB metastatic mammary
carcinoma cells are invading the 1M guanidinium
hydrochloride extracted cartilage.   (H&E, x500)

Classically, neoplasms represent a group of cells (or tissue) that adopt a set of behavioral characteristics different than those of the tissue from which they arise. The main characteristics of this pattern are uncontrolled growth, invasiveness, and the potential to metastasize to distant sites. Singly, some of these characteristics may be expressed in processes involved in the "normal development" or "maintenance" of the organism. Alone none of these traits are pathognomonic for a malignant tumor. It is the total complement of characteristics that denotes the malignant neoplasm.

A major area in cancer biological research involves examination of mechanisms which permit malignant tumors to invade stroma and metastasize to distant sites in the body. There is considerable evidence that the invasive potential of tumors is determined by both the intrinsic properties of tumor cells and host factors such as tumor vascularization. Efforts by investigators to determine criteria which enable cells to become aggresive have been frustrated in part because of the multiplicity of tissue alterations which occur concomitantly in the course of malignant transformation and which may account for the essential properties of malignant growth.

With increased knowledge in DNA biochemistry most of the efforts to study and influence a malignant tissue have focused on the facets of uncontrolled, sometimes rapid growth and anaplasia. If one, however, reflects on various life processes, one can somewhat arbitrarily divide their normal manifestations into either developmental or homeostatic instances. Most current chemotherapeutic agents are directed at abnormal cell growth and/or proliferation. Considering adverse effects of these agents upon the rapidly dividing bone marrow and gut cells one realizes the importance of cell proliferation as a normal adult homeostatic process. Thus, intervention in malignancy at the level of cell growth and proliferation endangers processes needed for normal metabolism and survival of the host.

The ultimate pragmatic implications that our investigations hold for altering the natural history of malignancies remain to be known. Theoretically attractive, however, is the possibility of controlling local and metastatic tumor invasion. If one examines the specific normal instances of invasion, the vast majority of these are developmental and have occurred by early adulthood. Hence, invasion, except in certain instances as in wound healing and sperm penetration, is not as significant to homeostatic processes in the adult as cell proliferation. Thus, therapy directed at abnormal invasion may offer a more benign course for the afflicted invididual.

ACKNOWLEDGEMENTS

Appreciation is expressed to the following research assistants, who are presently involved with the research concerning the cartilage-derived inhibitor, Mr. L.W. Soble, Mr. R.L. Croxen, Mrs. A.F. Croxen and Mrs. M. Chow. Particular thanks is due to R. Eisenstein, M.D., without whose collaboration many of the initial investigations on vascular invasion and current concepts would never have developed. The authors also wish to thank J. Bastien, M.D., for his initial involvement in the tumor cell invasion work and A.M. Sadove, M.D., for his collaboration on the biochemical aspects of primary human mammary carcinoma invasion. The work on the normal and tumor collagenases and their inhibition would not have been possible without the extensive and close collaboration and cooperation of E. Harper, Ph.D., University of California at San Diego and his gradute student, J. Hiti. The authors also wish to thank Drs. V.C. Hascall, J. Galante, H. Sky-Peck and R. Weinstein for helpful discussions and advice during these investigations, and Dr. F. Wezeman for his critical review of this manuscript. The author is very greatful to Miss V. Hearon for preparation of the manuscript.

This work was supported by NIH grant CA-21566 and in part by NIH grants AM-09132, GRS-RR-05477 and CA-17086 and grants from the Illinois Chapter of the Arthritis Foundation and the Hulbert Fund, Rush Presbyterian St. Luke's Medical Center.

Mechanisms of Localized Bone Loss

REFERENCES

1. Foulds, L.: Neoplastic Development. Vol. 1, Academic Press, London and New York, pp. 106-112, 1969.

2. Wilsman, N.J., and Van Sickle, D.C. 1972. Cartilage Canals, Their Morphology and Distribution. Anat. Rec., 173: 79-94.

3. Zinkernagel, R. Riede, U., and Schenk, R. 1972. Ultrastrukturelle Untersuchungen der juxtaepiphysalen Kapillaren nach Perfusionsfixation. Experientia, 28: 1205-1206.

4. Eisenstein, R., Sorgente, N., Soble, L.W., Miller, A. and Kuettner, K.E. 1973. The Resistance of Certain Tissues to Invasion: Penetrability of Explanted Tissues by Vascularized Mesenchyme. Amer. J. Pathol., 73: 765-774.

5. Sorgente, N., Kuettner, K.E., Soble, L.W., and Eisenstein, R. 1975. The Resistance of Certain Tissues to Invasion. II. Evidence for Extractable Factors in Cartilage which Inhibit Invasion by Vascularized Mesenchyme. Lab. Invest., 32: 217-222.

6. Kuettner, K.E., Soble, L.W., Sorgente, N., and Eisenstein, R.: The Possible Role of Protease Inhibitors in Cartilage Metabolism. In: Protides of the Biological Fluids (Peeters, H., ed.). Vol. 23, Pergamon Press, Oxford, pp. 221-225, 1976.

7. Folkman, J., and Cotran, R.: Relation of Vascular Proliferation to Tumor Growth. In: International Review of Experimental Pathology, (Richter, G.W. and Epstein, M.A., eds.). Vol. 16, Academic Press, New York, pp. 207-248, 1976.

8. Brem, H., Arensman, R. and Folkman, J.: Inhibition of Tumor Angiogenesis by a Diffusible Factor from Cartilage. In: Extracellular Matrix Influences on Gene Expression, (Slavkin, H.C. and Greulich, R.C., eds.). Academic Press, New York, pp. 767-772, 1975.

9. Kaminski, M., Kaminska, G., Jakobisiak, M., and Brzezinski, W. 1977. Inhibition of Lymphocyte-Induced Angiogenisis by Isolated Chondrocytes. Nature, 268: 238-240.

10. Sorgente, N., Hascall, V.C., and Kuettner, K.E. 1972. Extractability of Lysozyme from Bovine Nasal Cartilage. Biochim, Biophys. Acta, 284: 441-450.

11. Kuettner, K.E., Pita, J.C., Howell, D.S., Sorgente, N. and Eisenstein, R.: Regulation of Epiphyseal Cartilage Maturation. In: Extracellular Matrix Influences on Gene Expression (Slavkin, H.C., and Greulich, R.C., eds.). Academic Press, New York, pp. 435-440, 1975.

12. Kuettner, K.E., Sorgente, N., and Eisenstein, R. 1975.

Lysozyme in Calcifying Tissues (A Review). Clin. Orthop. Rel. Res., 112: 316-339.

13. Schoefl, G.I. 1963. Studies on Inflammation. III. Growing Capillaries: Their Structure and Permeability. Virchows Arch. Pathol. Anat. Physiol. Klin. Med., 337: 97-141.

14. Schoefl, G.I. 1964. Electron Microscopic Observations on the Regeneration of Blood Vessels After Injury. Ann. N.Y. Acad. Sci., 116: 789-802.

15. Eisenstein, R., Kuettner, K.E., Neopolitan, C., Soble, L.W., and Sorgente, N. 1975. The Resistance of Certain Tissues To Invasion. III. Cartilage Extracts Inhibit and Growth of Fibroblasts and Endothelial Cells in Culture. Amer. J. Pathol., 81: 337-348.

16. Eisenstein, R., Sorgente, N., and Kuettner, K.E. 1975. Studies on Cartilage Vascularization. Ann. Rheum. Dis., 34: (supplement), 76.

17. Eisenstein, R., Kuettner, K.E., Soble, L.W., and Sorgente, N.: Tissue Inhibitors Are Cell Growth Regulations. In: Protides of the Biological Fluids (Peeters, H., ed.). Vol. 23, Pergamon Press, Oxford, pp. 217-219, 1976.

18. Tokes, Z.A. and Sorgente, N. 1976. Cell Surface-Associated and Released Proteolytic Activities of Bovine Aorta Endothelial Cells. Biochem. Biophys. Res. Comm., 73: 965-971.

19. Kuettner, K.E., Harper, E.J., and Eisenstein, R. 1977. Protease Inhibitors in Cartilage. Arthr. & Rheum., 20: (supplement), S124-S129.

20. Kuettner, K.E., Croxen, R.L., Eisenstein, R., and Sorgente, N. 1974. Proteinase Inhibitor Activity in Connective Tissues. Experientia, 30: 595-597.

21. Sharkey, M., Veis, A., and Kuettner, K.E. 1974. Isolation and Characterization of Dentinal Phosphoproteins. J. Dent. Res., 52: 301.

22. Sorgente, N., Kuettner, K.E., and Eisenstein, R.: The Isolation, Purification and Partial Characterization of Proteinase Inhibitors from Bovine Cartilage and Aorta. In: Protides of the Biological Fluids (Peeters, H., ed.). Vol. 23, Pergamon Press, Oxford, pp. 227-230, 1976.

23. Harper, E., Hiti, J., Kuettner, K.E., and Goodman, M. 1976. Inhibition of Collagenase Activity by a Proteinase Inhibitor Derived From Cartilage. Fed. Proc., 35: 1961.

24. Kuettner, K.E., Hiti, J., Eisenstein, R., and Harper, E. 1976. Collagenase Inhibition by Cationic Proteins Derived From Cartilage and Aorta. Biochem. Biophys. Res. Comm., 72: 40-46.

25. Kuettner, K.E., Soble, L., Croxen, R., Hiti, J., Harper, E., and Pauli, B. 1977. Inhibition of Tumor Collagenases by a Cartilage-Derived Inhibitor. Fed. Proc., 36: 2138.

26. Horton, J.E., Wezeman, F.H., and Kuettner, K.E.: Regulation of Osteoclast-Activating Factor (OAF)-Stimulated Bone Resorption In Vitro with an Inhibitor of Collagenase. In: Mechanisms of Localized Bone Loss, (Horton, J.E., Tarpley, Jr., T.M., and Davis, W.E., eds.). Information Retrieval Inc., Arlington, VA, (in press, 1978).

27. Horton, J.E., Wezeman, F.H., and Kuettner, K.E. (in press, 1978). Inhibition of In Vitro Bone Resorption by a Cartilage Derived Anti-Collagenase Factor. Science.

28. Bennet, G.A. Bones. In: Pathology, Sixth Edition, (Anderson, W.A.D., ed.). Vol. 2, C.V. Mosby Co., St. Louis, pp. 1684-1754, 1971.

29. Robbins, S.L. In: Pathologic Basis of Disease. W.B. Saunders Co., Philadelphia, London, Toronto, pp. 1452-1455, 1974.

30. McAllister, R.M., Gardner, M.B., Greene, A.E., Bradt, C., Nichols, W.W., and Landing, B.H. 1971. Cultivation in vitro of Cells Derived From a Human Osteosarcoma. Cancer, 27: 397-402.

31. Reed, M.V. and Gey, G.O. 1962. Cultivation of Normal and Malignant Human Lung Tissue. I. The Establishment of Three Adenocarcinoma Cell Strains. Lab. Invest., 11: 638-652.

32. Kuettner, K.E., Soble, L.W., Croxen, R.L., Marczynska, B., Hiti, J., and Harper, E. 1977. Tumor Cell Collagenase and Its Inhibition By a Cartilage Derived Protease Inhibitor. Science, 196: 653-654.

33. Werb, Z. and Burleigh, M.C. 1974. A Specific Collagenase From Rabbit Fibroblasts in Monolayer Culture. Biochem. J., 137: 373-385.

34. Goldhaber, P.: Bone Resorption Factors, Cofactors, and Giant Vacuole Osteoclasts in Tissue Culture. In: The Parathyroid Glands, (Gaillard, J.P., Talmage, R.V. and Budy, A.M., eds.). The University of Chicago Press, Chicago and London, pp. 153-171, 1965.

35. Kaufman, E.J., Glimcher, M.J., Mechanic, G.L., and Goldhaber, P. 1965. Collagenolytic Activity During Active Bone Resorption in Tissue Culture. Proc. Soc. Exp. Biol. Med., 120: 632-637.

36. Sakamoto, S., Sakamoto, M., Goldhaber, P., and Glimcher, M. 1975. Collagenase and Bone Resorption: Isolation of

Collagenase From Culture Medium Containing Serum After Stimulation of Bone Resorption by Addition of Parathyroid Hormone Extract. Biochem. Biophys. Res. Comm., 63: 172-178.

37. Ozzello and Speer, F.D. 1958. The Mucopolysaccharides in the Normal and Diseased Breast. Their Distribution and Significance. Amer. J. Pathol., 34: 993-1009.

38. Sadove, A.M., and Kuettner, K.E.: Inhibition of Mammary Carcinoma Invasiveness with Cartilage-Derived Inhibitor. In: Surgical Forum, (Schulenberg, R.M., ed.). Vol. 28, The American College of Surgeons, Chicago, pp. 449-501, 1977.

39. Kuettner, K.E., Pauli, B.U., and Soble, L.W. (in press, Feb., 1978). Morphologic Studies on the Resistance of Cartilage to Invasion by Osteosarcoma Cells In Vitro and In Vivo. Cancer Research.

40. Moss-Salentijn, A.G.M.: The Epiphyseal Vascularization of Growth Plates. A Development Study in Rabbits. Rijks Universitet, Utrecht. Dept. of Cell Biol, Doctoral Dissertation, 1976.

Immunologically Mediated Bone Resorption in Periodontal Disease.

Mirdza E. Neiders and Russell J. Nisengard

Departments of Oral Pathology, Periodontics and Microbiology, School of Dentistry and Medicine, SUNY at Buffalo, Buffalo, N.Y. 14214

INTRODUCTION

Chronic inflammatory periodontal disease is a progressive disease that involves the supporting structures of teeth. Clinically, it is characterized by inflammation of gingival tissues followed by the detachment of periodontal tissues from teeth and loss of bone. The progress of the disease is slow, however, it is the major cause for loss of teeth after forty. (1)

Histologically, Page and Schroeder (2) have divided periodontal disease in four stages: initial, early, established and advanced lesions. This is useful for considering the extent of involvement and the characteristics of the pathological process. In the initial stages, the involvement consisting of vasculitis and minimal lymphocytic infiltrate is restricted to tissues adjacent to junctional epithelium. (3) The early lesion is characterized by a dense lymphoid cell infiltrate. The lymphoid cells make up approximately 75% of the total infiltrate and immunoblasts appear throughout the inflammation. Collagen loss is more extensive than in the initial lesion. (3-5) The established lesion is characterized by the appearance of plasma cells that eventually predominate in the inflammatory infiltrate. (6) The predominant immunoglobulin in the plasma cells is IgG. A small number of cells contain IgA, and cells containing IgM and IgE are rare. (7,8)

Clinically, the initial, early and established lesions represent stages of progressive inflammation limited to the gingiva surrounding the teeth and, therefore, can be designated as gingivitis. The damage produced during gingivitis is minimal and usually reversible. Treatment produces resolution of inflammation with minimal or no loss in the gingival contour.

The advanced lesion is characterized by inflammation extending into the periodontal ligament and alveolar bone. Clinically, the advanced lesion represents periodontitis. Epithelial proliferation and subsequent detachment of periodontal tissues produces periodontal pockets, which may ulcerate and suppurate. The extension of inflammation in bone is associated with bone resorption. Progressive involvement may require extraction of teeth due to abscess formation or excessive mobility of teeth. Treatment at any stage prior to extraction may arrest the disease, but regeneration of lost tissue is minimal. (9,10)

BONE RESORPTION

Loss of alveolar bone is considered to be the most critical aspect of inflammatory periodontal disease with regard to tooth loss. (11) The bone loss is usually evaluated clinically on radiographic examination. Bone loss is considered to be present when the alveolar crest is found to be more than 1 mm. from the cementoenamel junction. (12) The determination of bone loss on histologic examination is also based on comparing the height of alveolar crest with the height that would be present in normal disease-free individuals.

Studies on progress and mechanisms of bone loss in human inflammatory disease have been limited because specimens can be obtained only at autopsy or at surgical resection. It has been demonstrated that in the advance lesion, the inflammatory exudate extends along blood vessels into bone marrow. (13-15) Loss of bone is first seen in the marrow spaces of the alveolar crest. (15) The resorption eventually results in either a horizontal decrease of alveolar crest or in a wide variety of defects adjacent to the root of the tooth. (1) Histologic examination of specimens with bone loss may show active osteoclastic resorption. (16-19) In other instances, active bone resorption cannot be demonstrated, but only loss of alveolar bone height or decrease in the number of bone trabeculae. (20-21) It can therefore be concluded that once osteoclastic resorption is initiated, it is not continuous, but may undergo periods of remission.

While the conditions that promote osteoclastic resorption are not known, it usually occurs in proximity to inflammatory infiltrates. (18,19,22) Correlation of osteoclastic resorption or remission of resorption with the degree and/or the type of inflammatory cell infiltrate has not yet been made.

While the progress from initial to early lesion, and early lesion to established lesion is well documented, (3,6) such progression cannot be easily demonstrated for the progress of the established lesion to advanced lesion. (2) It appears that at least in some cases, the extension of inflammation in the underlying tissue does not occur for a long time. This observation has led to speculation that progress to advanced lesions may be due to differences in host response or changes in the etiologic agent. (2) The evidence supporting the progression of the established lesion into advanced lesion is that pocket formation and bone loss usually are associated with involvement of the gingiva. Also, the inflammatory infiltrate of the advanced lesion is similar to the inflammatory infiltrate of the established lesion. In addition, extended studies in animals have shown that an established lesion is followed by bone loss. (23,24)

ETIOLOGY OF PERIODONTAL DISEASE

There is abundant evidence implicating microorganisms as the primary etiologic agent in chronic inflammatory disease of gingiva. (25-29) Epidemilogical studies have correlated the presence of microbial plaque on teeth with the inflammation of the gingiva. (30) Withdrawal of oral hygiene measures in healthy persons with clinically normal gingivae which allows microbial plaque accumulation results in the development of marginal gingivitis. (3,6,31-33) Removal of plaque with re-institution of oral hygiene (34) or with bacteriocidal agents (35) results in the resolution of the gingival inflammation. The association of plaque deposition on clean teeth and the production of gingival inflammation has also been demonstrated in monkeys (36,37) and the beagle dog. (38)

The relationship between microorganisms and the advanced lesions cannot be as readily demonstrated as in gingivitis. In cross-sectional epidemiological studies, the severity of alveolar bone loss has been correlated with the decreasing efficiency in maintaining teeth free of microbial deposits. (12) It has been shown in longitudinal studies, that good oral hygiene may retard or arrest bone loss in man. (9,10,39-41) Bone regeneration has been observed if meticulous oral hygiene is maintained after surgical treatment. (42,43) Bone loss will occur in dogs if plaque is allowed to deposit, and this loss can be retarded with maintaining good oral hygiene. (24,44)

Another group of studies that associate bacteria with bone loss are the studies on induction of periodontal disease in gnotobiotic animals with organisms isolated from the oral cavity. (45-47) Extensive bone destruction occurs around teeth. Although it has been speculated that this bone may not be mediated by osteoclasts, (48) other studies clearly indicate that resorption in this model is mediated by osteoclasts. (49,50)

IMMUNOLOGIC MECHANISMS IN PERIODONTAL DISEASE

Recent reviews document evidence implicating immunological responses in periodontal disease. (8,51-54) Hypersensitivity reactions mediated by antibodies to microorganisms or cells sensitized by microbial antigens may produce tissue damage. (55-58) Such damage may also occur in periodontal disease. The classical hypersensitivity reactions include immediate hypersensitivity, Arthus reaction and delayed hypersensitivity. (59)

Diverse approaches have been used to demonstrate the role of immunological mechanisms in periodontal disease. Some of the approaches will be discussed in the next sections.

Humoral and cellular responses to oral microorganisms.

Presence of antibody to oral bacteria has been demonstrated by investigating antibody titers to oral microorganisms. (60-64)

The increase of antibody titers may be related to the increase in the severity of periodontal disease, (61,62,64) but this is not always the rule. (63) Some of the antibodies are produced locally in the gingival tissues. (65) Therefore, it appears that at least some of the immunoglobulin seen in plasma cells infiltrating the gingival tissues (8) may be specific for antigens of oral microorganisms. These antibodies may be protective in the pathogenesis of periodontal disease (66) but they also may participate in local immediate hypersensitivity or Arthus reactions.

Lymphocytes obtained from individuals with periodontal disease show a blastogenic response with plaque or antigens derived from plaque microorganisms, (67-71) indicating previous sensitization to these antigens. (72) It has been possible to make some correlation between the increased blastogenic response to preparations of plaque and severity of periodontal disease. (68,73) In addition, supernatants of antigen-stimulted cultures contain a variety of lymphokines including macrophage inhibition factor, lymphotoxin and monocyte chemotactic factor. (74-76) These soluble products are thought to mediate the local events of cell-mediated immunity. (77,78) Products released from sensitized cells following antigen stimulation may mediate tissue destruction seen in periodontal disease.

Hypersensitivity reactions to oral microorganisms.

Studies that indicate that oral microorganisms elicit hypersensitivity in patients with periodontal disease are few. Immediate hypersensitivity and delayed hypersensitivity have been demonstrated in humans with an extract of Actinomyces using skin tests. (79) A statistically significant correlation was found between the incidence of immediate hypersensitivity and severity of periodontal disease. Skin testing with extracts of three other organisms has also shown the presence of immediate hypersensitivity in patients with periodontal disease. (80) Immediate hypersensitivity has also been demonstrated to sonicated gingival plaque in 3 out of 5 periodontitis patients by passive cutaneous anaphylaxis reactions in monkeys. (81)

The testing of hypersensitivity reactions to oral microorganisms has not been extensive. This may be partially due to the inability to select the proper microorganisms for testing. Although there is evidence that the etiologic agent in periodontal disease is microbial plaque, the pathogenic microorganism or microorganisms have not yet been identified. (29)

Experimental induction of hypersensitivity reactions.

A number of studies have compared experimentally-induced hypersensitivity reactions in periodontal tissues to the pathological changes seen in human periodontal disease.

Early studies demonstrated that hypersensitivity reactions

of Arthus or delayed hypersensitivity type can be induced in the oral mucosa of guinea pigs and hamsters. (82-85)

The role of local hypersensitivity in periodontal disease was considered by Rizzo and Mergenhagen. (86) They demonstrated similarities between the inflammatory cell infiltrate in human periodontal disease (established or advanced lesion) and that seen in the gingiva of sensitized rabbits challenged with antigen five days prior to sacrifice. This infiltrate consisted of lymphocytes and plasma cells. The relatively late appearance of plasma cells in hypersensitivity reactions and their increase in number with subsequent challenges was documented. In a later study, (87) it was demonstrated that sensitization can occur by repeated deposition of antigen in the gingival sulcus. The observations in these two studies suggested that microbial antigens may also sensitize the animal via the gingival sulcus, and that subsequent challenge may produce a cellular infiltrate similar to periodontal disease. Therefore, studies on hypersensitivity reactions in gingiva appear relevant to periodontal disease.

Ranney and Zander (88) studied hypersensitivity reactions produced by sensitizing squirrel monkeys with subcutaneous injections of ovalbumin emulsified with complete Freund's adjuvant. Antigenic challenge in these animals yielded predominantly an Arthus-type reaction. Animals challenged with multiple doses of antigen in the gingival sulcus produced an infiltrate of lymphocytes and plasma cells that was similar to the established lesion in human periodontal disease.

Reactions predominantly of the delayed hypersensitivity type show small numbers of plasma cells when examined 3 or 6 days after beginning daily challenges. (89) When specimens are taken from monkeys 48 hours after challenge, only a few plasma cells are seen. (90) Since this infiltrate resembles the early lesion in periodontal disease, it has been concluded that it is unlikely that delayed hypersensitivity reactions play a significant role in the advanced stages of periodontal disease. (90) This conclusion is premature because the study did not evaluate the cellular infiltrate at longer intervals after challenge with antigen or following repeated challenges of sensitized animals.

More extensive studies are needed to determine the possible role of a particular type of hypersensitivity reaction in the various stages of periodontal disease.

BONE RESORPTION IN EXPERIMENTAL PERIODONTITIS INDUCED BY HYPERSENSITIVITY REACTIONS

A series of studies were undertaken to investigate the bone changes associated with classical hypersensitivity reactions: Arthus-type reactions, immediate hypersensitivity and delayed hypersensitivity. The experimental animal in all these studies was the Rhesus monkey (Macaca mulatta). Antigen in the sensitized animal was administered by injection to assure proximity of the hypersensitivity reaction to bone and challenge with a known amount of antigen. The bone changes were evaluated by routine histologic techniques.

Arthus-type reactions.

Monkeys were sensitized with crystalline bovine serum albumin (BSA, Armour Pharmaceutical Company) and crystalline egg albumin (OA, Pfalz and Bauer, Inc., Flushing, NY.) using multiple intradermal injections of 1 mg. of antigen with complete Freund's adjuvant once a week for 14 weeks. (91)

The hypersensitivity induced in the monkey was classified as Arthus reaction because: 1. the antibody titers to homologous immunizing antigen were high; 2. skin test reactions were maximal 8 hours after challenge; 3. histopathology of skin test biopsies were similar to Arthus reaction; 4. immunofluorescent tests for localization of IgG and C4 revealed maximum perivascular deposits 4 to 8 hours after challenge.

The gingival challenge was administered by injections of 1, 10 or 100 μg of the homologous sensitizing antigen in the dental papilla. Control sites received 100 μg of the heterologous antigen. Monkeys were sacrificed 72 hours after gingival injection.

Examination of decalcified tissues revealed that injections with 10 or 100 μg of homologous sensitizing antigen produced chronic inflammatory response, while 1 μg of homologous antigen or 100 μg of heterologous antigen did not produce inflammatory changes. Bone resorption was evident in specimens that showed chronic inflammatory infiltrate (Fig. 1). This bone resorption was seen in the marrow spaces that showed sparce infiltration with inflammatory cells.

Reverse passive Arthus reactions can also elicit osteoclastic bone resorption. (92) Monkey antisera to BSA and OA were injected in gingival papilla in doses of 4,8 and 16 units in 0.02 ml of antisera and following intravenous administration of 5,000 mg. of BSA. The gingival sites were injected once a day for one, four and seven consecutive days prior to sacrifice at various times after injection.

Inflammatory response was noted in specimens challenged with anti-BSA and not with anti-OA. A significant increase in the numbers of osteoclasts was noted in sites receiving single or multiple injections three days after the last challenge with BSA (Table 1). The optimum time for demonstration of osteoclasts was 3 or 4 days after challenge (Table 2).

The above studies demonstrate that direct and reverse passive Arthus reactions elicited in gingiva can produce an increase in osteoclastic activity. These observations may correspond to reports on bone resorption in vitro by antigen-antibody complexes. Fell et al. (93) demonstrated an increase

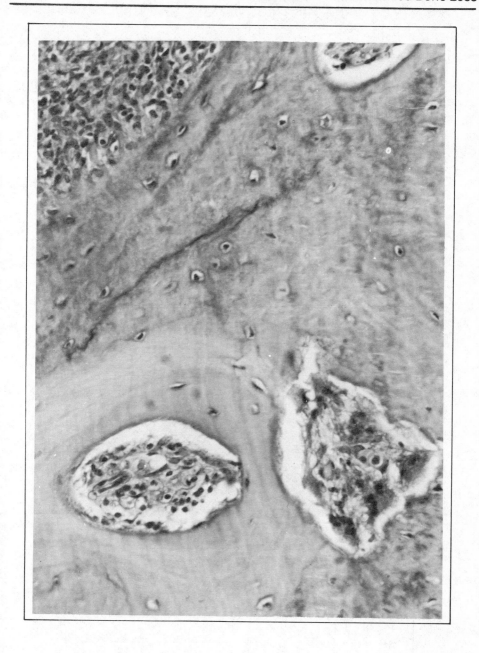

Fig. 1 Arthus reaction. Bone resorption seen in the marrow cavity of alveolar process of a monkey that was sensitized with BSA and challenged with 100 μg of BSA, 72 hours prior to sacrifice. 250X, Hematoxylin and eosin.

Table 1

REVERSE PASSIVE ARTHUS REACTION

Average number of osteoclasts observed in the alveolar crest of monkeys receiving 5000 mg. of BSA systemically, challenged with multiple doses of antisera or PBS in gingiva and sacrificed 3 days after last injection.[1]

Number of Injections[2]	Challenging Solution			
	Anti-BSA		Anti-OA	PBS
	8 U/ml[3]	4 U/ml[3]	8 U/ml[3]	
1	5.3 ± 2.0[4]	2.2 ± 2.6	0	0.3 + 0.9
4	4.2 ± 2.6	1.9 ± 0.4	0	0.5 ± 0.7
7	5.8 ± 2.0	5.7 ± 2.8	0	1.1 ± 0.2

1. Adapted from Asaro, et al.[(92)]

2. .02 ml of antisera or PBS were injected in the gingival tissue overlying the alveolar bone daily for number of times specified.

3. Units of antiserum per ml. Units were determined as outlined by Beutner, et al.[(99)]

4. Number of osteoclasts ± standard deviation in 6-18 sections in an area extending 10 mm. from base of soft tissue inflammation into bone.

Table 2

REVERSE PASSIVE ARTHUS REACTION

Average number of osteoclasts ± standard deviation observed in the alveolar crest of monkeys receiving 5000 mg of BSA systemically, challenged with a single dose of 8 units of antisera and sacrificed at various times after injection.[1]

Days of Examination of Specimen[2]	Challenge	
	Anti-BSA	Anti-OA
1	0[3]	3.3 ± 4.4
2	2.5 ± 2.9	0
3	10.3 ± 2.5	1.2 ± 1.5
4	9.0 ± 2.5	0
5	1.2 ± 1.5	0

1. Adapted from Asaro, et al.[(92)]
2. The number of days between the challenge and sacrifice of the animal.
3. Number of osteoclasts ± standard deviation in 6-18 sections in one area extending 10 mm. from base of soft tissue inflammation into bone.

of osteoclasts in explants of chick bone incubated with anti-Forssman antibodies. Hausman et al.(94) has demonstrated increased resorption of bone explants after incubation with antigen-antibody precipitates. Examination of histologic sections from Arthus reactions cannot determine whether the bone resorption is mediated directly by antigen-antibody complexes and the inflammatory cells are an innocent bystander or that the inflammatory cells mediate osteoclast formation. (95)

Immediate Hypersensitivity.

Immediate hypersensitivity was induced by sensitizing monkeys with the enzyme Nova alcalase. (96) Immediate hypersensitivity was verified by positive Prausnite-Kustner test, histamine release by antigenic challenge of leukocytes and gingiva from sensitized monkeys, and histamine release from passively sensitized rat mast cells following antigenic challenge. Gingival challenge consisted of injections of 0.1 to 10 μg of antigen daily for 1,3,5 or 7 consecutive days. Animals were sacrificed one to ten days after the last injection.

The inflammatory infiltrate in the gingival specimens after multiple injections consisted of chronic inflammatory cells, primarily lymphocytes and plasma cells. Increased numbers of osteoclasts were not seen in these specimens, regardless of whether the specimens were taken early (1 day) or later (3,5, or 7 days) after the last challenge with antigen. The findings within this model system suggest that multiple immediate hypersensitivity reactions may be responsible for soft tissue changes seen in periodontal disease, but do not play a role in the formation of osteoclasts.

Delayed hypersensitivity.

Delayed hypersensitivity was induced in monkeys by a series of three intradermal injections of 0.1 ml of a commercial preparation of Bacillus Calmette-Guerin vaccine (BCG, Parke-Davis, Detroit, Mich.) over a period of five weeks. The specificity of this sensitization was determined by skin testing with veterinary Old Tuberculin (OT, Department of Agriculture, Albany, N. Y.) and histologic examination of skin biopsy sites at 48 hours. The gingival tissues of sensitized animals were challenged with 0.1 ml of OT repeatedly injected 1 or 5 times a week for 1 to 7 weeks. Papilla injected with phosphate buffered saline (PBS) were used as controls. The animals were sacrificed 5,7 or 10 days after receiving the last injection.

Decalcified sections showed a mononuclear cell infiltrate in all specimens, except those sites injected once a week for less than 5 weeks. The inflammatory infiltrate showed either a perivascular distribution or was diffuse. The perivascular distribution was most often seen in the connective tissue overlying the periosteum. The diffuse pattern was the predominant type of inflammation seen within the marrow cavities of bone. Osteoclastic bone resorption was seen in all specimens injected 5 times for 1 week with the last injection 5 days prior to sacrifice (Fig. 2 and 3). If the specimens were sacrificed 10 days after the last injection, osteoclastic activity was absent. Bone formation was extensive in specimens that received 5 injections of OT. per week for 5 weeks or one injection for 7 weeks (Fig. 4 and 5). The histologic observations in specimens injected 5 times a week are summarized in Table 3.

Levy et al.(97) have also investigated the role of delayed hypersensitivity in alveolar bone loss. Massive bone loss was seen in specimens 21 and 30 days after challenge of sensitized monkeys with complete Freund's adjuvant. Direct comparisons between our studies and this study cannot be made because differences exist in the antigen preparation, frequency of administration of the challenging antigen and time of examination of specimens after challenge. However, as in our study, bone resorption and regeneration was seen in Rhesus monkeys associated with delayed hypersensitivity reactions.

Supernatants of mononuclear cells from periodontal patients stimulated by plaque antigens contain a bone resorbing activity, the osteoclast activating factor. (98) This factor induces formation of osteoclasts in fetal bones in vitro. The formation of osteoclasts in delayed hypersensitivity may be mediated by products released from sensitized cells.

CONCLUSIONS

The chronic cell infiltrate described in periodontal disease consists of lymphocytes, plasma cells and macrophages. Such inflammatory cell infiltrates are also seen in the gingiva with experimentally-induced hypersensitivity reactions. As examined with light microscopy, the inflammatory infiltrates of Arthus reaction 3 days after challenge and immediate and delayed hypersensitivity after multiple challenges appear remarkably similar. However, this type of inflammatory infiltrate is associated with osteoclast formation only in Arthus reactions and delayed hypersensitivity.

Several questions concerning the relationship between the inflammatory cell infiltrate and osteoclast formation in localized inflammatory lesions cannot yet be resolved.

First, it cannot be determined whether osteoclast formation is in all instances mediated by inflammatory cells in the area. Page and Schroeder (2) refer to studies in which bone resorption occurs some distance from the inflammatory cell infiltrate. It is feasible that some types of etiologic agents or biologic products stimulate osteoclast production directly. (95) The inflammatory cell infiltrate seen may only represent the connective tissue reaction to the etiologic agent and may not be involved in the osteoclast formation.

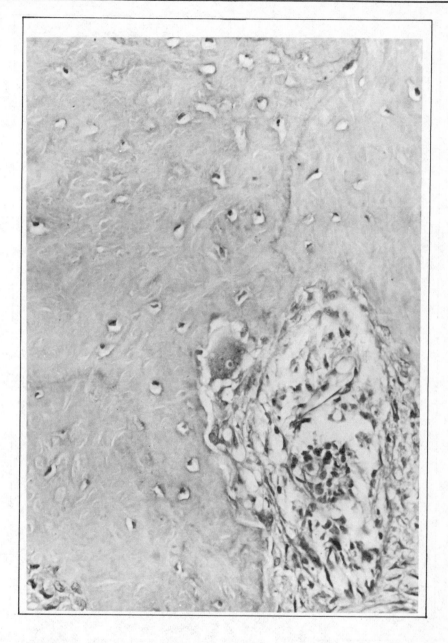

Fig. 2 Delayed hypersensitivity. Bone resorption in the
marrow cavity of the alveolar process of anterior maxilla
of a monkey that was sensitized with BCG and challenged
5 times a week with OT for one week. The animal was
sacrificed 5 days after last challenge. 250X, Hematoxylin and eosin.

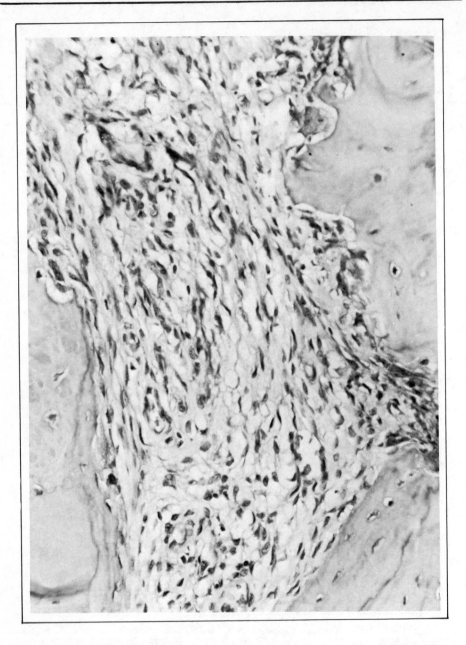

Fig. 3 Delayed hypersensitivity. Bone resorption seen in the
marrow cavity of the alveolar process in the posterior
mandible of a monkey that was sensitized with BCG and
challenged with OT 5 times a week for 1 week. The animal
was sacrificed 5 days after last challenge. 250X,
Hematoxylin and eosin.

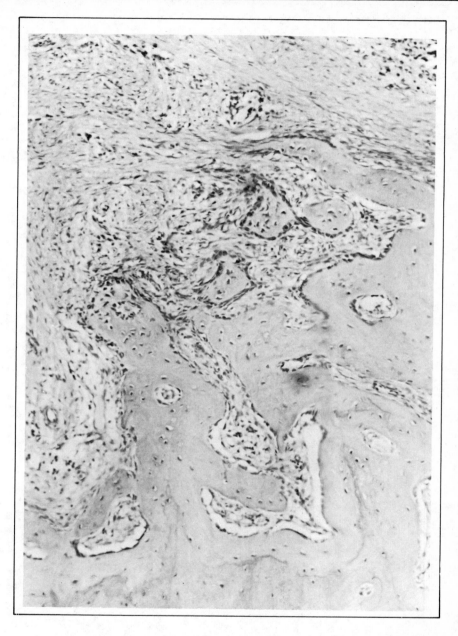

Fig. 4 Delayed hypersensitivity. Bone formation on the alveolar crest of a monkey that was sensitized with BCG and
challenged of OT 5 times a week for 5 weeks. The animal
was sacrificed 10 days after last challenge. Irregular
trabeculae of bone are surrounded by osteoblasts. 100X,
Hematoxylin and eosin.

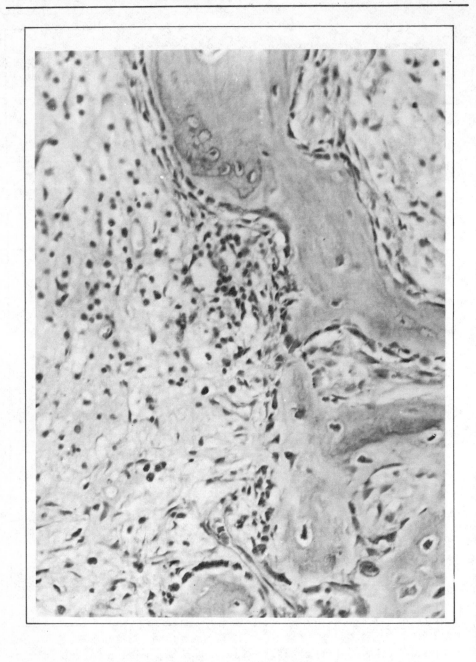

Fig. 5 Delayed hypersensitivity. Bone formation on the
alveolar crest of the posterior maxilla of a monkey that
was sensitized with BCG and challenged with OT 5 times
a week for 5 weeks. The animal was sacrificed 10 days
after last challenge. 250X, Hematoxylin and eosin.

Table 3

DELAYED HYPERSENSITIVITY

Tissue reactions in monkeys sensitized with BCG, injected in gingiva with
0.1 ml. of OT five times a week for 1 or 5 weeks and sacrificed 5 or 10
days after challenge.[1]

Number of Weeks Injected	Days Between Challenge and Sacrifice	Inflammation[2]	Bone Resorption[3]	Bone Regeneration[4]
1	5	++	+++	+
1	10	+	0	0
5	5	+++	0	+++
5	10	++	0	+++

1. Neiders, et al., unpublished data.

2. Inflammation was scored using the following scale: 0 = no inflammation; + = inflammation in the connective tissue overlying the alveolar
   process; ++ = inflammation extending into marrow spaces; +++ = similar
   to ++ but more dense in character.

3. Bone resorption was scored: 0 = same number of osteoclasts as seen in
   PBS controls; +++ = resorption involving large areas with erosion of
   normal cortical or trabecular architecture.

4. Bone regeneration was scored: 0 = same amount of osteoblastic activity
   as seen in normal or PBS injected specimens; + = increased number of
   osteoblasts lining existing trabeculae; +++ = extensive formation of
   new bone on surface of cortical outlines of the alveolar process.

Second, if inflammatory cells mediate bone resorption, the type of cell or cells which are of primary importance in the bone resorption in vivo have not yet been identified. In the experimentally-induced hypersensitivity reactions, a mixed chronic cell infiltrate was associated with bone resorption. In other studies, bone resorption has been reported to occur in proximity to an acute inflammatory cell infiltrate. (100) It is quite possible that several inflammatory cell types have the potential to mediate bone resorption in vivo. Thus, B and T-cells may mediate resorption by osteoclast activating factor. (101) Macrophages produce a considerable amount of prostaglandin (102) and prostaglandin has been shown to produce bone resorption. (103) In addition, there may be other substances produced by inflammatory cells that induce osteoclast formation not yet described. It is quite likely that the agents that mediate osteoclast formation are not the same in all experimentally induced periodontal disease models. In addition, many mechanisms may operate simultaneously or singly at various stages in naturally occurring periodontal disease.

Third, it cannot be determined what differences exist between the inflammatory cell infiltrates that are associated with bone resorption and those that are not associated with bone resorption. The chronic inflammatory cell infiltrate seen in multiple immediate hypersensitivity reactions did not differ significantly from reactions that were associated with bone resorption. Careful analysis of cell types involved in the various hypersensitivity reactions may reveal subtle differences between the inflammatory cell infiltrate. It may be that analysis of cell types in the proximity of bone will give some insight not only into the relevence of the experimental models, but also into human periodontal disease. This may help identify the characteristics of established lesions in periodontal disease that progress to advanced lesions and those that do not. (2)

Another point of interest in the studies on immunological mechanisms of bone loss is the time interval at which osteoclasts can be demonstrated after challenge. In Arthus reactions the optimum time for demonstrating the osteoclasts was 3 to 4 days after challenge. Osteoclasts were observed 5 days after challenge in delayed hypersensitivity, but not at 7 or 10 days. Studies on mechanical injury to bone, such as extraction (104) demonstrate that osteoclasts are abundant 3 days after surgery.

At the present time, we do not have any information about whether the kinetics of the osteoclast appearance is different in Arthus reactions or delayed hypersensitivity. In addition, it is not known whether the osteoclast appearance in vivo after mechanical trauma or following injection of various biological substances, antigens, or chemicals differs from immunologically-mediated bone resorption. Studies that are designed to test the osteoclast formation in vivo by particular agents, therefore, cannot yet be designed using a single examination period after administration of the test agent. Lack of osteoclast presence may only indicate that the examination of tissue was done too early or too late.

The experimental periodontitis models described in the presented studies may be useful in further elucidation of inflammatory cell and osteoclast interactions, as well as the study of osteoclast kinetics in vivo.

Abbreviations:

BSA	Bovine serum albumin
OV	Egg albumin
BCG	Bacillus Calmette-Guerin
OT	Old tuberculin
PBS	Phosphate buffered saline

REFERENCES

1. Manson, J.D. 1976. Bone morphology and bone loss in periodontal disease. J. Clin. Periodont., 3, 14-22.

2. Page, R.C. and Schroeder, H.E. 1976. Pathogenesis of inflammatory periodontal disease. Lab. Invest., 33, 235-249.

3. Payne, W.A., Page, R.C., Ogilvie, A.L. and Hall, W.B. 1975. Histopathologic features of the initial and early stages of experimental gingivitis in man. J. Periodontal Res., 10, 51-64.

4. Schroeder, H.E. and Page, R.C. 1972. Lymphocyte-fibro-blast interaction in the pathogenesis of inflammatory gingival tissue. Experientia, 28, 1228-1231.

5. Schroeder, H.E., Munzel-Pedrazelli, S. and Page, R. 1973. Correlated morphometric and biochemical analysis of gingival tissue in early chronic gingivitis in man. Archs. oral Biol., 18, 899-923.

6. Zachrisson, B.U. 1968. A histologic study of experimental gingivitis in man. J. Periodontal Res., 3, 293-302.

7. Nisengard, R.J., Beutner, E.H. and Gauto, M. 1971. Immunofluorescence studies of IgE in periodontal disease. Ann. New York Acad. Sci., 177, 39-47.

8. Genco, R., Mashino, P., Krygier, G. and Ellison, S. 1974. Antibody-mediated effects on the periodontium. J. Periodont., 45, 330-337.

9. Ramfjord, S.P., Knowles, J.W., Nissle, R.R., Shick, R.A. and Burgett, F.G. 1973. Longitudinal study of periodon-tal therapy. J. Periodont., 44, 66-77.

10. Lindhe, J. and Nyman, S. 1975. The effect of plaque con-trol and surgical pocket elimination on the establishment and maintenance of periodontal health. A longitudinal study of periodontal therapy in cases of advanced disease. J. Clin. Periodont., 2, 67-79.

11. Schluger, S., Youdelis, R.A. and Page, R.C. 1977. Periodontal Disease. Lea & Febiger, Philadelphia, p. 227.

12. Schei, O., Waerhaug, J., Lovdal, A. and Arno, A. 1959. Alveolar bone loss as related to oral hygiene and age. J.Periodont., 30, 7-16.

13. Goldman, H.M. 1957. Extension of exudate into supporting structures of the teeth in marginal periodontitis. J. Periodont. 28, 175-183.

14. Melcher, A.H. 1962. The pathogenesis of chronic gingivitis I. The spread of the inflammatory process. Dent.Practnr. 13, 2-7.

15. Akiyoshi, M., and Mori, K. 1967. Marginal peridontitis: A histological study of the incipient stage. J. Periodont. 38, 45-52.

16. Hopewell-Smith, A. 1918. Normal and Pathological Histology of the Mouth. 2nd Ed. P. Blakiston's Son & Co., Philadelphia, p. 284.

17. Macphee, T. and Cowley, G. 1969. Essentials of Periodontology and Periodontics. Blackwell Scientific Publications, Oxford, p. 30.

18. Glickman, J. 1972. Clinical Periodontology. 4th Ed. W.B. Saunders Company, Philadelphia, p. 223.

19. Baer, P.N. and Morris, M.L. 1977. Textbook of Periodontics. J. B. Lippincott Company, Philadelphia, p. 66.

20. Grant, D.A., Stern, I.B. and Everett, F.G. 1968. Orban's Periodontics. 3rd ed. The C.V. Mosby Company, St. Louis, p. 182.

21. Stahl, S.S. 1968. In Periodontal Therapy. H.M. Goldman and D.W. Cohen, Eds. The C.V. Mosby Company, St. Louis, p. 133.

22. Glickman, J. and Smulow, J.B. 1974. Periodontal Disease: Clinical, Radiographic and Histopathologic features. W.B. Saunders Company, Philadelphia, p. 123.

23. Kennedy, J.E., and Polson, A.M. 1973. Experimental marginal periodontitis in squirrel monkeys. J. Periodont. 44, 140-144.

24. Lindhe, J., Hamp, S.E. and Löe, H. 1975. Plaque induced periodontal disease in beagle dogs. A 4-year clinical roentgenographical and histometrical study. J. Periodontal Res. 10, 243-255.

25. Genco, R.J., Evans, R.T. and Ellison, S.A. 1969. Dental research in microbiology with emphasis on periodontal desease. J. Am. Dent. Assoc., 78, 1016-1036.

26. Socransky, S.S. 1970. Relationship of bacteria to the etiology of periodontal disease. J. Dent. Res. 49, 203-222.

27. Kelstrup, J. and Theilade, E. 1974. Microbes and periodontal disease. J. Clin. Periodont. 1, 15-35.

28. Taichman, N.S. and McArthur, W.P. 1975. Current concepts in periodontal disease. Ann. Rep. Medic. Chem. 10, 228-239.

29. Socransky, S.S. 1977. Microbiology of periodontal disease-present status and future considerations. J. Periodont. 48, 497-504.

30. Russell, A.L. 1967. Epidemiology of periodontal disease. Int. Dent. J. 17, 282-296.

31. Löe, H., Theilade, E. and Jensen, S.B. 1965. Experimental gingivitis in man. J. Periodontal Res. 36, 177-187.

32. Theilade, E., Wright, W.H., Jensen, S.B. and Löe, H. 1966. Experimental gingivitis in man. II. A longitudinal clinical and bacteriological investigation. J. Periodontal Res. 1, 1-13.

33. Holm-Pedersen, P., Agerback, N., and Theilade, E. 1975. Experimental gingivitis in young and elderly individuals. J. Clin. Periodont. 2, 14-24.

34. Löe, H. 1970. A review of the prevention and control of plaque. In Dental Plaque. W.D. McHugh, ed. E&S Livingstone, Edinburgh, p. 259.

35. Löe, H., Schiott, and Rindom, E. 1970. The effect of mouthrinses and topical application of chlorhexidine on the development of dental plaque and gingivitis in man. J. Periodontal Res. 5, 79-83.

36. Krygier, G., Genco, R., Mashimo, P. and Hausman, E. 1973. Experimental gingivitis in Macacca speciosa monkeys. Clinical, bacteriological and histologic similarities to human gingivitis. J. Periodont. 44, 454-463.

37. Johnson, N.W. and Hopps, R.M. 1975. Cell dynamics of experimental gingivitis in macaques. J. Periodontal Res. 10, 177-190.

38. Lindhe, J., Hamp, S.E. and Löe, H. 1973. Experimental periodontis in the beagle dog. J. Periodontal Res. 8, 1-10.

39. Lövdal, A., Arno, A., Schei, O. and Waerhaug, J. 1961. Combined effect of subgingival scaling and controlled oral hygiene on the incidence of gingivitis. Acta Odont. Scand. 19, 537-555.

40. Lightner, L.M., O'Leary, T.J., Drake, R.B., Crump, P.P. and Allen, M.F. 1971. Preventive periodontic treatment procedures: Results over 46 months. J. Periodont. 42, 555-561.

41. Suomi, J.D., Greene, J.C., Vermillion, J.R., Doyle, J., Chang, J.J. and Leatherwood, E.C. 1971. The effect of controlled oral hygiene procedures on the progression of periodontal disease in adults: Results after third and final year. J. Periodont. 42, 152-160.

42. Nyman, S., Rosling, B. and Lindhe, J. 1975. Effect of professional tooth cleaning on healing after periodontal surgery. J. Clin. Periodont. 2, 80-86.

43. Rosling, B., Nyman, S. and Lindhe, J. 1976. The effect of systematic plaque control on bone regeneration in infrabony pockets. J. Clin. Periodont. 3, 38-53.

44. Greene, J.C. and Vermillion, J.R. 1971. Oral hygiene research and implication for periodontal care. J. Dent. Res. 50. Suppl. 2, 184-193.

45. Gordan, H.V., Fitzgerald, R.J. and Stanley, H.R. 1965. Plaque formation and periodontal pathology in gnotobiotic rats infected with an oral Actinomycete. Am. J. Path. 47, 1157-1167.

46. Gibbons, R.J., Berman, K.S., Knoettner, P. and Kapsimalis, B. 1966. Dental caries and alveolar bone loss in gnotobiotic rats infected with capsule forming streptococci of human origin. Archs. oral Biol. 11, 549-560.

47. Socransky, S.S., Hubersak, C. and Propas, D. 1969. Induction of periodontal destruction in gnotobiotic rats by a human strain of Actinomyces naeslundii. Archs. Oral Biol. 15, 993-995.

48. Irving, J.T., Socransky, S.S. and Heely, J.O. 1974. Histological changes in experimental periodontal disease in gnotobiotic rats and conventional hamsters. J. Periodontal Res. 9:73-81.

49. Garant, P.R., 1976. An electron microscopic study of periodontal tissues of germfree rats and rats monoinfected with Actinomyces naeslundii. J. Periodontal Res. Suppl. 15, 1-79.

50. Garant, P.R. 1976. Light and electron microscopic observations of osteoclastic alveolar bone resorption in rats monoinfected with Actinomyces naeslundii. J. Periodont. 47, 717-723.

51. Snyderman, R. 1973. Immunological mechanisms of periodontal tissue destruction. J. Am. Dent. Ass. 87, 1020-1026.

52. Horton, J.E., Oppenheim, J.J. and Mergenhagen, S.E. 1974. A role for cell-mediated immunity in the pathogenesis of periodontal disease. J. Periodont. 45, 351-360.

53. Lehner, T. 1975. Immunological aspects of oral disease. In Clinical Aspects of Immunology 3rd Ed. P.G.H. Gell, R.R.A. Coombs and F.J. Lachmann, eds. Blackwell Scientific Publications, Oxford, p. 1387.

54. Nisengard, R.J. 1977. The role of immunology in periodontal disease. J. Periodont. 48, 505-516.

55. McCluskey, R.T. and Leber, P.O. 1974. Cell-mediated reactions in vivo. In Mechanisms of cell-mediated immunity. R.T. McCluskey and S. Cohen, eds. John Wiley & Sons, New York. pp. 1-24.

56. Turk, J.L. 1975. The mechanism and mediators of cellular hypersensitivity. In Clinical Aspects of Immunology. P.G.H. Gell, R.R.A. Coombs and P.J. Lachmann, eds. Blackwell Scientific Publications, Oxford, pp. 987-1019.

57. Coombs, R.R.A., Gordon Smith, C.E. and Lachman, P.J. 1975. The allergic reactions as factors determining and influencing microbial pathogenicity. In Clinical Aspects of Immunology. P.G.H. Gell, R.R.A. Coombs and P.J. Lachmann, eds. Blackwell Scientific Publications, Oxford, pp. 987-1018.

58. Wells, J.V. Immune Mechanisms in tissue damage. 1976. In Basic and Clinical Immunology. H.H. Fudenberg, P. Stites, L. Caldwell and J. Wells, eds. Las Altos, California, Lange Medical Publications, pp. 225-241.

59. Coombs, R.R.A. and Gell, P.G.H. 1975. Classification of allergic reactions responsible for clinical hypersensitivity and disease. In Clinical Aspects of Immunology. P.G.H. Gell, R.R.A. Coombs and P.J. Lachmann, eds. Blackwell Scientific Publications, Oxford, pp. 762-781.

60. Evans, R.T., Spaeth, S. and Mergenhagen, S.E. 1966. Bacteriocidal antibody in mammalian serum to obligatory anaerobic gram-negative bacteria. J. Immunol. 97, 112-119.

61. Steinberg, A.I. and Gershoff, S.N. 1968. Quantitative differences in spirochetal antibody observed in periodontal disease. J. Periodont. 39, 286-289.

62. Nisengard, R.J. and Beutner, E.H. 1970. Immunologic studies of periodontal disease. V. IgG type antibodies and skin test responses to Actinomyces and mixed oral flora. J. Periodont. 41, 149-152.

63. Gilmour, M.N. and Nisengard, R.J. 1974. Interactions between serum titers to filamentous bacteria and their relationship to human periodontal disease. Arch. Oral Biol. 19, 959-968.

64. Orstavik, D., and Brandtzaeg, P. 1977. Serum antibodies to plaque bacteria in subjects with dental caries and gingivitis. Scand. J. Dent. Res. 85, 106-113.

65. Berglund, S.E. 1971. Immunoglobulins in human gingiva with specificity for oral bacteria. J. Periodont. 42, 546- 551.

66. Rylander, H., Lindhe, J., and Ahlstedt, S. 1976. Experimental gingivitis in immunized dogs. J. Periodont. Res. 11: 339-348.

67. Ivanyi, L. and Lehner, T., 1970. Stimulation of lymphocyte transformation by bacterial antigens in patients with periodontal disease. Arch. Oral Biol. 15, 1089-1096.

68. Horton, J.E., Leikin, S., and Oppenheim, J.J. 1972. Human lymphoproliferative reaction to saliva and dental plaque-deposits: An in vitro correlation with periodontal disease. J. Periodont. 43, 522-527.

69. Patters, M.R., Genco, R.J., Reed, M.J. and Mashimo, P. 1976. Blastogenic response of human lymphocytes to oral bacterial antigens: comparison of individuals with periodontal disease to normal and edentulous subjects. Infect. Immun. 14, 1213-1220.

70. Patters, M.R., Sedransk, N. and Genco, R.J. 1977. Lymphoproliferative response during resolution and recurrence of naturally occurring gingivitis. J. Periodont. 48, 373-380.

71. Lang, N.P. and Smith, F.N. 1977. Lymphocyte blastogenesis to plaque antigens in human periodontal disease. 1. Populations of varying severity of disease. J. Periodontal Res. 12, 298-309.

72. Ling, N.R. 1968. Lymphocyte Stimulation. North-Holland Publishing Co. Amsterdam, pp. 147-174.

73. Ivanyi, L. and Lehner, T. 1971. Lymphocyte transformation by sonicates of dental plaque in human periodontal disease. Archs. Oral Biol. 16, 1117-1121.

74. Ivanyi, L., Wilton, M.M.A. and Lehner, T. 1972. Cell-mediated immunity in periodontal disease; cytotoxicity, migration inhibition and lymphocyte transformation studies. Immunol. 22, 141-145.

75. Horton, J.E., Oppenheim, J.J. and Mergenhagen, S.E. 1973. Elaboration of lymphotoxin by cultured human peripheral blood leukocytes stimulated with dental plaque deposits. Clin. Exp. Immunol. 13, 383-390.

76. Mackler, B.F., Altman, L.C., Wahl., S., Rosenstreich, D.L., Oppenheim, J.J. and Mergenhagen, S.E. 1974. Blastogenesis and lymphokine synthesis by T and B lymphocytes from patients with periodontal disease. Infect. Immunity 10, 844-850.

77. Remold, H.G. and David, J.R. 1974. Migration inhibition factor and other mediators in cell-mediated immunity. In Mechanisms of Cell-Mediated Immunity. T. McCluskey and S. Cohen, eds. John Wiley & Sons, New York pp. 25-42.

78. Rocklin, R.E. 1976. Mediators of cellular immunity. In Basic and Clinical Immunology. H.H. Fundenberg, P. Stites, L. Caldwell and J. Wells, Lange Medical Publications, Los Altos, California, pp. 102-113.

79. Nisengard, R.J. and Jarrett, G. 1974. Hypersensitivity reactions to four oral microorganisms. J. Dent. Res. 54: 137.

80. Nisengard, R.J., Buetner, E.H. and Hazen, S.P. 1968. Immunologic studies of periodontal disease III. Bacterial hypersensitivity and periodontal disease. J. Periodont. 39, 329-332.

81. Jayawardene, A., and Goldner, M. 1977. Reagin-like activity of serum in human periodontal disease. Infect. Immun. 15, 665-667.

82. Hyman, H.M. and Zeldow, B.J. 1963. A comparison of cutaneous and mucosal Arthus reaction in the guinea pig and hamster. J. Immunol. 91, 701-708.

83. Spowge, J.D. and Cutter, B.S. 1963. Hypersensitivity reactions in mucous membranes. Oral Surg., Oral Med., Oral Path. 16, 539-550.

84. Terner, C. 1965. Arthus reaction in the oral cavity of laboratory animals. Periodontics 3, 18-22.

85. Adams, D., Williamson, J.J. and Dolby, A.E. 1969. Delayed hypersensitivity response in guinea-pig oral mucosa. J. Path. 97, 495-501.

86. Rizzo, A.A. and Mergenhagen, S.E. 1965. Studies on the significance of local hypersensitivity in periodontal disease. Periodontics 3, 271-274.

87. Rizzo, A.A., and Mitchell, C.T. 1966. Chronic allergic inflammation induced by repeated deposition of antigen in rabbit gingival pockets. Periodontics 4, 5-10.

88. Ranney, R.R. and Zander, H.A. 1970. Allergic periodontal disease in squirrel monkeys. J. Periodont. 41, 12-21.

89. Nobreus, N. and Attström, R. 1974. Experimental contact hypersensitivity in the gingiva of dogs. J. Periodont. Res. 9, 245-254.

90. Wilde, G., Cooper, M.and Page, R.C. 1977. Host tissue response in chronic periodontal disease. VI. The role of cell-mediated hypersensitivity. J. Periodontal Res. 12, 179-196.

91. Nisengard, R., Beutner, E.H., Neugeboren, N., Neiders, M. and Asaro, J. 1977. Experimental induction of periodontal disease with Arthus-Type Reactions. Clin. Immunol. Immuno-path. 8, 97-104.

92. Asaro, J.P., Nisengard, R., Beutner, E.H. and Neiders, M. Experimental periodontal disease: reverse passive Arthus reactions. Clin. Immunol. Immunopath. In Press.

93. Fell, H.B., Coombs, R.R.A. and Dingle, J.T. 1966. The breakdown of embryonic (chick) cartilage and bone cultivated in the presence of complement-sufficient antiserum. Int. Arch. Allergy 30, 146-176.

94. Hausman, E., Genco, R., Weinfeld, N. and Asaro, R. 1973. Effects of sera on bone resorption in tissue culture. Calcif. Tissue Res. 13: 311-317.

95. Hausman, E. 1974. Potential pathways for bone resorption in human periodontal disease. J. Periodont. 45, 338-343.

96. Asaro, J., Nisengard, R., Neiders, M. and Beutner, E. 1977. The role of IgE mediated immediate hypersensitivity reactions in periodontal disease. J. Dent. Res. 56B: 90.

97. Levy, B.M., Robertson, P.B., Dreizen, S., Mackler, B.F. and Bernick, S. 1976. Adjuvant induced destructive periodontitis in nonhuman primates. A comparative study. J. Periodontal Res. 11, 54-60.

98. Horton, J.E., Raisz, L.G., Simmons, H.A., Oppenheim, J.J. and Mergenhagen, S.E. 1972. Bone resorbing activity in supernatant fluid from cultured human peripheral blood leukocytes. Science 177, 793-795.

99. Beutner, E., Wick, G., Sepulveda, M. and Monin, K. 1970. A reverse immunodiffusion assay for antibody protein concentration in antisera or conjugates to human IgG. In Standardization of Immunofluorescence. Ed. E. J. Holborow. Blackwell Scientific Publications, Oxford, pp. 165-169.

100. Heijl, L., Rifkin, B.R. and Zander, H.A. 1976. Conversion of chronic gingivitis to periodontitis in squirrel monkeys. J. Periodont. 47, 710-716.

101. Chen, P., Trummel, C., Horton, J., Baker, J.J. and Oppenheim, J.J. 1976. Production of osteoclast-activating factor by normal human peripheral blood rosetting and non-rosetting lymphocytes. Eur. J. Immunol. 6, 732-736.

102. Gordon, D., Bray, M.A. and Morley, J. 1976. Control of lymphokine secretion by prostaglandins. Nature 262, 401-402.

103. Goodson, J.M., McClatchey, K., and Revell, C. 1973. Prostaglandin-induced resorption of the adult rat calvarium. J. Dent. Res. 53, 670-677.

104. Green, L.J., Gong, J.K. and Neiders, M.E. 1969. Relationship between Sr85 uptake and histological changes during the healing in dental extraction wounds in rats. Archs. Oral Biol. 14, 865-871.

Connective Tissue Resorption and Rheumatoid Arthritis: Synovial Cell Culture as a Model.

Jean-Michel Dayer, Steven R. Goldring and Stephen M. Krane

Department of Medicine, Harvard Medical School and the Medical Services (Arthritis Unit), Massachusetts General Hospital, Boston, Massachusetts 02114

Destruction of the diarthrodial joint is a major problem in chronic rheumatoid arthritis. Erosions of cartilage and bone, rupture of tendons and weakening of the joint capsule and ligaments all may occur (1). Even if remission ensues, one may still be left with irreversible changes in these structures since the process of repair is never complete.

Although the etiology of rheumatoid arthritis is unknown, there is considerable information now available on the pathogenesis of the destructive process. The predominant feature of the early rheumatoid lesion is a diffuse "proliferation" of the synovial lining cells (1, 2). If remission does not occur there is further increase in synovial lining cells, neovascularization and infiltration of the deeper synovial layers with a variety of cells including lymphocytes, plasma cells, macrophages, fibroblasts and other cells not yet identified. Most of the destructive changes in the articular cartilage and adjacent bone take place in regions where cells of the advancing granulations (pannus) are in direct contact with these articular structures (Fig. 1). In addition, there may be loss of proteoglycan in portions of articular cartilage not directly in contact with pannus (3). The magnitude of the bone resorption may be intense with large sections of bone destroyed rapidly over a period of months. In the regions of bone undergoing resorption, giant cells are often found blending into the mass of cells of the pannus. In such instances it may be difficult to ascertain whether the cells responsible for the connective tissue destruction are derived from preexisting bone cells or from the invading inflammatory cell mass.

We have examined rheumatoid synovial tissue obtained at the time of surgical synovectomy to determine what possible role each of the component cells and cell products might play in the degradation of joint structures. Substances which could be involved in this destructive process are several, but we have chosen to measure primarily two factors: collagenase, which can degrade collagens of the joint (4, 5, 6) and prostaglandins which might have a number of effects on the inflammatory process including stimulation of bone resorption (6, 7). Previously fragments of synovium have been shown to release typical animal collagenase in organ culture capable of degrad-

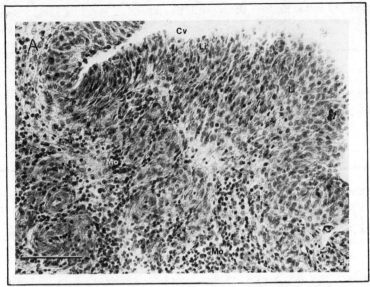

Fig. 1.A.   Portion of a synovial villus from the knee of a
patient with active, classical rheumatoid arthritis.
Increase in numbers of synovial lining cells (Li)
are seen at the surface adjacent to the synovial
cavity (Cv). Mononuclear cells (Mo) are abundant in
regions deep to the lining cells. Hematoxylin and
eosin. Bar = 100 μm.

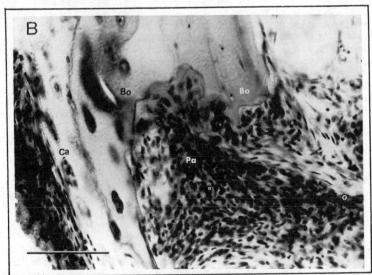

Fig. 1.B.   Junction of pannus (Pa) with bone (Bo) and cartilage
(Ca) from a metacarpophalangeal joint of a patient
with active, classical rheumatoid arthritis. Hematoxylin and eosin. Bar = 100 μm.

ing types I, II and III collagens (5). Such fragments also synthesize and release prostaglandins, particularly PGE_2, as measured by radioimmunoassay of culture media (7, 8). These synovial fragments contain a heterogeneous cell population and study of the interaction between specific cells and cell products is not possible in this system. Alternative methods using conventional explant techniques are also limited since these cultures usually yield cells most closely resembling dermal fibroblasts. Such fibroblasts produce little or no detectable collagenase and only small amounts of PGE_2.

Properties of Cultured Adherent Synovial Cells.

In order to isolate cells which retained the high levels of collagenase and PGE_2 production that presumably occur in vivo, we utilized the proteolytic enzymes, clostridial collagenase and trypsin, to disperse the synovial cells of the superficial layers of synovectomy specimens (9). Of the dispersed cells a heterogeneous population adhered to the culture vessel surface; we found that the PGE_2 and collagenase production was associated with these adherent cells. The majority of the adherent synovial cells (ASC) were large cells often assuming a stellate character, with abundant cytoplasm, several large dendritic processes and large nuclei (Fig. 2). These cells which did not possess conventional macrophage markers (lysozyme production, Fc receptor, phagocytosis) released typical animal collagenase in large amounts, in early cultures up to 70µg of collagen lysed/min at 37° (70 units)/10^6 cells/day. Some adherent cell cultures continued to release detectable collagenase for prolonged periods (weeks to > 18 months) (9). Since the cells had been cultured in Dulbecco's medium (DMEM) containing 10% fetal calf serum (FCS), it was necessary to pretreat the medium with trypsin, followed by excess soybean inhibitor to detect collagenase activity. During the first two weeks in culture (Fig. 3), the cells usually produced large amounts of PGE_2 as well (up to 1200 ng/10^6 cells/day) (8). Secretion of PGE_2 usually declined rapidly after 7-10 days, although collagenase production usually continued at close to initial levels for weeks in non-passaged cells. However, with continued age in culture or after passage by trypsinization and dilution, the levels of collagenase released declined. In general, the levels decreased more rapidly when cells were passaged at high dilution (low density), similar to the situation for dermal fibroblasts as shown by Bauer (10). Another cell type was frequently present in primary cultures. These cells were round, smaller than the stellate cells, and possessed markers characteristic of monocyte-macrophages (Fc and complement receptors and phagocytosis). The presence of these cells probably accounts for the lysozyme production detected in primary culture.

Production of a Stimulating Factor by Blood Mononuclear Cells.

Only the heterogeneous population of adherent cells produced collagenase and PGE_2. Spontaneous collagenase pro-

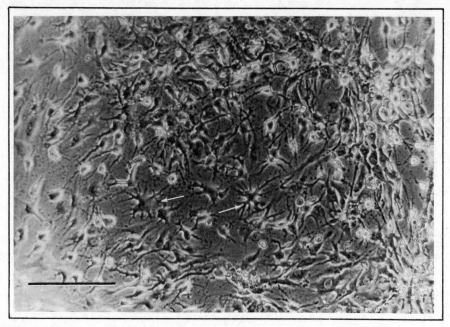

Fig. 2 Photomicrograph from a primary culture of adherent rheumatoid synovial cells (ASC) 3 days after plating and 2 days after washing and replacing with fresh medium. Arrows indicate stellate cells referred to in the text. Phase contrast. Bar = 200 μm.

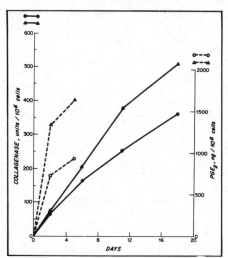

Fig. 3 Cumulative collagenase and prostaglandin production by rheumatoid cells in primary culture, 1 day after plating and removal of most nonadherent cells by washing. Values shown are for 2 separate 6 cm diam. petri dishes from the same cultured specimen.

duction decreased with passage and since the passage of the adherent cells was accompanied by the disappearance of the small cells possessing monocyte-macrophage markers we considered the possibility that these small cells (monocyte-macrophages) as well as the nonadherent cells (lymphocytes) could be a potential source of substances which might modulate collagenase and PGE_2 production by the adherent stellate cells. All of these mononuclear cells are characteristic components of the deeper synovial infiltrates (1, 2, 11, 12) and it has been suggested that lymphocyte products are critical in the genesis of certain aspects of the rheumatoid lesion (13). Furthermore, it has been shown by Wahl et al. that guinea pig lymphocytes stimulated with Concanavalin A or specific antigen could increase collagenase production by cultured guinea pig macrophages (14).

In order to study the interaction between mononuclear cell products and cultured synovial cells we isolated mononuclear cells from the peripheral blood of normal and rheumatoid subjects using sodium metrizoate/Ficoll gradients and cultured these cells in DMEM with 10% FCS for varying periods (15). The medium was then separated by centrifugation and added, in dilutions of 1:5 to 1:40, to the adherent rheumatoid synovial cells in 6 cm diam. polystyrene petri dishes or more commonly in trays containing 24 wells each of 16 mm diam.. Following exposure to the mononuclear cell supernatant (LM) the synovial cell medium was removed and assayed for collagenase and PGE_2 (15, 16).

The addition of the LM markedly increased production of both collagenase and PGE_2, the magnitude of the stimulation depending upon the particular specimen of target synovial cells and the culture age and density selected. In general, primary cultures could be stimulated two-to three-fold whereas in cells examined after the second or third passage, when basal levels of collagenase and PGE_2 had decreased, stimulation of several hundred-fold was occasionally obtained. The LM could be removed, the cells washed and fresh medium added, yet continued stimulation could be observed in some instances for 10-15 days. The stimulation could still be detected even after trypsinization and passage of the cells. It was also possible to restimulate the cells with fresh LM. The factor which stimulated both collagenase and PGE_2 production could be eluted in the same fractions from AcA 54 columns and had an apparent molecular weight between 10,000 to 20,000 Daltons. It was possible to observe a log-dose response for both collagenase and PGE_2, although the slope for these factors was not the same using different target cell preparations (15, 16).

In the absence of lectins, we have regularly observed that cultures of the mononuclear cells from the sodium metrizoate/ Ficoll gradients released LM which increased collagenase and PGE_2 production by synovial cells. Addition of several different lectins to the mononuclear cell cultures, including Concanavalin A, phytohemagglutinin (PHA) and pokeweed mitogen (PWM), always increased the amount of LM.

In collaboration with Drs. L. Chess and J. Breard (in preparation), we attempted to further characterize the mononuclear cells in human peripheral blood which might be responsible for the production of LM, utilizing techniques (17) which separate cells on the basis of adherence, phagocytic properties, and the presence or absence of surface immonoglobulins (Ig). We have regarded lysozyme secretion as a marker for macrophages (18) since the other lysozyme-secreting circulating cells (the poly- morphonuclear leukocytes) are separated from the original mono- nuclear cell layer in the sodium metrizoate/Ficoll gradients. The purest populations of phagocytic, adherent, surface Ig⁻ cells (monocyte-macrophages) that we have isolated secreted LM in culture in the absence of lectins (Table I). Adding lectins did not increase the amount of LM released but did decrease the secretion of lysozyme by these cells. Increasing the number of these monocyte-macrophages (0.01-2.2×10^6/ml) in culture was associated with a linear increase in the rate of production of LM and lysozyme. In contrast, the population of T cells (non- adherent, surface Ig- lysozyme negative) produced only 1-2% as much LM as a comparable number of monocyte-macrophages. As with the monocyte-macrophages, lectins did not alter factor produc- tion by the T cells. Addition of 5% monocyte-macrophages to the T cells resulted in $\sim$ 60 fold increase in production of LM, but only when PWM was added concomitantly. We assume that the popu- lations of "B" lymphocytes (nonadherent, Ig+) which we obtained were contaminated with monocyte-macrophages since the culture media always contained lysozyme. Such B cell populations did se- crete LM, amounts of which were increased by lectins. We cannot be certain whether this is due to the presence of other mononu- clear cells or is a property of the B cell itself. Thus the monocyte-macrophage emerges as the important cell of orgin of LM which acts on synovial cells, but important interactions with lymphocytes, particularly T cells, may also markedly affect the magnitude of LM production.

In the adherent synovial cell cultures more than one cell type may be the target for LM. We have no data which provide proof that the same target cell produces both collagenase and PGE_2. Since the ASC cultures represent a closed system in which the concentration of both collagenase and PGE_2 increase drama- tically with exposure to LM, the possibility therefore exists that these and other cell products may significantly affect other cell functions. With respect to PGE_2 the response could be manifested in several ways such as an alteration in the re- lease of other cell products or changes in cell growth and replication. Many different cells increase adenylate cyclase and cAMP levels upon exposure to prostaglandins (19, 20, 21). In several culture systems, the prostaglandin-induced increases in cAMP levels have been associated with decreases in cell pro- liferation (19, 22, 23). In order to define the relationship between PGE_2 production and various synovial cell functions we examined the effect of endogenous and exogenous PGE_2 on ASC proliferation and collagenase production (24).

Relationship between PGE_2 and cAMP levels.

Adherent synovial cells exposed to exogenous PGE_2 for 10 min increased cAMP levels. With continued presence of PGE_2 in

Table I

Effects of media from cultured lymphocyte and monocyte populations on production of factor (LM) which stimulates collagenase and PGE_2 production by ASC.

	Cultured Mononuclear Cells		Products released by ASC	
Step	Population	Lysozyme	Collagenase	PGE_2
		$\mu g/ml$	units/10^6 cells	ng/ml
1	Unfractionated	72	12.5 ± 1.4	110 ± 12
2	After iron carbonyl + magnet	0	1.6 ± 0.1	46 ± 7
3	T lymphocytes	0	1.6 ± 0.1	11 ± 2
4	B lymphocytes	12	18.3 ± 0.7	168 ± 41
5	Monocyte-macrophages	82	142.3 ± 8.9	405 ± 12
	No mononuclear cell	--	0.2 ± 0.1	6 ± 2

Lymphocytes or monocytes after separation (see text) were incubated in RPMI-1640 containing 10% heat inactivated FCS for 4 days. The media were then removed, centrifuged at 1500 rpm for 15 min and the supernatant solution diluted 1:11 in DMEM, 10% FCS, to be assayed on ASC. Lysozyme was measured using suspensions of Micrococcus lysodeikticus in 10 % agar (29). Incubations with ASC were for 3 days, following which the media were removed and assayed for collagenase and PGE_2. In the undiluted supernatant solutions of the monocyte-macrophage cultures, no collagenase activity was detected and the PGE_2 level was < 4 ng/ml. Values shown for ASC collagenase and PGE_2 assays represent the mean ± S.E..

the medium, the levels of cAMP remained elevated for several hours and then began to decline, so that by 24-72 hours of continous exposure, cAMP levels had returned to those observed prior to PGE_2 exposure (25). Similarly, after 72 hours of exposure to LM, when the endogenous PGE_2 levels had increased > 100-fold, the cAMP levels were not significantly different from controls. Although we have not detected a rise in cAMP during the first 2-3 hours in cells exposed to LM, coincident with the first detectible increase in PGE_2 ($\sim$ 6 hours) there was an increase in cAMP. As in the cells exposed to exogenous PGE_2 this initial increase was followed by a decrease in cAMP levels towards control. Thus, we concluded that the mononuclear cell factor does not increase cAMP levels directly but does so secondarily through stimulation of prostaglandin production.

Other investigators have shown that preexposure of cells to a given hormone may result in a state of refractoriness (desensitization) in which no response to this hormone can be elicted. This phenomena has been termed "down regulation" (21, 26, 27). Based on these observations, we therefore tested the cAMP response to exogenous PGE_2 in cells exposed for 72 hours to LM. As expected, we found that the cAMP response to exogenous PGE_2 was blunted in synovial cells exposed to LM, since the medium from these cultures at the end of 72 hours contained high concentrations of endogenous PGE_2 (Fig. 4). In contrast, in cultures treated with indomethacin alone there was an augmented response to exogenous PGE_2, presumably related to the absence of prostaglandin in the medium secondary to inhibition of prostaglandin synthesis by this drug. Of interest was the observation that the cells exposed to LM plus indomethacin had the greatest cAMP response to PGE_2, in excess of that observed with indomethacin alone. Moreover, not only did LM in the presence of indomethacin increase the magnitude of the cAMP response to exogenous PGE_2 but an augmented response to low concentrations (10 ng/ml PGE_2) was also seen in such cells. The shape of the dose-response curve suggested the possibility that the mononuclear cell factor increased the number of PGE_2 receptors as well as the affinity of the receptors for the PGE_2.

Cell Proliferation.

Many investigators have shown that PGE_2 inhibits cell proliferation. This has been attributed in part to PGE_2-induced increases in cAMP (19, 22, 23). In ASC, LM decreased cell proliferation presumably by increasing PGE_2 release into the medium, whereas inhibition of PGE_2 synthesis by indomethacin increased replication. Furthermore, the partially purified LM plus indomethacin increased replication more than indomethacin alone (24). We assume that the increased production of PGE_2 by the factor was responsible for the decreased cell proliferation since the addition of exogenous PGE_2 to the cultures abolished the stimulation by indomethacin with or without LM. Only by negating the effects of increased PGE_2 production by inhibiting its synthesis with indomethacin could the growth-

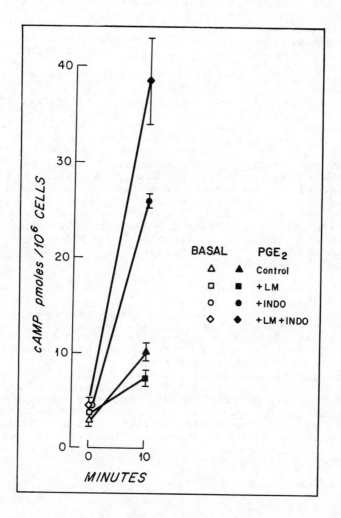

Fig. 4. cAMP response to exogenous PGE₂ of ASC previously incubated under various conditions. ASC at first passage were
plated at 10 x 10⁴ cells/well, 3 days before the experiment. At day 3, cells were incubated in a total volume
of 300 µl/well in DMEM, 10% FCS, alone (control), or with
LM, indomethacin (Indo) + LM or indomethacin, 10 µm,
alone for an additional 2 days. At day 5 media were removed and cells were exposed to buffer alone (basal) or
PGE₂, 1 µg/ml, for 10 min at 37° C. Each symbol indicates mean ± S.E.

Interactions of Prostaglandins and Collagenase.

In primary cultures of synovial cells concentrations of indomethacin, which inhibited PGE_2 synthesis, did not inhibit collagenase release. On the contrary, in some experiments collagenase production was increased in the presence of indomethacin (9). Furthermore, when indomethacin, $14\mu M$, was added to synovial cell cultures in the presence of LM, in most cultures collagenase stimulation by the factor was not affected (16). We have explored further, in other synovial cell cultures, the effects of inhibition of PGE_2 synthesis on collagenase production. Using unstimulated cells in primary culture and several concentrations of indomethacin we found that the ID_{50} for PGE_2 synthesis was about 1-5 nM. At these concentrations of indomethacin, collagenase levels were either increased or unaffected. At higher concentrations of indomethacin (> 10nM) when PGE_2 production was almost completely blocked, $\sim50\%$ inhibition of collagenase production was observed. In some ASC stimulated by LM, addition of indomethacin, $14\mu M$, decreased the magnitude of collagenase stimulation. This blunting effect could be overcome and collagenase stimulation restored by the addition of low concentrations (10 ng/ml) of PGE_2, whereas higher concentrations of PGE_2 (100-1000 ng/ml) in some cultures tended to be inhibitory (Table II).

We can thus tentatively formulate a model in cell culture for some features of the joint lesions of rheumatoid arthritis as follows: The large stellate synovial cells which are distinct from macrophages or conventional fibroblasts, are a source of collagenase and prostaglandins. These cells are influenced by mononuclear cells, particularly macrophages, which themselves interact with lymphocytes, also present in the hyperplastic synovium. The mononuclear cells release soluble factor(s) which can turn on the production of both collagenase and prostaglandins, particularly PGE_2. PGE_2 influences the metabolism and proliferation of the target synovial cells and modulates collagenase production. The chemical structure of the soluble factor and the nature of its interaction with the synovial cells remain to be elucidated. The relationship of this factor to other putative mediators also requires clarification.

Table II

Effects of PGE_2 and stimulating factor from mononuclear cells on

collagenase production by adherent rheumatoid synovial cells (ASC)

Exogenous PGE_2

ng/ml	0	10	50	100	1000
		Collagenase production by ASC			
		units/well			
Control	0.01	0.01	0.01	0	0.02
LM	0.42 ± 0.04	0.24 ± 0.03	0.08 ± 0.01	0.07 ± 0.01	0.01± 0.01
LM + indomethacin	0.22 ± 0.04	1.87 ± 0.24	0.48 ± 0.27	0.42 ± 0.13	0.13± 0.05
Indomethacin	0.01	0.01	0.01	0.01	0.01

ASC were plated for a second passage at 8×10^4 cells/well 6 days before

the experiment. At day 6 cells were incubated under various conditions:

DMEM, 10% FCS alone (control), partially purified LM, LM + indomethacin, 10μM,

and indomethacin alone. Exogenous PGE_2 was added simultaneously on day 6

at the concentrations shown. On day 9 media were removed and assayed for

collagenase.

In the control wells and in those containing indomethacin alone,

ASC collagenase activities were at the lower limit of the assay and therefore

S.E. was not calculated.

Summary.

It is possible to culture cells dispersed with proteolytic enzymes from synovectomy specimens of rheumatoid synovium. These cells release large amounts of latent collagenase and PGE_2, substances which are likely to play an important role in the degradation of joint structures in rheumatoid arthritis. When the levels of these effectors decrease, they can be restored (stimulation up to several hundred-fold) by a factor (molecular weight 10,000-20,000) released from peripheral blood mononuclear cells. The monocyte-macrophage is the major source of this factor, although interactions of the macrophage with T lymphocytes may also be important in regulating production of this factor. Endogenous PGE_2 production stimulated by the mononuclear cell factor has profound effects on the target stimulating effects of the mononuclear cell factor be unmasked. The possibility also arises that release of proteases could be factors affecting cell replication as has been shown in other systems (23, 28).

synovial cells including modulating rates of replication, possibly mediated by activation of adenylate cyclase and increases in cellular cyclic AMP. The mononuclear cell factor alters the response to the prostaglandins presumably by "down-regulation". When the effects of the mononuclear cell factor are examined under conditions in which prostaglandin synthesis is inhibited (i.e. exposure to indomethacin) then an increased sensitivity to prostaglandins is observed, possibly due to an increase in number of receptors as well as an increase in affinity for PGE2. Parallel effects on cell replication can be seen, i.e. decrease in replication of the target cells exposed chronically to high levels of prostaglandin, and increased replication in cells exposed to the mononuclear cell factor when prostaglandin synthesis is blocked by indomethacin. The mitogenic effect revealed by blocking PGE2 synthesis could also be due to the increase in protease released into the medium. Altering the levels of prostaglandins in some synovial cells alters collagenase production as well, i.e. decreased PGE2 synthesis (indomethacin) is accompanied by decreased collagenase, the levels of which can be restored partially or completely by adding low concentrations of exogenous PGE2. The synovial cell culture system serves as a possible model for rheumatoid arthritis in which the detrimental effects of a number of cell-derived mediators seem critical in pathogenesis.

ACKNOWLEDGMENTS

We are grateful to D. Bastian, W. Karge, P. Rogers, E. Schmidt and L. Servello for expert technical assistance, to the orthopaedic surgeons who provided us with tissue and to Dr. D. R. Robinson for helpful advice. Supported by USPHS grants AM-03564, AM-05067, grants from the Massachusetts Chapter and The National Arthritis Foundation and a grant from the Surtman Foundation. J.-M. Dayer has been partially supported by grants from Fondation Suisse de Bourses en Medecine et Biologie. This is publication number 740 of the Robert W. Lovett Memorial Group for the study of Diseases Causing Deformities.

ABBREVIATIONS

PGE_2, Prostaglandin E_2; FCS, Fetal calf serum; DMEM, Dulbecco's modification of Eagle's medium; ASC, Adherent synovial cells; LM, Collagenase and prostaglandin stimulating factor from blood mononuclear cells; cAMP, Cyclic adenosine 3', 5' monophosphate.

REFERENCES

1) Collins, D.H. 1955. The pathology of spinal and articular disease. Edward Arnold and Co., London, England.

2) Kulka, J.P., Bocking, D., Ropes, M.W., Bauer, W. 1955. Early joint lesions of rheumatoid arthritis. A.M.A. Arch. Path., 59, 129-150.

3) Janis, R., Hamerman, D. 1969. Articular cartilage in early arthritis. Bull, Hosp. Joint Diseases, 30, 136-152.

4) Krane, S.M. 1975. Collagnase production by human synovial tissues. Ann. N.Y. Acad. Sci., 256, 289-303.

5) Harris, E.D., Jr., Krane, S.M. 1974. Collagenases. N. Engl. J. Med., 291, 557-563, 605-609, 652-661.

6) Woolley, D.E., Crossley, M.J., Evanson, J.M. 1977. Collagenase at sites of cartilage erosion in the rheumatoid joint. Arthritis Rheum., 20, 1231-1239.

7) Robinson, D.R., Tashjian, A.H., Jr., Levine, L. 1975. Prostaglandin-induced bone resorption by rheumatoid synovia. J. Clin. Invest., 56, 1181-1188.

8) Robinson, D.R., McGuire, M.B. 1975. Prostaglandins in rheumatic diseases. Ann. N.Y. Acad. Sci., 256, 318-329.

9) Dayer, J.-M., Krane, S.M., Russell, R.G.G., Robinson, D.R. 1976. Production of collagenase and prostaglandins by isolated adherent rheumatoid synovial cells. Proc. Nat. Acad. Sci. U.S.A., 73, 945-949.

10) Bauer, E.A. 1977. Cell culture density as a modulator of collagenase expression in normal human fibroblast cultures. Exp. Cell. Res., 107, 269-276.

11) Van Boxel, J.A., Paget, S. A. 1975. Predominantly T-cell infiltrate in rheumatoid synovial membranes. N. Engl. J. Med., 293, 517-520.

12) Ishikawa, H., Ziff, M. 1976. Electron microscopic observation of immunoreactive cells in the rheumatoid synovial membrane. Arthritis Rheum., 19, 1-14.

13) Stastny, P. Rosenthal, M., Andreis, M. Ziff, M. 1975. Lymphokines in the rheumatoid joint. Arthritis and Rheum., 18, 237-243.

14) Wahl, L.M., Wahl, S.M., Mergenhagen, S.E., Martin, G. R. 1975. Collagenase production by lymphokine-activated macrophages. Science (Wash. D.C.), 187, 261-263.

15) Dayer, J.-M., Russell, R.G.G., Krane, S.M. 1977. Collagenase production by rheumatoid synovial cells: Stimulation by a human lymphocyte factor. Science (Wash. D.C.), 195, 181-183.

16) Dayer, J.-M., Robinson, D.R., Krane, S.M. 1977. Prostaglandin production by rheumatoid synovial cells: Stimulation by a factor from human mononuclear cells. J. Exp. Med., 145, 1399-1404.

17) Chess, L., MacDermott, R.P., Schlossman, S.F. 1974. Immuno-logic functions of isolated human lymphocyte subpopulations. I. Quantitative isolation of human T and B cells and response to mitogens. J. Immunology, 113, 1113-1121.

18) Gordon, S., Todd, J., Cohn, Z.A. 1974. In vitro synthesis and secretion of lysozyme by mononuclear phagocytes. J. Exp. Med., 139, 1228-1248.

19) Pastan, I.H., Johnson, G.S., Anderson, W.B. 1975. Role of cyclic nucleotides in growth control. Ann. Rev. Biochem., 44, 491-522.

20) Samuelsson, B., Granstrom, E., Green, K., Hamberg, M., Hammerstrom, S. 1975. Prostaglandins. Ann. Rev. Biochem., 44, 669-695.

21) Lefkowitz, R.J., Mullikin, D., Wood, C.L., Gore, T.B., Mukherjee, C. 1977. Regulation of prostaglandin receptors by prostaglandins and guanine nucleotides in frog erythro-cytes. J. Biol. Chem., 252, 5295-5303.

22) Polgar, P., Taylor, L. 1977. Effects of prostaglandins on substrate uptake and cell division in human diploid fibro-blasts. Biochem. J., 162, 1-8.

23) Makman, M.H., Morris, S.A., Ahn, H.S. 1977. Cyclic nucleo-tides. In Growth, Nutrition and Metabolism on Cells in Culture, eds. Rothblat, G.H., Cristofalo, V.J. Vol. III, 295-336.

24) Dayer, J.-M., Goldring, S.R., Robinson, D.R., Krane, S.M. 1977. Modulation of synovial cell growth by mononuclear cell factor. Clin. Res., 25, 482A.

25) Newcombe, D.S., Gosek, C.P., Jr., Ishikawa, Y., Fahey, J.V. 1975. Human synoviocytes: Activation and desensitization by prostaglandins and 1-epinephrine. Proc. Nat. Acad. Sci. U.S.A., 72, 3124-3128.

26) Raff, M. 1976. Self regulation of membrane receptors. Nature, 259, 265-566.

27) Swillens, S., Dumont, J.E. 1977. The mobile receptor hypo-thesis in hormone action: A general model accounting for desensitization. J. Cyclic Nucleotide Research, 3. 1-10.

28) Cunningham, D.D., Ho, T. 1975. Effects of added proteases on Concanavalin A-specific agglutinability and proliferation of quiescent fibroblasts. In Proteases and Biologic Control,, eds. Reich, E., Rifkin, D.B., Shaw, E. (Cold Spring Harbor Laboratory, Cold Spring Harbor, N.Y.), 795-806.

29) Osserman, E.F., Lawlor, D.P. 1966. Serum and urinary lysozyme (muramidase) in monocytic and monomyelocytic leuke-mia. J. Exp. Med., 124, 221-252.

Multiple Myeloma: Clinical Staging and Role of Osteoclast Activating Factor in Localized Bone Loss.

Brian G.M. Durie[1], Sydney E. Salmon, Gregory R. Mundy[2].

Section of Hematology and Oncology, University of Arizona Health Sciences Center, Tucson, Arizona.
[1] Scholar Leukemia Society of America.
[2] Division of Endocrinology and Metabolism, University of Connecticut Health Center, Farmington, Connecticut.

Introduction

A characteristic feature of multiple myeloma is the development of lytic lesions in bone. It has long been felt that this was a direct result of the infiltration with malignant plasma cells (myeloma cells) though the exact mechanisms have been unclear. In a previous study of short term cultures of myeloma cells obtained by direct bone marrow aspiration, Mundy et al.(1) found substantial amounts of osteoclast activating factor (OAF) in supernant fluids. They were able to show that this factor was biologically and chemically similar to OAF produced by phytohemagglutinin activated normal peripheral blood leukocytes (2,3). Supernatants from cultures of cells not associated with bone destruction did not contain increased levels of OAF. Morphologic examination of autopsy and biopsy samples of bone from 37 patients with myeloma confirmed osteoclast activity at bone-resorbing surfaces adjacent to areas of myeloma cell infiltration.

In the current study we have attempted to correlate the OAF production in short term myeloma cell cultures with the extent of bone lesions, serum calcium level and other clinical features in a series of 33 patients with multiple myeloma. All patients also had direct measurement of myeloma cell mass based upon synthetic rate and metabolic studies as previously reported,(4,5). Levels of OAF production have been evaulated with respect to stage of disease, (4) measured myeloma cell mass, a graded scale of extent of bone involvment, presence or absence of hypercalcemia and other features such as immunoglobulin type and subsequent response to therapy. Marrow cultures from normal people and patients with non-myelomatous bone marrow diseases were also examined for comparison.

Materials and Method

Patients Studied

Patients with myeloma and macroglobulinemia were well characterized clinically and immunologically. The diagnosis of myeloma was made on the basis of immunochemical analysis of blood and urine, morphologic examination of marrow smears, and skeletal

radiology, (6). Serum and urine M components were defined by
cellulose acetate electrophoresis (Microzone System: Beckman
Instruments, Palo Alto, California) and immunoelectrophoresis
with antiserums to IgG, IgA, IgM, IgD, IgE, and κ and λ light
chains. Marrow aspirates were also cultured for quantitative
measurements of the M-component synthesis rate in vitro with the
sandwich radioimmunoassay technic described elsewhere, (4). Total
body tumor cell number was calculated in all patients, (5).

Myeloma Cell Cultures

Cells were obtained by direct bone marrow aspiration. The
cells were washed six times in a balanced salt solution and
cultured at a concentration of 1 to 2 x 10^6 cells per milliter.
Differential counts of the washed cells were done on slides
stained with Wright's technic prepared with a Shandon cytocen-
trifuge, as previously described, (7). The cells were cultured
either directly in Falcon plastic tissue cultured tubes (7) or
in an in vitro "Marbrook" diffusion chamber in which cells grow
in suspension separated from a larger volume of medium by a
dialysis membrane, (8). The culture mediums employed and found
suitable were McCoy's, Eagle's minimal essential medium, and
RPMI 1640 supplemented with fetal calf serum or human autologous
or homologous plasma. Cultures were maintained in a water-
jacketed incubator at 37ºC with an atmosphere of 5 percent carbon carbon dioxide in air. Each culture was performed at least
three-four weeks after the previous course of pulse chemotherapy.
Supernatants were harvested for assay for bone-resorbing
activity after 24 hours of culture for the tissue culture tube
samples and after one week for the diffusion chamber samples.
In both systems the viability of myeloma cells was well maintained.

Marrow cells obtained from seven patients with a variety of
other hematologic disorders were cultured in the same manner.
Unstimulated peripheral blood leukocyte cultures were also
obtained from two patients with chronic lymphocytic leukemia,
and the supernatants tested for bone-resorbing activity.

Bioassay for Bone-Resorbing Activity

The supernatant fluid from marrow cell cultures were assayed for bone resorbing activity with a quantitative bioassay that
has been fully described elsewhere, (9). Bone resorption was
measured by the release of previously incorporated ^{45}Ca from
fetal rat long bones in organ culture. Female rats were injected with 0.4 mCi of ^{45}Ca on the 18th day of pregnancy and
killed on the following day. The radii and ulnae of each fetus
were dissected, and the cartilaginous ends removed. Each long-
bone shaft was cultured in modified BGJ medium (10) (Grand
Island Biological Company, Grand Island, New York) for 24 hours
to permit equilibration of readily exchangeable calcium, and then
transferred to the solution to be assayed or to a control medium
containing the appropriate concentration of serum or plasma. The
bones were cultured at 37ºC in an atmosphere of 5 percent carbon
dioxide and air.

The period of culture in the test medium was either 48 or 96 hours; the longer period was used to detect small amounts of bone-resorbing activity or factors that act slowly such as prostaglandins, (11). At the end of culture, the bones were dissolved in 5 percent trichloroacetic acid, and the ^{45}Ca content of medium and bone was measured by liquid scintillation counting. Resorption was quantitated as the percentage of total radioactivity released into the medium from treated and control cultures. Statistical differences were analyzed with use of Student's t-test. Bone resorbing activity was considered to be present when the treated-to-control ratio was significantly greater than 1.0 or when the percent release was significantly greater ($p<0.05$) than that for bones cultured in control mediums that had not been used for cell culture.

Calculation of OAF per Plasma Cell and "Total OAF"

Since cultures contained different percentages of plasma cells, to allow comparision between patients, the osteoclast activating factor (OAF) treated/control ratio was expressed per plasma cell. In addition, to obtain some measure of the total body production of OAF to correlate with extent of bone lesions, "total OAF" was determined representing the product of OAF/plasma cell and the measured myeloma plasma cell number (cells $X \ 10^{12}/M^2$).

Statistical Methods

Presented clinical features and measured myeloma cell mass were correlated singly and in combination with OAF, OAF/plasma cell and "total OAF". Results are expressed in terms of the Pearson correlation coefficient for which values of $\geqslant 0.28, > 0.4$, and > 0.6 are statistically significant with p values of $<0.05, < 0.01$, and (at least) < 0.001, respectively.

Stepwise multivariate regression analysis was carried out using several routines available from the Vogelback Computing Center, Northwestern University, Chicago (Statistical Package for Social Sciences, version 5.5, Oct. 1973)* The resultant regression equations had the format: $Y = X + Av_1 + Bv_2 + Cv_3 \ldots Nv_m$, where Y= total OAF value (see prior section) X = constant; A, B, C . . . N = derived values; and v_1, v_2, v_3 . . . v_4 = introduced variables (e.g. presenting clinical features). Most preliminary regressions were "step-up"; final regressions were preset. Optimal models were chosen according to the value of the multiple correlation coefficient (R^2).

Results

Supernatant fluids from bone marrow cultures derived from

---

* Revision of routines published in Statistical Package for the Social Sciences, Norman Nie, Dale H. Bent, and C. Hadlai Hull. New York, McGraw, 1970.

thirty three patients with multiple myeloma were assayed for bone-resorbing activity. The finding of no significant bone-resorbing activity in supernatants from bone marrow and peripheral blood cultures from patients with non-myelomatous conditions including, Waldenstrom's macroglobulinemia, non Hodgkin's lymphoma, refractory anemia and chronic lymphocytic leukemia, has been previously published (1) and forms the basis for this current report on OAF levels in different stages of myeloma.

The exact types of myeloma patient studies and their treatment status are indicated in Table I. Since the data are the most reliable in patients with active myeloma before any treatment has been initiated, results in the twenty one untreated patients are listed separately in Table II which also includes the details of extent of bone lesions, serum calcium levels, measured myeloma cell mass and immunoglobulin type. It can be seen that all but two of the patients with high or intermediate tumor cell mass had demonstrable bone-resorbing activity. However only one of five patients with low cell mass had a clearly increased OAF (treated/control) ratio. The derived values of OAF/plasma cell and "total OAF" are also shown and summarized in figures 1 and 2. There was a definite correlation between "total OAF' and the extent of bone disease demonstrable radiographically. The difference between patients with extensive as compared to those with no or minimal bone lesions was highly significant (P<0.01). Of interest there was more scatter in the amounts of OAF/plasma cell (Fig. 1). Patients who had limited bone disease and low to intermediate cell mass in some instances had quite high levels of OAF/plasma cell. However, the difference between the high and low cell mass categories was still statistically significant (P<0.05).

More detailed correlations were carried out between the total OAF values for all the patients and the specific clinical features and measured myeloma cell mass. (Fig. 2) In Table III results of bivariate correlation are listed. The significant association of total OAF production and extent of bone disease is again evident. The clearly higher levels of bone-resorbing patients with IgA myeloma as compared to IgG or the Bence Jones only types was statistically significant (P<0.05). Negative associations with κ as opposed to λ light chain type, amount of Bence Jones protein (Gms/day) and hemoglobin. In a multivariate regression analysis summarized in Table IV, the same features were the major correlates with total OAF. A minor, but significant, determinant in the equation was response to chemotherapy which had a positive correlation with total OAF level.

A somewhat surprising finding seen in Table II and summarized, for all thirty three patients, in Table V, was the general lack of correlation between hypercalcemia and bone-resorbing activity. In the high cell mass category, for example, (Table II) patients with and without hypercalcemia had similar levels of OAF, OAF per plasma cell and total OAF. In Table V, in which

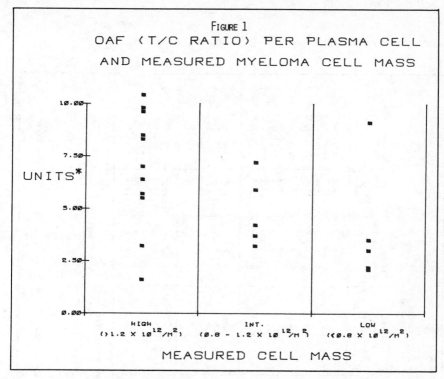

Figure 1: The levels of OAF per plasma cell (see materials and methods) are plotted for three measured myeloma cell mass categories. The units represent the T/C ratio of ^{45}Ca release per plasma cell. Difference between high and low cell mass categories significant ($P<0.05$).

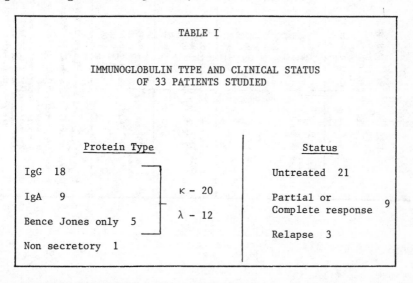

TABLE I

IMMUNOGLOBULIN TYPE AND CLINICAL STATUS
OF 33 PATIENTS STUDIED

Protein Type

IgG   18
IgA   9   κ – 20
Bence Jones only 5   λ – 12
Non secretory 1

Status

Untreated   21
Partial or
Complete response   9
Relapse   3

TABLE II

SUMMARY DATA ON THE 21 UNTREATED PATIENTS

	OAF* (Treated/Control Ratio)	OAF/** Plasma Cell	Total** OAF	Measured Myeloma Cell Mass (cells X 10^{12}/M²)	Extent of Bone Lesions[†] (scaled 0-3)	Serum Calcium Level (Mg%)	M-component Type
1. High Cell Mass (>1.2 X 10^{12}/M²)	1.08 ± 0.10	8.3	24.9	3.0	3	18.0	IgA κ
	1.31 ± 0.07	1.6	4.8	3.0	3	17.0	IgG κ
	1.65 ± 0.09	3.2	11.2	3.5	3	15.4	IgA κ (B.J. only)
	1.18 ± 0.07	5.7	19.5	3.3	3	14.9	λ (B.J. only)
	1.13 ± 0.06	7.0	21.0	3.0	3	14.7	IgG κ
	1.69 ± 0.15	8.5	21.3	2.5	3	12.4	IgG κ
	2.60 ± 0.35	10.4	26.0	2.5	3	9.9	IgG κ
	1.69 ± 0.09	9.6	31.7	3.3	3	10.1	IgA κ
	2.25 ± 0.41	9.8	20.6	2.4	3	10.2	IgA κ
	1.60 ± 0.11	6.4	16.0	2.5	3	9.8	λ (B.J. only)
2. Intermediate Cell Mass (0.6-1.2 X 10^{12}/M²)	1.42 ± 0.14	5.9	11.8	2.0	2	10.0	IgG κ
	1.52 ± 0.29	7.2	10.4	1.5	2	9.9	IgG κ
	1.12 ± 0.08	3.7	7.4	2.0	2	10.1	IgG κ
	1.60 ± 0.11	3.2	7.0	2.2	2	10.0	IgA κ
	1.25 ± 0.10	4.2	6.0	1.7	1	9.8	IgG κ
3. Low Cell Mass (<0.6 X 10^{12}/M²)	1.36 ± 0.03	9.1	9.6	1.0	0	10.0	IgA λ
	1.11 ± 0.10	2.1	4.4	1.7	0	10.1	IgG κ
	1.04 ± 0.10	3.5	3.5	1.0	0	9.8	IgG κ
	1.08 ± 0.10	2.2	2.9	1.3	0	10.0	IgG λ
	1.13 ± 0.06	3.0	4.5	1.5	1	10.0	IgA κ

* 96 hr. ^{45}Ca release. Mean ± SEM of 4 to 12 bone marrow cultures

** See materials and methods for derivation

[†] Scaling system for bone lesions
 0 = normal bones
 1 = mild osteoporosis or solitary lytic lesion
 2 = multiple lytic bone lesions
 3 = extensive skeletal destruction (lytic or osteoporotic) with or without major fractures

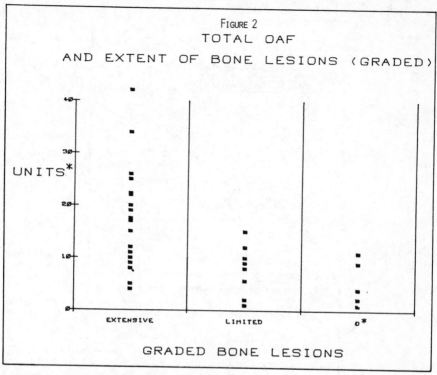

Figure 2: The values of total OAF are plotted for graded categories of bone disease. 0 = normal bones; Limited = limited number lytic lesions or mild osteoporosis; Extensive = extensive bone destruction. Difference between extensive and 0 highly significant (P<0.01).

TABLE III

BIVARIATE CORRELATIONS WITH
TOTAL OSTEOCLAST ACTIVATING FACTOR (OAF)

	PEARSON COEFF.	P
EXTENT OF BONE LESIONS	+ 0.82	<.01
WHETHER IgA	+ 0.45	<.05
WHETHER κ /λ	− 0.28	<.05
AMOUNT B.J. PROTEIN	− 0.28	<.05
HEMOGLOBIN	− 0.23	.06

TABLE IV

MULTIVARIATE REGRESSION ANALYSIS AND
TOTAL OSTEOCLAST ACTIVATING FACTOR (OAF)

TOTAL OAF = 6.9 + 3.5 X BONE LESIONS[*]
+ 2.7 IF IgA
- 1.9 IF κ
- 0.28 X CORRECTED CALCIUM[**]
+ 0.73 X RESPONSE TO Rx[T]

OVERALL P <0.001 (R^2 = 0.84)

[*] BONE LESIONS SCALED 0-3; SEE TABLE II

[**] SERUM CALCIUM CORRECTED FOR SERUM ALBUMIN; SEE TABLE VI AND REFERENCE 15.

[T] TREATMENT RESPONSE GRADED 0-2 : 0 = NO RESPONSE
1 = PARTIAL RESPONSE ($\geq$50%)
2 = COMPLETE RESPONSE

TABLE V

TOTAL OSLEOCLAST ACTIVATING FACTOR (OAF) LEVEL
AND CORRECTED CALCIUM*

	NORMOCALCEMIC	HYPERCALCEMIC (>11.0)
	N = 25	N = 8
TOTAL OAF		
MEAN	11.5	12.7
S.D.	5.5	6.5
	P = 0.7	

*CORRECTED CALCIUM VALUE = SERUM CALCIUM - SERUM ALBUMIN + 4.0
SEE REFERENCE 15.

the serum calcium level is corrected for any abnormality in serum albumin level, there is no difference between the eight hypercalcemic and twenty five normocalcemic patients. Clearly other factors besides OAF must have determined serum calcium levels.

In the group of patients studied other assays and extraction procedures were carried out to distinguish the bone-resorbing activity from prostaglandin E, vitamin-D-like sterols and para-thyroid hormone as previously reported. (1) Dose response curves for OAF were also carried out and indicated a steep curve resembling that of osteoclast activating factor and bone-resorbing factor produced by lymphoid cell lines.

Discussion

This study shows a definite relationship between bone-resorbing or osteoclast activating factor (OAF) production by bone marrow cells from a series of patients with multiple mye-loma and the extent of bone disease and measured myeloma cell mass in these same patients. Although there are exceptions, i.e. patients without demonstrable OAF production, yet extensive bone disease, the calculated total body production of OAF correlates very well with the amount of measureable disease. There is, therefore, strong support for the contention that OAF is an important substance in the bone destruction which occurs in patients with myeloma. The prior concomitant observation by Mundy, et al. (1) that large multinucleated osteoclasts are present in increased numbers in resorption lacunae in bone, lying adjacent collections of myeloma cells, further supports this conclusion.

However, the findings do not preclude the participation of other substances and/or cells (e.g. monocytes, (12) tumor cells (13)) in the bone resorption process. Clearly, further studies will be necessary to clarify the situation. With the develop-ment of more sensitive immunoassay procedures for OAF (14) it should be possible to more accurately and reproducibly measure OAF levels in supernatant and other fluids. Inhibition of OAF production in vitro and prevention of bone destruction in patients would give more direct proof of the role of OAF in the pathogenesis of localized bone loss in myeloma.

The lack of association between OAF production and serum calcium level is of considerable interest. Clearly the fate of mobilized calcium and serum calcium levels are controlled by a complex homeostatic mechanism of which OAF may only be a small part.

References

1. Mundy, G.R., Raisz, L.G., Cooper, R.A., Schecter, G.P., Salmon, S.E.: Evidence for the secretion of an osteoclast stimulating factor in myeloma. N. Engl. J. Med. 291: 1041-1046, 1974.

2. Horton, J.E., Raisz,L.G., Simmons, H.A., et al: Bone resorbing activity in supernatant fluid from cultured human peripheral blood leukocytes. Science 177: 793-795, 1972.

3. Luben, R.A., Mundy, G.R., Trummel, C.L., et al: Partial purification of osteoclast-activating factor from phytohemagglutinin-stimulated human leukocytes. J. Clin. Invest. 53:1473-1480, 1974.

4. Durie, B.G.M. and Salmon, S.E.; A clinical staging system for multiple myeloma. Cancer 36:842-854, 1975.

5. Salmon, S.E. and Durie, B.G.M.: Cellular kinetics in multiple myeloma--A new approach to staging and treatment. Arch. Intern. Med. 135:131-138, 1975.

6. Salmon, S.E. and Smith, B.A.: Immunoglobulin synthesis and total body tumor cell number in IgG multiple myeloma. J. Clin, Invest. 49:1114-1121, 1970.

7. Idem: Sandwich solid phase radioimmunoassays for the characterization of human immunoglobulins synthesized in vitro. J. Immunol. 104:665-672, 1970.

8. Golde, D.W. and Cline, M.J.: Growth of human bone marrow in liquid culture. Blood 41:45-57, 1973.

9. Raisz, L.G.: Bone resorption in tissue culture: factors influencing the response to parathyroid hormone. J. Clin. Invest. 44:103-116, 1965.

10. Raisz, L.G. and Niemann, I.: Effect of phosphate, calcium and magnesium on bone resorption and hormonal responses in tissue culture. Endocrinology 85:446-452, 1969.

11. Klein, D.C. and Raisz, L.G.: Prostaglandins: stimulation of bone resorption in tissue culture. Endocrinology 86:1436-1440, 1970.

12. Mundy, G.R., Altman, A.J., Gondek, M.D., Bandelin, J.G.: Direct resorption of bone by human monocytes. Science 196(4294):1109-1110, 1977.

13. Editorial: Osteolytic metastases. Lancet 1062-1064, November 13, 1976.

14. Luben, R.A.: Development of an assay for osteoclast activating factor in biological fluids. The First Scientific Evaluation Workshop on Mechanisms of Localized

Bone Loss, Washington, D.C., November 13-14, 1977.

15. Payne, R.B., Little, A.J., Williams, R.B., et al: Interpretation of serum calcium in patients with abnormal serum proteins. Br. Med. J. iv:643-646, 1973.

Discussion for Session IV: Disorders of Bone Associated with Inflammation and Neoplasia.

DR. RAISZ: Dr. Kuettner, I think certainly the osteosarcoma and I suspect the breast cancer cell lines are collagen-synthesizing lines, are they not?

DR. KUETTNER: Yes.

DR. RAISZ: My question is: does heparin do this by helping those cells degrade the collagen around them, and thus spread more easily; or behave in a different way? Have you any evidence for that?

DR. KUETTNER: I don't have any evidence, but the work of Heuson showed that the primary mammary carcinoma seems to be often surrounded with mast cells, particularly in the area where you have destruction of the collagen, which would fit the same concept. Probably the mast cell is a "helper" cell for the destruction of the collagen in the area; and I am talking about a scirrhous carcinoma, where there is a lot of collagen.

DR. SAKAMOTO: Have you seen a possible antagonistic action of AIF versus heparin in the collagenase assay system?

DR. KUETTNER: If we mix heparin and AIF together, there is no collagenolytic activity.

DR. MINKIN: Dr. Kuettner, did I see multinucleated cells eating the cartilage that arose from the breast tumor in the last slide?

DR. KUETTNER: No. These were osteosarcoma cells which pile up, not multinucleated cells. There were several cells sitting right directly next to each other, which you see quite often in the osteosarcoma.

DR. ROBINOVITCH: Have you tested any other polyamines to see if they have heparin-like activity?

DR. KUETTNER: We are just in the process. Dextran sulfate, originally tested by Goldhaber, has the same effect, and can also induce the tumor cell lines to secrete collagenase.

DR. MILLER: Dr. Kuettner, would you care to speculate what happens to AIF or any of these factors during the normal development of the growth plate, i.e., the hypertrophic and then the calcification and the subsequent invasion?

DR. KUETTNER: When we look at the calcified cartilage, the total amount of AIF is very, very minimal. There is a decrease. How it is disappearing we don't know. I have one speculation. It may be somehow absorbed through the calcified matrix; because if we take our AIF material and pass it through a column of hydroxyapatite, we get a large amount of the protease inhibitor absorbed to hydroxyapatite at neutral pH. Whether or not this is the mechanism, I don't know; but there is at least a possibility.

DR. KLEINMAN: Do you have any evidence that heparin enters the cell to serve its function?

DR. KUETTNER: No. I have no evidence yet.

DR. KUETTNER: Dr. Neiders, you showed your infiltrating cells close to the bone. What is happening if these infiltrating cells reach the tooth? Are they capable of destroying the tooth, invading the tooth, or is the tooth resistant to this process?

DR. NEIDERS: We produced the inflammation on the surface of the alveolar process away from the tooth; so our inflammatory infiltrate never even reached the periodontal ligament.

If you judge on studies of normal periodontal disease, the tooth does not get resorbed. It is the bone, and the tooth gets exfoliated.

DR. HIRSCH: Dr. Neiders, are you trying to have a model here that would represent that which occurs during periodontal disease?

DR. NEIDERS: At the moment, direct implications of specific immunological mechanisms in periodontal disease are fairly difficult. One method of study is to create reactions in gingiva that are similar to those seen in periodontal disease; namely, characterized with chronic cell infiltrate and bone resorption, and then extrapolate whether such mechanisms can take part in periodontal disease.

This type of approach has been used for some time, and various hypersensitivity reactions have been induced in the soft tissue. At this time, I did not use an antigen that produces or is involved in periodontal disease. This model can only state that bone resorption can be mediated by classic hypersensitivity reactions.

DR. SONIS: In your Arthus model, did you have an acute inflammatory response preceding your round cell?

DR. NEIDERS: Yes; that is classical at eight hours. In many studies inducing immune mechanisms in the gingiva, people have restricted themselves to very short periods of time. However, those studies that have looked at any kind of reaction after three days, or following multiple injections, have shown the classic chronic inflammatory cell infiltrate.

DR. SONIS: Would you care to speculate that there might be some mediator or something going on between the acute infiltrate and the chronic infiltrate? There have been reports in the literature regarding the role of proteases in this regard.

DR. NEIDERS: I cannot speculate from the in vivo studies.

DR. TRUMMEL: Could you be a little more specific about your methods of quantitating osteoclasts; how you counted per high power field?

DR. NEIDERS: We selected an area that measured 10 milli- meters from the tip of the alveolar crest; we then drew a parallel line and counted this tip of the alveolar crest in six to 18 sections, averaged the number between sections, and expressed as osteoclasts per section.

DR. MERGENHAGEN: Many years ago, Rizzo and myself approached this problem with similar techniques in the rabbit. We challenged the same area with bacterial endotoxin, and within a period of 24 hours, giving a systemic challenge, produced a Schwartzman reaction and found essentially what you saw in terms of osteoclastic resorption of bone.

So the idea of a specific immunologic challenge to this tissue as it is associated with bone loss is fine, but the idea that this is the way that you have to produce the osteoclastic resorption of bone may be misleading in some minds. I think if you induce any inflammatory situation, you will eventually lead to the same type of resorption.

DR. NEIDERS: We were aware of your studies, but did them differently. We put the emphasis on attempting to show which classically-described immune mechanisms can mediate bone resorption.

However, I do agree that bone resorption can be mediated by various other damage to bone. For example, if you examine extraction sites, at three days after extraction you also see osteoclasts. The kinetics of these osteoclasts' appearance and disappearance may be quite similar to your model and our model.

But, I think this is a question that still has to be answered: whether the kinetics of osteoclastic activity are different in different hypersensitivity reactions, whether they are different in other types of injury.

DR. LUBEN: Dr. Durie, exactly how did you quantitate total OAF, and what were the units?

DR. DURIE: It is an abstraction. You begin with the

treated to control ratio for calcium-45, which is per one times 10^6 cells. You correct that for the percentage of those cells that are plasma cells, then multiply that by the known number of plasma cells in the body, which we have calculated from our metabolic studies based upon immunoglobulin production, and that gives you total OAF.

DR. LUBEN: So it is, in fact, a dimensionless unit.

DR. DURIE: Correct.

DR. LUBEN: I would like to point out that Dr. Mundy and myself showed earlier, in Dr. Raisz's lab, and have shown again quite reliably in my laboratory: that OAF has a dramatic biphasic dose response curve. It is almost impossible in any given sample in our hands to determine, from a single measurement of the treated to control ratio, what the relative OAF concentrations are.

In any of this work, did you take measures to identify OAF as separate from other things that might be present in the culture medium which could cause bone resorption; e.g., prostaglandins, br-A, etc.?

DR. DURIE: Some of the patients involved in this study are part of the earlier study that Dr. Mundy has published, so that the supernatants were subjected to lipid extraction and measurements for PTH. Perhaps Dr. Mundy might like to comment further.

DR. MUNDY: I can't agree that every given myeloma patient will have exactly the same bone resorbing substances in his culture cell medium.

DR. DURIE: Not at all. All I am saying is that this particular substance correlates with the extent of bone lesions. That does not mean that there is some other combination of stimulators and inhibitors that might also be present.

DR. MUNDY: The basic points Dr. Luben is making are right. This is an abstraction. We are measuring a bioassay, and it is semi-quantitative phenomenon that we are observing.

The other thing: these are crude samples; and we are using control media each time which isn't conditioned with cells. In our samples, we haven't found a sharp biphasic dose response curve. It is when we get pure samples that we find problems of doing multiple dilutions.

But that is not really to take away from the major point which you are making, which is that this bioassay is semi-quantitative, and not absolute.

DR. DURIE: I didn't show all the treated to control ratios. In the patients with high tumor cell mass, there is a wide scatter. However, that scatter is clearly above the scatter that you see in patients with low cell mass statistically.

DR. LUBEN: I would agree with your point that there is a tremendous scatter. We have looked at OAF concentrations in patients using a specific purification technique for OAF. Quantitating against highly purified OAF, we find between 50 and 500 nanograms of OAF per milliliter in the serum of different myeloma patients.

DR DURIE: Let me just add one other thing. A patient who has a low cell mass can have a high secretion rate, and have a low total OAF production in the body.

DR. LUBEN: Right. Our findings agree with that too.

DR. HORTON: In regard to this discussion, and possibly Dr. Mundy would be the one to answer, were the culture fluids from the myeloma cells all tested at one or several dilutions? In people with different stages of myeloma, either in regression, or in exacerbation, or in relation to their number of lytic lesions, if the OAF within the supernatants from their cultured cells was able to be diluted to a greater or lesser extent, it would show that the cells from very active patients are producing a greater quantitation. Is this information available?

DR. MUNDY: A very small amount of material is produced by these cultured cells, and there aren't a lot of cells in the marrow aspirate. We finally do have a few dose response curves, which is probably the best way that we can try and quantitate how much biological activity is present in those supernatants, with the limitations of the bioassay. At present it is only on a very small number of patients. I don't think we could correlate it with anything.

DR. TEITELBAUM: Dr. Krane, I am disturbed that you didn't find any collagenase in monocytes per se, particularly since Mundy and Kahn and I have found the organic matrix of dead bone is resorbed by monocytes.

When you looked at collagenase in these monocytes, was it directly off of the gradient or were the monocytes cultured and stimulated in some way?

DR. KRANE: We were looking at monocyte macrophages that are taken by culturing adherent cells from the lymphocyte-monocyte layer from a Ficoll-Hypaque gradient, keeping them in culture for variable periods of time, concentrating the media, and looking for the enzyme produced, either with or without phagocytosis.

DR. TEITELBAUM: But these were plated cells?

DR. KRANE: That is right. We know the genetic machinery for making anything is present in every somatic cell. It is just a matter of turning it on; and we haven't been able to turn it on under conditions we can turn on other things.

DR. PARFITT: I have three questions for Dr. Durie. The

first has to do with methodology. You told us how M component was made in the cultured marrow cells; you did not explain how the total body M component synthesis was measured.

DR. DURIE: From the marrow material you can calculate the synthetic rate of immunoglobulin per cell. Now, from knowledge of the serum M component level, and a knowledge of its catabolism, you can calculate what the total production of M component in the body must be to produce that level of a serum M component. So if you divide that number by the amount that we measure per cell, you can calculate the number of cells.

DR. PARFITT: Thank you. Secondly, you mentioned that many myeloma patients have what you called "diffuse osteoporosis of the spine." I wonder if you or anyone else has good data demonstrating that the apparent incidence of this is significantly greater than in age and sex-matched controls? There are many diseases that are alleged to be causes of spinal osteoporosis on the basis of lack of an adequate control study.

DR. DURIE: The patients that I am referring to have myeloma; and I am not being facetious in the sense that there are very rigid criteria for making that diagnosis which depend on the percentage of plasma cells, the presence of an M component, and the like. This disease clearly develops over a very brief period of time, with the rapid development of osteoporosis, collapse of vertebra, and fracture of bones, which I don't think could be accounted for by some other type of osteoporosis, of aging, or the like. Also, studies have shown the presence of plasma cells in those bones.

DR. PARFITT: In the vertebrae?

DR. DURIE: Yes. At the time of laminectomy, for example, when the vertebra has been collapsed, there is no doubt that these bones contain plasma cells.

DR. PARFITT: The final question: your data show quite clearly that a critical cell mass of myeloma cells is a necessary, but not a sufficient, condition for the development of hypercalcemia. I wonder if your data permits you to say what the other factors have to be for hypercalcemia to develop?

DR. DURIE: For some reason, in this group of patients, the ones that were hypercalcemic tended to be osteoporotic rather than having multiple lytic lesions. I don't know. This is probably too small a sample to draw any conclusions.

One factor is renal function. If you have abnormal renal function, then of course calcium excretion is impaired. I am sure there are many other factors which just haven't been measured which could be influencing the actual calcium level.

DR. MARKS: I find it very difficult, Dr. Durie, to understand why you mentioned a correlation coefficient in a small period of time, when it seems to be clear from what you said that the total body burden of tumor correlates with a number of the clinical features of the disease, and that is not too surprising. However, it wasn't clear whether any of these correlations were improved by adding into your regression equation the OAF production per cell. Were any of these correlations, in fact, improved? In other words, correlates with tumor mass, with the presence of bone disease, with the presence of hypercalcemia.

If you add into that equation OAF production per cell, does that improve the correlation in any of these things?

DR. DURIE: The multivariate regressions which I showed you weren't set up in that way. In other words, the cell mass was calculated by the methods I have described; the multivariate regression with respect to total OAF was to take that as a firm number and try to correlate that number with the clinical features. It was not set up the other way, to see if you take OAF and add it in, can you predict what the cell mass is going to be.

DR. MARKS: I would suggest you could very easily compare one multivariate analysis to the other and see if your significance levels are improved by entering the OAF production per cell into the estimate of association with cell mass itself.

DR. DURIE: Right. It could be done; and my guess is that just taking the OAF value, you could predict the cell mass; you know, you could do exactly the opposite, and it could be a major determinant.

DR. MARKS: No, I am not saying that you want to take the OAF value to predict the cell mass; because your OAF value is the product of cell mass and OAF production per cell; so that is trivial. What I want to know is whether the OAF production per cell has any independent predictor of clinical consequences?

DR. DURIE: The OAF per cell also correlates with cell mass. The OAF; you are talking about the OAF production per plasma cell; it also correlates with myeloma cell mass. However, as I said, there are some patients with low cell mass that have a high synthesis rate.

DR. MERGENHAGEN: Dr. Krane, did any of the adherent cells that you worked with from the synovium showed any indication of C-3 or immunoglobulin receptors?

DR. KRANE: No. When you put out primary cultures of variable percentage, maybe up to 20 percent of the cells will make rosettes with immunoglobulin-coated red cells, so they have Fc receptors. They also make EAC rosettes. These are the small round cells; and these cultures make lysozyme for the first week or 10 days.

After about 10 days, whether you passage them or not, the number of those cells then markedly decreases, for one reason or another; by passage, we see zero and none of the larger cells that make any of these markers.

DR. MERGENHAGEN: Yes, then that is consistent. Drs. Koopman and Sandberg in my lab have been working with peritoneal exudate macrophages. In primary culture, you will see about 40 to 60 percent of the cells that will rosette with the EAC-1 through 4. And then, upon passage, you can go all the way down to nil cells with the C-3 receptors.

So unlike the lymphocyte, the B cell, these receptors are modulated on the surface of the macrophages quite readily.

DR. KRANE: Do they continue to put out large amounts of lysozyme in culture?

DR. MERGENHAGEN: We don't know about the lysozyme. We were just concerned with the C-3b receptor and its function on the macrophage; as I say, with the B cell, it is no problem. Any time in culture, you can demonstrate the same proportion of C-3b receptors; but the macrophage modulates that receptor all over.

DR. SHERWOOD: Dr. Durie, on a more basic level, are you aware of any data, either in cultured human cells or experimental plasmacytoma, that the genome that codes for the M protein might be related to OAF production in any way? Is there any data on that subject?

DR. DURIE: I don't know. I can tell you that there isn't any correlation between the synthetic rate of immunoglobulin and OAF production.

DR. RAISZ: Dr. Durie, can you think, offhand, whether your patients, the osteoporotic ones, tended to be males or females, and what their age range was?

DR. DURIE: I can think of one 65-year-old woman, but I hadn't appreciated any major abnormal distribution in the osteoporotic patients.

DR. RAISZ: Then, there are not more females. If Parfitt's comment were correct, then the osteoporotic group would be a post-menopausal female group, subgroup, within the myeloma population.

DR. DURIE: Yes.

DR. RAISZ: It was at least our clinical impression that that was not true, and I thought that was also not true of your series.

DR. DURIE: Right. I don't think that the osteoporosis in those myeloma patients has any direct relationship to other types of osteoporosis. I don't see any reason why there should be.

DR. SCHECTER: Dr. Durie, Dr. Horton and I have studied about 10 myeloma and four patients with reactive plasmacytosis.

We were puzzled by the fact that there were occasional patients with myeloma in whom we could not demonstrate OAF. One patient in particular that I can recall, the mass was taken from a huge osteolytic lesion in the arm in which the culture showed 100 percent plasma cells. We have also seen, in two of four patients with reactive plasmacytosis, bone-resorbing activity that did not seem to be correlated with high levels of prostaglandin. I wonder whether you have also had similar experience?

DR. DURIE: Yes. On the table which I showed with high, intermediate, and low tumor burden, there were two patients at the bottom of the left column with high cell mass that had very low levels of OAF. The initial treated-to-control ratios were very low; so that my statement would be that there are definitely patients who have demonstrable, widespread bone disease in whom we didn't find high OAF production.

DR. HORTON: Dr. Krane, the synovial cells which elaborate collagenase are elaborating it in tremendously high concentrations, more than any other cell type that I am aware. My understanding is that the collagenolytic activity is measured in these cultures without any source of exogenous protein, for example, serum or plasma. Is that correct?

DR. KRANE: Most of the data I showed today were measurements that were made when cells were cultured in the presence of 10 percent fetal calf serum, or in 10 percent either heat-inactivated human or isologous serum.

DR. HORTON: Then this collagenase is activated in order to measure it?

DR. KRANE: Yes. If cultures are performed in the presence of serum, then we have to activate it; but if we take the same cultures in the absence of serum, we don't have to.

DR. HORTON: Given the high collagenase production, by these cells in a serum medium, which you can detect by activation, I wonder if you can push the system to whereby whatever is tying up the collagenase may be sufficiently saturated so that one could then detect free collagenase in the system?

DR. KRANE: It is possible that could be done. So far it has not. Now if we use the trick Sakamoto has used earlier, by treating the serum itself with trypsin and then inactivating that, then you can demonstrate the presence of activity in the presence of serum.

Our trick was to use trypsin beads, so we could get rid of the trypsin in the cultures by spinning the beads off. Under those circumstances, you could detect activity in the presence of serum.

DR. WERB: Dr. Krane, I need a hypothesis about the prostaglandins and collagenase secretions in the synovial cells. As I remember from your data, in early cultures, the cells must secrete collagenase not at all related to prostaglandin production, and indomethacin doesn't affect it. Are the prostaglandins being secreted by the same cell there as later, in the passed cells, where you get this sort of prostaglandin-mediated, collagenase secretion?

DR. KRANE: We can offer a lot of hypotheses. The data are that the level of prostaglandin in each of these cultures, per cell, is variable. Some cells make enormous amounts, up to, let's say, micrograms of prostaglandin per 10^6 cells per day, which is a huge quantity. Other cells make much less. David Newcomb is here, and he has shown in the past that the response of a cell to prostaglandin depends upon what the cell's exposure to the prostaglandin has been. You can probably turn off receptors, as other people have shown, with prostaglandin; so what you see in the cultures is a complex mix of the amount made and the amount to which the cells have responded. Now, we have no direct information as yet as to whether the same cell that makes the collagenase is making the prostaglandin, even in our later cultures. We do know that we can turn them on, and we have to look at this. Dr. Robinson has access to an antibody to the cyclo-oxygenase, and we have just begun to explore this to see if we could use this. We can't look at prostaglandins on cells, because you don't know whether they have been made by the cell or are hitting a receptor on the cell. Dr. Williams' lab has reported, in synovial specimens using large amounts of antibody, that he can demonstrate prostaglandin in cells from rheumatoid synovium, removed and examined in the synovial specimen, rather than the culture. Similarly, David Wooley has been able to demonstrate that only certain cells of the rheumatoid synovium are making collagenase at any one time; that it is the stellate cell that seems to be making the collagenase. Whether the stellate cell will also make the prostaglandin, we don't know yet.

DR. PARFITT: Dr. Durie, I would like to go back to the question that Dr. Marks raised concerning the relative contribution of total cell mass and secretion or synthesis per cell in the calculation of total OAF.

If I understood the answer correctly, what you said was that the more cells there were, the higher was the secretion of OAF per cell, indicating that the same factors would tend to regulate cell number and cell activity. I wonder if that really is what you meant to say.

DR. DURIE: No. There was a tendency; I can't give you the statistics, but I can tell you two things. One was that in general, the patients who had a higher percentage of plasma cells, there were higher levels of OAF in the supernatants.

DR. PARFITT: Yes; but OAF per cell is the question.

DR. DURIE: OAF per cell.

DR. PARFITT: I see.

DR. DURIE: However, there were two or three patients who had early myeloma with relatively small percentages of plasma cells who also had high levels of OAF per cell. However, when you calculated that out, the total amount of OAF in their system was considerably less than you would have if you had a larger number of cells producing even much lower levels.

So there was a range of OAF per plasma cell in each of the categories. However, there was a trend to higher OAF levels in the patients with higher percentages, but by no means complete at all. And I think the same observation applies to synthetic rate, if you are calculating the number of cells; there are some patients with high cell mass and low secretion rates, and vice versa. But in terms of the total amount in the body, there was no doubt the total amount was higher in the patients with advanced disease.

DR. HEERSCHE: Dr. Kuettner, it is well known that blood vessels do not penetrate cartilage. However, during the process of endochondral ossification, at some stage, blood vessels enter to form the secondary centers of ossification in the epiphyseal cartilage.

Now is there any explanation for that phenomenon, and is there any correlation of mast cells, for instance, with the blood vessels that do penetrate in these particular areas?

DR. KUETTNER: Let me describe it indirectly by an experiment which we did. If you place any kind of calcified matrix onto the chorioallantoic membrane, it will attract blood vessels; if you put just a piece of plaster of Paris on the chorioallantoic membrane, it will immediately attract blood vessels; so there is a kind of correlation right there.

And if you look at the embryogenesis of the bone, prior to blood vessels, you have some chondrocytes, which will hypertrophy and then calcify. Then the blood vessels are coming in. I think there is probably an indirect attraction of the blood vessels. How they get through the cartilage, I have no idea. But don't forget that in a very early phase of embryogenesis, we have blood vessels in the cartilage. As soon as the cartilage is mature, they are excluded or degenerated or whatever you want to call it.

DR. HEERSCHE: Yes, I accept that they are attracted. But these blood vessels penetrate non-calcified cartilage, as you know.

DR. KUETTNER: That is what I am saying.

DR. HEERSCHE: And that is the question.

DR. KUETTNER: Yes. I have no idea how; this is the only case where we have it. I can't answer how it happens in this particular situation.

SESSION V

PRIMARY DISORDERS OF
BONE CELL FUNCTION

Osteoporosis: Juvenile, Idiopathic and Postmenopausal.

Jenifer O.M. Jowsey[1] and Kenneth P. Offord[2].

[1]Director, Orthopaedic Research, Mayo Clinic, Rochester, Minnesota.
[2]Medical Research Statistics, Mayo Clinic, Rochester, Minnesota.

Important medical research is frequently stimulated by the existence of a large group of patients with chronic, unsolved problems. This is true of osteoporosis; the disease is common and likely to become more so. The purpose of this paper will be to summarize the bone morphometric findings in osteoporotic patients and to relate them to the biochemical values. Etiological factors important in the development of the disease will be discussed and finally the present status in the reversal of bone loss in patients with osteoporosis will be presented.

In 1948 Fuller Albright wrote that postmenopausal osteoporosis was the result of a defect in matrix formation (1). Based on studies in egg-laying pigeons in which estrogen promotes intermedullary bone formation, he felt estrogen deficiency was responsible for a failure of osteoblastic activity (2). More recently, it has been possible to directly measure bone formation and resorption in bone biopsies from patients with symptomatic bone disease and fractures and to compare these values with those from control, non-osteoporotic people. The data show that the abnormality in osteoporosis is one of increased bone resorption. This is true of juvenile and idiopathic osteoporosis as well as of postmenopausal osteoporosis (Fig. 1, Table 1).

A large amount of information is available from different investigators who have measured bone turnover in osteoporosis and it would be remiss not to review these since some differences are found in the data. The most frequent difference is in the levels of bone formation; Jowsey reports no decrease in formation using cortical and trabecular bone (Table 2) while Schenk's group, using trabecular bone only, have reported a decrease in bone formation with increasing age in normal individuals and also a lower value for bone formation in osteoporosis (3). The decrease in normals was only seen in Schenk's data when high values for bone formation were eliminated from the age groups older than 50 years; no basis for eliminating these values is given and in the "uncorrected" data there is no significant decrease in bone formation with age (4). Nevertheless, a decrease in osteoblasts in bone samples from osteoporotic individuals compared with normal appear to be a clear difference. Osteoblast numbers and bone formation do tend to be lower in

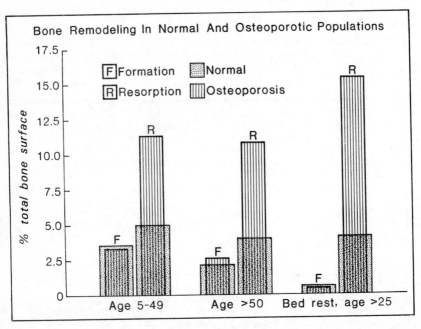

Figure 1--Values for bone resorption and formation in patients
with osteoporosis. The three groups are: juvenile
and idiopathic osteoporosis, postmenopausal osteoporosis and osteoporotic patients who have been at
bed-rest, each with age-matched non-osteoporotic controls. Bone resorption is higher than normal in all
three groups while formation is not different from
normal and is decreased in both the osteoporotic and
control groups with bed-rest.

Table 1

Bone Formation and Resorption in Different

Groups of Osteoporotic Patients

	Age in years	% total bone surface Formation	% total bone surface Resorption
Normal (n=77)	5-49	3.6 $\pm$ 2.6	5.0 $\pm$ 2.0
Osteoporotic (n=20)	5-49	3.3 $\pm$ 2.3	11.3* $\pm$ 4.5
Normal (n=67)	>50	2.1 $\pm$ 1.5	4.0 $\pm$ 1.3
Osteoporotic (n=147)	>50	2.6** $\pm$ 1.8	10.8* $\pm$ 5.4
Normal + bed-rest (0-14 days) (n=21)	>25	0.7 $\pm$ 0.5	4.1 $\pm$ 2.3
Osteoporotic + bed-rest (?days) (n=6)	>25	0.3 $\pm$ 0.2	16.4* $\pm$ 5.6

Values are mean $\pm$ 1S.D.

*p < 0.005

** p < .05

Table 2

Percent Bone Formation in Cortical and Trabecular Bone in Control
and Osteoporotic Individuals of Different Ages in the Anterior Iliac Crest

(values are mean percent)

	0-19	20-29	30-39	40-49	50-59	60-69	70-79	80
Trabecular bone								
control	4.4	3.9	2.4	1.4	1.5	2.1	2.4	1.3
osteoporosis	2.1	3.6	1.9	2.4	2.3	1.8	2.5	0.9
Cortical bone								
control	14.5	4.7	6.2	3.8	5.9	6.6	4.2	5.1
osteoporosis	15.0	3.6	2.9	5.4	7.1	5.3	5.7	2.1
Total bone								
control	7.9	4.0	3.7	3.2	3.1	3.5	2.8	2.7
osteoporosis	5.9	3.6	2.1	3.8	4.1	2.9	3.6	1.2
control	14	9	11	11	10	13	12	14
osteoporosis	5	1	4	4	15	19	15	6

trabecular bone in older individuals; certainly both in osteoporotic and normals the values are all less after the age of 30 than before 30 years of age (Table 2). But in trabecular bone quantitative microradiography does not demonstrate a decrease in bone formation in osteoporotic individuals compared with controls in contrast to the work of Schenk and Bordier (4). The reason may be in the activity level of the patients. All patients studied at the Mayo Clinic are ambulatory and are not hospitalized but are studied under outpatient conditions using a Clinical Study Unit. Bone responds rapidly to bed-rest (Table 1); a decrease in bone formation can be seen after 24 hours of bed-rest in normal people and it is probable that when a decrease in osteoblast activity is seen in either normal or osteoporotic groups, it represents a response to inactivity.

There may also be other differences in the population of patients used. Investigators have included patients who are already receiving a form of treatment that can be expected to alter bone remodeling, such as calcium supplements (5, 6). The mean age of the population may also be different; the patients in the combined studies in investigations at the Mayo Clinic have a mean age of 59.3 years which is younger than the group studied by Schenk (mean age 73) or by Meunier (3, 7). Bordier's experience substantiates the importance of the age of the osteoporotic population, particularly with regard to bone resorption; in a group of 11 patients of an average age of 37, bone resorption, urinary hydroxyproline and other parameters of resorption were approximately twice normal (Table 3) (8); in a similar group with a mean age of 56, resorption was also increased in osteoporosis (9). However, in older patients resorption was not increased above normal (10).

The major difference in morphological data is the type of bone on which the morphometric analysis has been carried out. One of the earliest investigators, H. Frost, studied cortical bone in the rib and clavicle, where he found increases of threefold in bone formation between age 30 and 60 (11). In iliac crest specimens trabecular bone shows a decline in formation while if cortical and trabecular bone are evaualted no change is seen (Table 2). In considering bone resorption it is evident from bone density measurements of trabecular and cortical bone or of bones composed predominantly of trabecular or cortical bone, that loss of tissue occurs more rapidly in the cortex (Table 4) (12, 13). Therefore, if in a disease characterized by bone loss such as osteoporosis, where elevated resorption must be considered as a cause of the bone loss, it is necessary to make quantitative measurements in the area of bone where the loss is occurring most rapidly. Trabecular bone loss, in fact, appears to be negligible after the age of 50 to the point that the percentage of trabecular to total bone actually increases while cortical bone continues to decrease (12).

The majority of bone density data suggest that bone loss begins at an age previous to the menopause and since decrease in the mass of mineralized tissue and osteoporosis also occur in

Table 3

Bone Resorption in Control and Young

Osteoporotic Individuals, mean age 37 years

(n=11, age-matched controls)

	Control*	Osteoporotic**
Osteoclasts, per mm^2	0.15 ± 0.10	0.30 ± 0.20
Active resorption, %total surface	0.59 ± 0.5	0.95 ± 0.86
Urinary hydroxyproline, mg/24 hours	25 ± 10	50 ± 13

*mean ± 2S.D.

**mean ± 1S.D.

From Bordier, et al.(8)

Table 4

Linear Regression Equations (Y=A + Bx) for % Bone

Volume (Y) on Age (X) in the Iliac Crest

	A	B	Sy.x
Cortical bone	61.77	-0.09	1.94
Trabecular bone	38.10	+0.09	1.98

From Giroux, et al.(12)

men, other factors must be important in causing bone loss. Calcium deficiency has been suggested as a cause of osteoporosis but there is little data to support this suggestion unless the phosphorus level is taken into account (14, 15). In animals a phosphorus to calcium ratio of greater than one will result in stimulation of bone resorption and diminution of bone mass (16, 17, 18). The animal data includes studies on many different species and in dogs serum parathyroid hormone assay was possible; the values were higher after a period of high phosphate supplementation (19). In man the calcium to phosphorus ratio is 0.54 in patients with osteoporosis which is similar to that which will stimulate increased parathyroid hormone secretion and bone resorption in man (Table 5) (20, 21).

Before the menopause and in men it appears that a dietary inbalance between calcium and phosphorus forms a stimulus to accelerated bone loss. Certainly the carefully carried out balance studies have shown that the calcium intake in both pre- and postmenopausal women is inadequate to prevent a negative calcium balance (22). Amounts of 1.0 to 1.4 grams of calcium per day are required to produce positive calcium balance. Since dietary studies have so far failed to show clear differences in calcium and phosphorus levels in individuals with and without osteoporosis, the predisposition to fracture must depend not only on continued bone loss with age but also on the amount of bone existing at skeletal maturity (22). Very little is known about the factors that dictate what this is, but again it may well be the calcium to phosphorus ratio in the diet. In addition the existence of a fracture, which is generally held to separate osteoporotic patients from non-osteoporotic individuals, obviously depends on stress.

Evidence of increased resorption as the abnormality of bone in osteoporosis is firm, if cortical and trabecular bone are evaluated; however the values for parathyroid hormone are still somewhat controversial. Published values have been reported as being higher in osteoporosis (24-27) or not statistically different (28), using the carboxyl-terminal assay of Arnaud, et al (21). If all the values in the number of studies carried out at the Mayo Clinic are pooled with normal values collected during the same period of time, then osteoporotic patients appear to have a value higher than normal.

It has been suggested that values collected over a long period are not comparable; however, the mean for the pooled 1970-1971 data is 29.1 and for 1972-1977 is 30.0 µlEq/dl suggesting that the results are consistent over this time; the same is true of the control values which have varied in published data between 17 and 22.4 µlEq/dl while recent unreported values average 20.9 µlEq/dl. The object was to compare the PTH (Y) on an Age (X) regression in normal subjects and osteoporotic patients (osteoporotics). In a comparison of this sort, it is highly desirable to have a comparable age range in the two groups. Since there were no osteoporotics under 40, two separate sets of analyses were performed. Approach I utilized all 143 normals,

Table 5

Serum Parathyroid Hormone and Bone Resorption

in Relationship to a High Phosphorus Intake

	n	Dietary Ca:P ratio	Bone resorption %total surface	Serum PTH
Adult cats				
13 mos. normal Ca	7	0.9	1.2*± 0.9	2.9**± 0.6
13 mos. high P	8	0.1	11.8 ± 3.9	6.5 ± 2.0
Adult dogs (same animals in Ca P period)				
11 mos. normal Ca	6	1.07	2.7 ± 1.4	55.3 ± 14.1
5 mos. high P	6	0.33	16.7 ± 3.5	142.5 ± 53.2
Man				
normal adults, > 50 yrs.	67	--	4.0 ± 1.3	20.9 ± 3.8 (n=16)
osteoporotic adults, >50 yrs.	147	--	11.3 ± 4.5	29.5 ± 12.5(n=86)

In man the resorption and PTH data are from different groups; in normals there was no overlap and in the osteoporotics the 86 PTH values were among the 147 in whom bone resorption was measured.

*resorption spaces

**A/B index from Jowsey and Raisz. (20)   All other values are serum immunoreactive iPTH using the C-terminal assay of Arnaud, et al (21)

while approach II included only the 95 normals of 40 years and
above.

Results of Approach I (All Normals (n=143), Osteoporotics (n=86))

When the 143 normals were considered alone, the estimated
slope was 0.082, which was significantly greater than zero at
P=.04. The slope for the 86 osteoporotic patients was not significantly different from zero at P>.10. The hypothesis of a common
line for both groups was rejected (P<.001). The hypothesis of a
common slope was not rejected (P>.10). The hypothesis of a
common intercept assuming a common slope was rejected (P<.001).
The estimated overall common slope of 0.088 was not significantly different from zero (P=.07). The conclusion based on this
approach is that the regression lines in the two groups are
parallel but separate in that the osteoporotic patients line is
shifted up, meaning they have a significantly higher mean PTH
for all ages. The regression on age is not very striking and
one might choose to compare the PTH values in the two groups
using a two-sample T-test, while ignoring age. The conclusions
from this two-sample T-test are the same. The mean PTH in the
osteoporotics is significantly greater than in normals (T=6.6,
df=227, P<.001).

There is a somewhat increased variability in PTH in the
osteoporotic group. If the PTH is transformed to $\ln_e$ PTH (Fig
2) in an effort to make the variability more comparable in the
two groups, the same conclusions are reached, except the slope
in the regression of $\ln_e$ PTH on age in the normals alone is no
longer significantly different from zero (P=.084).

Results of Approach II (Normals $\geq$ 40 yrs. (n=95) Osteoporotics
(n=86)).

The same conclusions hold as above except the slope of the
regression in normals alone is not significantly different from
zero. If the PTH is transformed to $\ln_e$ PTH is an effort to
make the variability more comparable in the two groups, the same
conclusions are reached and again the slope of the regression in
normals alone is not significantly different from zero.
Regardless of whether normals < 40 are included or whether
PTH or $\ln_e$ PTH is used or analysis of covariance or two-sample
T-test is employed, the same conclusion is reached. Mean PTH
values in osteoporotics are higher than in normals.

Understanding of the etiology of bone loss has been helpful in deciding what forms of treatment could be considered
useful in osteoporosis. It should be fully understood, though,
that a therapeutic agent which returns the bone turnover to
normal will not result in increased bone mass but will only
restore bone loss to normal.

If a relatively low dietary calcium intake compared with
phosphorus is effective in increasing bone resorption and
causing osteoporosis in man, calcium supplements should reverse

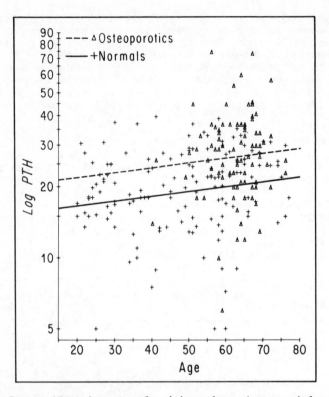

Figure 2--Serum iPTH in normals (+) and patients with symptomatic osteoporosis (Δ) in relation to age. Plotted are the lines obtained when a common slope is assumed.
Normals $\log n_e$ iPth = 2.7834 + 0.0039 x age (yrs)

Osteoporotics $\log n_e$ iPTH = 3.0595 + 0.0039 x age (yrs)
The individual lines for -normals: Logn_e iPTH = 2.7930 +0.0037 x age (yrs) -osteoporotics: Logn_e iPTH = 2.9414 +0.0058 x age (yrs)

this ratio and suppress parathyroid hormone and return resorption to normal. Long-term studies have shown this to be the case (Table 6) (29). Vitamin D formed part of the treatment and was felt to be somewhat more effective in high doses (50,000 units twice a week) than in low doses (400 units per day) but the high doses produced significant hypercalcuria and was felt to be more of a hazard than a benefit. Bone mass, however, remained unchanged (Jowsey, personal communication); therefore, although calcium with or without vitamin D may halt bone loss, it cannot be expected to restore bone to normal density.

There is some evidence that low levels of 1,25 vitamin D may be important in the etiology of osteoporosis (30). The decrease may be the result of estrogen lack in the postmenopausal state since estrogens have been shown to be effective in stimulating 1-hydroxylase activity (31). Therefore, unlike phosphorous-calcium ratios, 1,25 vitamin D can be expected to play a role in the etiology of bone loss only in the older postmenopausal age-group. Administration of 1,25 vitamin D in doses high enough to increase the intestinal adsorption of calcium have produced no significant changes in bone resorption or formation (Tables 7 & 9). "This finding is explicable in terms of the pathology of osteoporosis and suggests that 1,25-$(OH)_2D_3$ is unlikely to be useful in the treatment of this disorder." (32).

Albright correctly implicated estrogen deficiency as an important etiological factor in the osteoporosis of postmenopausal or oophorectomized women and later investigators have shown that estrogens mediate the effect of parathyroid hormone on bone causing a suppression of osteoclastic activity and a decrease of bone loss (33). In estrogen deficient, osteoporotic patients estrogen replacement causes a decrease in serum calcium, the expected response of a rise in serum parathyroid hormone, and a decrease in bone resorption (Table 8). With this information it has been suggested that estrogens will be useful for slowing the process of bone resorption. Short-term administration results in calcium retention and a decrease in bone resorbing surfaces but long-term studies have shown that the favorable effects are not maintained since bone formation also decreases (Table 8) (33). The side effects are significant. Riggs and colleagues reported that "estrogens were poorly tolerated and that half the patients experienced regular withdrawal bleeding; breakthrough bleeding and menopathia hemorrhagica...are not uncommon. Breast tenderness and dependent edema are other troublesome effects" (33). As with calcium and vitamin D, estrogens resulted in no change in bone mass and therefore can only be expected to slow the progress of bone loss (Table 8).

It is obvious that osteoporosis is a multifactoral disease. The role of estrogens in postmenopausal osteoporosis is well established. But the recent determinations of rates of bone loss have shown that there is a significant decrease in skeletal mass before the menopause and this paper has concentrated somewhat on this period by documenting the bone pathology of patients before age 50 and by examining the part played by the

Table 6

Bone Turnover in Osteoporotic Patients Before and After

Calcium or Calcium and Vitamin D Treatment

(mean $\pm$ S.D.)

	n	Bone Formation, %	Bone Resorption, %	Serum iPTH, μleq/ml
Osteoporosis				
before treatment	12	1.6 $\pm$ 0.5	8.4 $\pm$ 3.9	31.0 $\pm$ 11.0
Oral calcium & vitamin D				
treatment (3 mos)	12	0.6 $\pm$ 0.5	4.0 $\pm$ 1.6	26.7 $\pm$ 14.0
Change from pretreatment		-0.9 $\pm$ 0.5	-4.4 $\pm$ 3.4	-4.3 $\pm$ 8.2
values		$p < .001*$	$p < .001*$	$p > .05*$
Osteoporosis				
before treatment	10	1.5 $\pm$ 0.5	8.9 $\pm$ 3.9	32.9 $\pm$ 11.2
Oral Calcium and Vitamin D				
treatment (12 mos)	10	0.8 $\pm$ 0.6	4.5 $\pm$ 1.1	23.1 $\pm$ 10.5
Change from pretreatment		-1.0 $\pm$ 1.2	-4.4 $\pm$ 3.8	-8.8 $\pm$ 10.4
values		$p > .05*$	$p > .001*$	$p > .01*$
Osteoporosis				
before treatment	14	2.0 $\pm$ 1.3	9.4 $\pm$ 5.0	32.1 $\pm$ 20.0
Oral calcium				
treatment (3 mos)	14	1.2 $\pm$ 1.6	6.3 $\pm$ 3.3	33.1 $\pm$ 19.3
Change from pretreatment		-0.8 $\pm$ 1.6	-3.1 $\pm$ 3.5	+1.0 $\pm$ 10.4
values		$p > .50*$	$p > .005*$	$p > .70*$

*p values associated with two-tailed paired t-test.

Table 7

The Effect of Vitamin D or Placebo on Bone

Turnover in Osteoporosis

(mean ± S.D.)

	n	Bone Formation, %	Bone Resorption, %
Osteoporosis			
before treatment	12	2.0 ± 1.1	8.5 ± 3.6
after 1,25 vitamin D (6 mos)	12	1.8 ± 1.3	6.9 ± 2.3
change from pretreatment values		-0.2 ± 1.7	-1.6 ± 3.9
		t=0.444	t=1.454
		p ⟩.60*	p ⟩.10*
Osteoporosis			
before treatment	9	2.1 ± 1.4	8.1 ± 3.0
after placebo administration (6 mos)	9	2.3 ± 1.7	7.4 ± 3.5
change from pretreatment values		0.2 ± 2.2	-0.7 ± 2.9
		t=0.241	t=0.70
		p ⟩.80*	p ⟩.50*

*p values associated with two-tailed paired t-test.

Table 8

Bone Turnover in Control, Osteoporotic and Estrogen

Treated Osteoporotic Women

(mean $\pm$ S.D.)

	n	Bone Formation, %	Bone Resorption, %	Serum iPTH, μleq/ml
Estrogen replete,				
(premenopausal control,				
20-45 yr. females)	10	1.8 $\pm$ 1.2	4.1 $\pm$ 1.8	
Estrogen deficient,				
(postmenopausal osteoporosis,				
50-70 yr. females)	104	2.5 $\pm$ 1.6	9.7 $\pm$ 4.6	33.0*
Pretreatment osteoporosis	19	3.3 $\pm$ 2.0	12.7 $\pm$ 3.4	23.0 $\pm$ 4.2 (n=9)
Estrogen treated (3 mos)	19	3.4 $\pm$ 2.3	7.1 $\pm$ 2.2	29.4 $\pm$ 8.4 (n=9)
Change from pretreatment				
values		0.04$\pm$2.4	-5.47 $\pm$ 4.0	6.0 $\pm$ 9.3
		p $>$.90**	p $<$.001**	p $>$.10*
Pretreatment osteoporosis	8	5.0 $\pm$ 0.8	15.1 $\pm$ 2.7	not available
Estrogen treated (12 mos)	8	0.7 $\pm$ 0.6	10.6 $\pm$ 2.5	29.0 (n=5)
Change from pretreatment				
values		-4.3 $\pm$ 0.6	-4.5 $\pm$ 3.2	not available
		p $>$.001*	p $>$.001*	

*From Riggs, et al. [33]

**p values associated with two-tailed paired t-test.

Table 9

The Effect of Various Therapeutic Agents on Bone Formation and

Resorption in Osteoporotic Individuals

(mean values)

	n	Pretreatment		Treatment (3-4 mos)		Treatment (1-2 yrs)	
		% Formation	% Resorption	% Formation	% Resorption	% Formation	% Resorption
Placebo	9	2.1	8.1	2.3	7.4 (6 mos)		
EHDP	4	1.7	10.0	0.7	10.0		
Estrogens	9	4.8	15.0	4.0	6.4*	0.7*,**	10.4**
Anabolic Hormones	9	2.5	11.1	3.2	9.5	0.8**	8.7
Calcitonin	5	2.2	11.6	1.7	14.9		
Calcitonin & Calcium	23	2.2	8.6	1.4	3.9*	1.1	5.2
Calcium Infusions	12	2.1	9.5	3.9	5.5* (1-6 mos)		
Oral Calcium & Vitamin D	9	1.6	9.8	0.5*	4.1*	0.7*	4.6*
Oral Calcium	14	2.0	9.4	1.2	6.3*		
1,25 Vitamin D	12	2.0	8.5	1.8	6.9 (6 mos)		
Oral Phosphate	8	3.8	11.0	2.3	17.4*	0.7*,**	16.8*,**
Growth Hormone	5	[1.7]	[2.4]			4.1	4.1
Fluoride & Calcium	12	[[2.2]]	[[8.1]]	5.9*	3.6*	5.4*	4.0*

*Significantly different from pretreatment value.

**Significantly different from short-term therapy.

[ ] On calcium previous to treatment with growth hormone.

[[ ]] On estrogens previous to fluoride and calcium treatment

dietary calcium to phosphorus ratio. Inactivity is also of importance and these two factors play key roles in bone loss in the adult; while etiological factors which cause the disease may be considered as being potentially useful as therapeutic regimes for reversing the bone abnormality. Some, such as exercise, do not succeed in restoring bone mass. Non-physiological agents, such as the diphosphonates, have been studied and have not proved useful with the single exception of fluoride which has been shown to increase bone formation while resorption is depressed by concomitant calcium administration (Table 9).

Acknowledgments

I would like to thank Drs. Kelly and Johnson for their assistance in taking the bone biopsies in the patients: Drs. Riggs and Hoffman have been most helpful in the clinical aspects and Dr. C. D. Arnaud and the Mayo Regional Laboratories for measuring the immunoreactive parathyroid hormone.

Abbreviations

PTH--parathyroid hormone

References

1. Albright, F. and Reifenstein, E.C. 1948. The Parathyroid Glands and Metabolic Bone Disease. Baltimore, Williams and Wilkins Company, 145-197.

2. Gardner, W.U. and Pfeffer, C.A. 1943. Influence of estrogens and androgens on the skeletal system. Physiol. Rev., 23, 139-165.

3. Schenk, R.K., Olah, A.J. and Merz, W.A. 1973. Bone cell counts. Excerpta Medica, International Congress Series, No. 270, 103-113.

4. Merz, W.A. and Schenk, R.K. 1970. A quantitative study on bone formation in human cancellous bone. Acta Anat., 76, 1-15.

5. Jett, S., Wu, K. and Frost, H.M. 1967. Tetracycline-based histological measurement of cortical-endosteal bone formation in normal and osteoporotic rib. Henry Ford Hosp. Med. J., 15(4), 325-344.

6. Aloia, J.F., Zanzi, I., Ellis, K., Jowsey, J., Roginsky, M., Wallach, S. and Cohn, S.H. 1976. Effects of growth hormone in osteoporosis. J. Clin. Endocrinol. Metab., 43(5), 992-999.

7. Meunier, P., Courpron, P., Edouard, C., Bernard, J., Bringuier, J. and Vignon, C. 1973. Physiological senile involution and pathological rarefaction of bone. Clinics Endocrinol. Metab., 2 (2), 239-256.

8. Bordier, Ph. J., Miravet, L. and Hioco, D. 1973. Young adult osteoporosis. Clinics Endocrinol. Metab., 2 (277-292)

9. Bordier, Ph. J., Matrajt, H., Miravet, L. and Hioco, D. 1965. Mesure histologique De La resorption osseuse dans l'osteoporose: Etude preliminaire. Calcified Tissues, European Symposium, University Liege, 1964. Publisher: University de Liege, 39-50.

10. Bordier, Ph. J. and Tun Chot, S. 1972. Quantitative histology of metabolic bone. Clin. Endocrinol. 1, 197-215.

11. Frost, H.M. 1961. Postmenopausal osteoporosis: A disturbance in osteoclasia. J. Am. Geriat. Soc., 9, 1078-1085.

12. Giroux, J.-M., Courpron, P. and Meunier, P. 1975. Histomorphometrie De L'Osteopenie Physiologique Senile. Lyon.

13. Jowsey,J. 1977. The Bone Biopsy. Plenum Publishing Corp., New York.

14. Nordin, B.E.C. 1971. Clinical significance and pathogenesis of osteoporosis. Brit. Med. J., 1, 571-576.

15. Smith, Jr., R.W. and Frame, B. 1965. Concurrent axial and appendicular osteoporosis: Its relation to calcium consumption. New Engl. J. Med., 272, 73.

16. Jowsey, J. and Balasubramaniam, P. 1972. The effect of phosphate supplements on soft tissue calcification and bone turnover. Clin. Sci., 42, 289-299.

17. Laflamme, G.H. and Jowsey, J., 1972. Bone and soft-tissue changes with oral phosphate supplements. J. Clin. Invest., 51(11), 2834-2840.

18. Krook, L., Barrett, R.B., Usui, K. and Wolke, R.E. 1963. Nutritional secondary hyperparathyroidism in the cat. Cornell Vet., 53, 224-240.

19. Jowsey, J., Reiss, E. and Cantebury,J.M. 1974. Long-term effects of high phosphate intake on parathyroid hormone levels and bone metabolism. Acta Orthop.Scand., 45(6), 801-808.

20. Jowsey, J. and Raisz, L.G. 1968. Experimental osteoporosis and parathyroid activity. Endocrinol., 82(2), 384-396.

21. Arnaud, C.D., Tsao, Hang S. and Littledike, T. 1971. Radioimmunoassay of human parathyroid hormone in serum. J. Clin. Invest., 50(1), 21-34.

22. Heaney, R.P., Recker, R.R. and Saville, P.D. 1974. Calcium balance and calcium requirements in middle-aged women. Clin. Res., 22, 649A.

23. Newton-John, H.F. and Morgan, D.B. 1968. Osteoporosis: disease or senescence? Lancet, i, 232.

24. Fujita, T., Orimo, H., Okano, K. and Yoshihawa, M. 1973. Clinical application of parathyroid hormone radioimmunoassay. Excerpta Medica International Congress Series No. 270, 274-280.

25. Berlyne, G.M., Ben-Ari, J., Galinsky, D., Hirsch, M., Kushelvesky, A. and Shainkin, R. 1974. The etiology of osteoporosis: the role of parathyroid hormone. JAMA, 229, 1904-1905.

26. Gallagher, J.C., Bulusu, L. and Nordin, B.E.C. 1973. Oestrogenic hormones and bone resorption. Excerpta Medica, International Congress Series No. 270, 266-273.

27. Teitelbaum, S.L., Rosenberg, E.M., Richardson, C.A. and Avioli, L.V., 1976. Histological studies of bone from normocalcemic postmenopausal osteoporotic patients with increased circulating parathyroid hormone. J. Clin. Endocrinol., 42, 537-543.

28. Riggs, B.L., Arnaud, C.D., Jowsey, J., Goldsmith, R.S. and Kelly, P.J. 1973. Parathyroid function in primary osteo-

porosis. J. Clin. Invest. 52, 181-184.

29. Riggs, B.L., Jowsey, J., Kelly, P.J., Hoffman, D.L. and Arnaud, C.D. 1976. Effects of oral therapy with calcium and vitamin D in primary osteoporosis. J. Clin. Endocrinol. Metab., 42(6), 1139-1144.

30. Gallagher, J.C., Riggs, B.L., Eisman, J., Arnaud, S.B. and DeLuca, H.F. 1976. Impaired production of 1,25-dihydroxy-vitamin D in postmenopausal osteoporosis. Clin. Res., 24, 580A.

31. Kenny, A.D. 1976. Vitamin D metabolism: Physiological regulation in egg-laying Japanese quail. Am. J. Physiol. 230, 1609-1615.

32. Davies, M., Mawer, E.B. and Adams, P.H. 1977. Vitamin D metabolism and the response to 1,25-dihydroxycholecalcife-rol in osteoporosis. Calc. Tiss. Res., Supplement to vol. 22, 74-77.

33. Riggs, B.L., Jowsey, J., Goldsmith, R.S., Kelly, P.J., Hoffman, D.L. and Arnaud, C.D. 1972. Short- and long-term effects of estrogen and synthetic anabolic hormone in postmenopausal osteoporosis. J. Clin. Invest., 51(7), 1659-1663.

Bone Resorbing Cells in Paget's Disease.

Frederick R. Singer*, Barbara G. Mills**, and Roger Terry*

University of Southern California Schools of Medicine* and Dentistry**, Los Angeles, CA

Paget's disease of bone is an excellent example of a localized disorder of bone resorption. This is not immediately apparent in each case since the diagnosis of this condition is most often made in the later stages of the disease when a secondary increase in bone formation has led to the typically enlarged and deformed bones characteristic of this disorder. Schmorl (1) first recognized that the disease began with localized osteolysis characterized by an increase in the number of osteoclasts in Howship's lacunae. Subsequent to this he noted an increase in blood vessels and the development of connective tissue within the marrow. Finally the proliferation of osteoblasts on the surface of previously resorbed bone and on the trabeculae of newly formed bone in the fibrous marrow completed the apparent cycle of pathologic events. This sequence of events is generally accepted as correct, although a minority opinion is that osteocytic osteolysis is the primary abnormality responsible for the early increase in bone resorption (2).

In this paper we review previous studies and present our observations of the light microscopic and ultrastructural characteristics of osteoclasts and osteocytes in patients with active Paget's disease of bone.

The Osteoclasts

Light microscopy

The observation of the classical pathologists that osteoclasts are present in large numbers in active Paget's disease has been amply confirmed by quantitative morphometry of bone. Bordier and colleagues (3) have reported an osteoclast count of 1.6-6.7 per mm^2 in 10 patients (normal 0.1 to 0.3). Khairi and colleagues have found 2.2 ± 1.1 osteoclasts/mm^2 in 14 patients who had biopsies of involved iliac crest bone (normal 0.37 ± 0.15). In nine patients we found 5.36 ± 1.08 osteoclasts/mm^2 in pagetic iliac crest biopsies (5). In our study approximately half of the osteoclasts were not attached to bone. Presumably this reflects the great mobility of these cells.

Rubenstein and colleagues (6) were the first to note that osteoclasts in patients with Paget's disease could attain a size of over 200 microns in the greatest diameter and contain as many as 100 nuclei. Subsequently, Bordier (7, 8) stressed the great variability of size of the osteoclasts and that a section across an osteoclast might reveal only a few nuclei or more than 100. He felt that these features were characteristic of osteoclasts in Paget's disease only and that even in patients with severe primary hyperparathyroidism there was relative uniformity of size and rarely more than a dozen nuclei on a section. Our examination of biopsies in over 20 patients provides confirmation of the previous observations (Fig 1). We have found more than 50 nuclei in a single section of some osteoclasts but the majority of osteoclasts are much smaller and have far less nuclei. In 9 patients prior to treatment with salmon or human calcitonin the mean number of osteoclast nuclei on a section ranged from 4.4 to 8.9, the mean ± S.E. of the group was 6.1 ±0.47 (5). After chronic treatment with calcitonin, no statistically significant decrease in the number of osteoclast nuclei on a section was observed. The relative paucity of large multinucleated osteoclasts in these 9 patients may have obscured an effect of calcitonin on osteoclast size since Bordier found that in two patients with Paget's disease calcitonin and oral phosphate therapy decreased the nuclei per osteoclast from 11.37 and 19.22 to 6.78 and 11.46, respectively (7). The interpretation of this latter study is made difficult by the coexistence of primary hyperparathyroidism in both patients and by the administration of oral phosphate.

Electron Microscopy

In general the osteoclasts of Paget's disease exhibit the features of normal osteoclasts. When attached to bone, they have well-developed ruffled borders with an adjacent clear zone (Fig.2). The cytoplasm contains abundant mitochondria, vacuoles, free ribosomes, a small Golgi apparatus generally associated with a nucleus and very little rough endoplasmic reticulum. The characteristic abnormalties found in osteoclasts of Paget's disease are primarily in the nucleus. In approximately 20-40% of the osteoclasts we have observed a nuclear inclusion which varies greatly in size and arrangement (9). The inclusions consist of clusters of microfilaments grouped in paracrystalline array (Fig2) or, more commonly, the individual microfilaments are scattered randomly over a wider area of the nucleus. They are distinct from chromatin and the nucleolus. In some cells a degeneration of the nucleus is present (Fig.3) and microfilaments may then be found not only in between the remnants of the nucleus but in the adjacent cytoplasm (9).

The individual microfilaments seen in the osteoclasts average approximately 15 nm in diameter and contain an electron-lucent central core measuring 5 to 7 nm in diameter. The microfilaments are in a hexagonal arrangement when tightly packed in the nucleus in paracrystalline array. In the cytoplasm of the cell they are frequently found in strands of four or in loose bundles with random orientation.

The origin of the microfilaments is not known. However, it

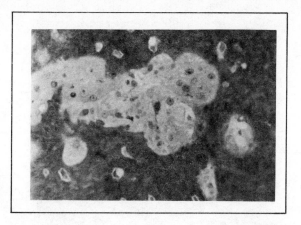

FIGURE 1

Large multinucleated osteoclasts in a Howship's lacuna. Note the adjacent osteocytes.

Decalcified, X1428

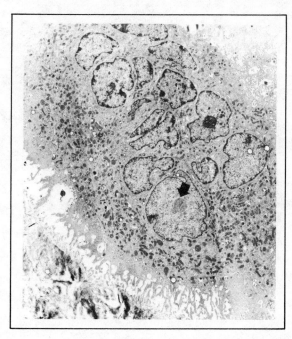

FIGURE 2

A pagetic osteoclast with 13 nuclei and a prominent nuclear inclusion (arrow). Note the well-developed ruffled border at the bone surface.

Decalcified, X5400

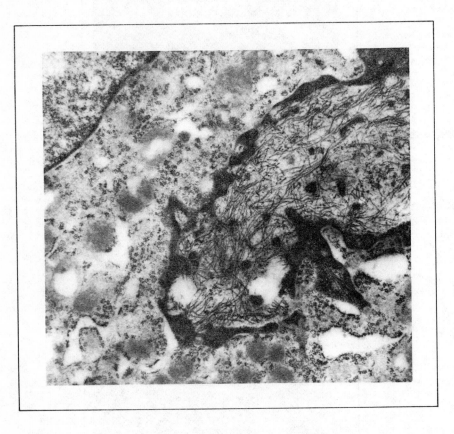

FIGURE 3

    A degenerating osteoclast nucleus with numerous randomly distributed microfilaments. Note a portion of a normal nucleus at the upper left.

Decalcified, X32,400

is now clear that they are a characteristic feature of osteoclasts in Paget's disease. Rebel and colleagues were the first
to report the existence of the osteoclast inclusions and have
found them in 35 biopsies of 23 patients (10-13). They have not
found a single patient who failed to demonstrate this ultrastructural feature. We also have found the inclusions in 24 of
24 patients evaluated by bone biopsy. Baldet has observed the
inclusions in Paget's disease but gave no indication of how many
patients were evaluated (14). The inclusions have not been seen
in other bone cells or in the osteoclasts of normal bone or of a
large variety of metabolic bone diseases including primary hyperparathyroidism, renal osteodystrophy, osteomalacia due to
intestinal malabsorption, vitamin D resistant rickets, fibrous
dysplasia, fibro-osseous dysplasia and multiple myeloma (9).
Although we have not had access to pathologic specimens of giant
cell tumors of bone, it does appear that identical nuclear inclusions are found in the multinucleated cells of some of these
tumors. Welsh and Meyer described nuclear inclusions and nuclear
fragmentation identical to that seen in pagetic osteoclasts in
two of three patients (15). In one patient microfilaments were
also found in the cytoplasm. A third documentation of typical
nuclear inclusions in a giant cell tumor has recently been
reported (16). In this tumor no nuclear fragmentation or cytoplasmic microfilaments were found. The origin of the multinucleated giant cells and their relationship to osteoclasts is
not known. It is of interest that nuclear inclusions of this
type have not been found in specimens of giant cell tumor of the
tendon sheath, giant cell reparative granuloma of bone, nonossi-
fing fibroma with giant cells, osteochondroma, chondroblastoma,
chrondrosarcoma and osteogenic sarcoma (15).

The morphologic characteristic of the nuclear and cytoplasmic inclusions in the pagetic osteoclasts bear a close
resemblance to the inclusions found in neurons and oligodendrog-
lial cells of patients with subacute sclerosing panencephalitis
(SSPE) (17). This disorder is now accepted as a slow virus infection resulting from exposure to a measles-like paramyxovirus.
The inclusions of SSPE are apparently viral nucleocapsids, incomplete forms of the fully developed virus which lack an envelope. In order to isolate infectious viruses from brain
specimens of these patients, it has been necessary to establish
cell cultures and utilize cell fusion techniques with susceptible cell lines (18, 19). We have utilized this information to
help test the hypothesis that Paget's disease is a slow virus
infection of bone. Bone specimens were obtained from five
patients with Paget's disease undergoing orthopedic surgery.
Fragments of bone were explanted on rattail tendon collagen and
grown in BGJ$_b$ medium. After cells migrated from the fragments,
they were passed at five weeks. Up to seven passages were
carried out over an 8-month period. Electron microscopic examination of the cultured cells revealed the presence of the
characteristic nuclear inclusions in the cells of two patients,
although no typical osteoclasts were seen (20). Cell fusion
experiments are being carried out in order to rescue any infectious virus which might be present in the cultured cells.

The nuclear inclusions of Paget's disease might also represent a marker of intense metabolic activity of the osteoclasts.
Since calcitonin given acutely (21) or chronically (3,5) can
reduce the rate of bone resorption and the number of osteoclasts
in bone it is of interest that patients treated in either manner
with calcitonin still have nuclear inclusions indistinguishable
from those found prior to calcitonin administration. These data
coupled with absence of nuclear inclusions in other metabolically active bone diseases suggest that the nuclear inclusions are
not a result of increased metabolic activity of the osteoclast.

The Osteocytes

Light Microscopy

Belanger has proposed that the early stage of Paget's
disease is initiated by an increase in osteolytic activity of the
osteocyte (2). Duriez and colleagues have also stressed the
large size of periosteocytic lacunae in Paget's disease (22).
This concept has been challenged by Meunier (23) who feels that
there is no adequate evidence to support the concept of a pathologic degree of periosteocytic "osteolysis" in Paget's disease.
He quantitated the size of the periosteocytic lacunae in both
lamellar and woven bone in 27 patients and found that the mean
cross-section surface of the lamellar lacunae was 51.8 ± 8.7 uM^2
as compared to 50.7 ± 5.5 uM^2 in 92 control subjects. In woven
bone there was a considerable increase in the mean cross-section
surface of the lacunae, 81.9 ± 15.3 uM^2. However, he stressed
that this is characteristic of woven bone in general and is a
constitutional feature of this type of bone. The possibility
that enlarged lacunae in woven bone result from periosteocytic
osteolysis has not been proven.

Our qualitative evaluation of osteocytes in the biopsies of
patients with Paget's disease revealed findings consistent in
some aspects with observations of both Belanger (2) and Meunier
(23). In most areas of lamellar bone the osteocytic lacunae
were indistinguishable in size from those in normal bone. However, enlarged osteocyte lacunae were occasionally observed
adjacent to Howship's lacunae (Fig 4). These Howship's lacunae
almost always contained one or more osteoclasts attached to the
bone surface. In woven bone the osteocyte lacunae were more
variable in size. Osteocytes underlying bone accretion surfaces
were large and filled their lacunae. Those which were more
centrally located within the matrix were in smaller lacunae and
had less cytoplasm and organelles. As in the case of lamellar
bone, osteocyte lacunae just below the surface of Howship's
lacunae sometimes were quite large (Fig 1). In areas of "burned
out" disease the osteocyte lacunae often contained degenerating
cells with pycnotic nuclei or were empty.

Electron Microscopy

Osteocytes near a bone accretion surface frequently retained

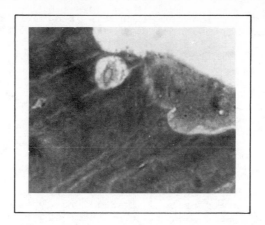

FIGURE 4

    A large osteocyte lacuna adjacent to an osteoclast in a Howship's lacuna in lamellar bone.

Decalcified, X1428

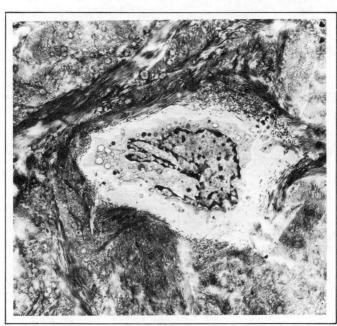

FIGURE 5

    An osteocyte in a lacuna which appears to be undergoing resorption. Numerous vacuoles are present in the sparse cytoplasm. Loose collagen fibrils are present within the lacuna.

Decalcified, X10,300

a well-developed endoplasmic reticulum, presumably reflecting their origin from osteoblasts. Other features of these cells which are common to active osteoblasts include a round nucleus containing euchromatin and abundant cytoplasm with mitochrondria, dense bodies and very little glycogen.

In only a relatively few osteocyte lacunae adjacent to active resorption surfaces in Howship's lacunae was there evidence of perilacunar resorption. In Figure 5 an osteocyte which may have resorbed bone is shown. Evidence that this cell may be stimulating perilacunar bone resorption is provided by the presence of loose collagen fibers within the lacuna, a feature not usually seen in more peripheral osteocyte lacunae adjacent to bone accretion surfaces. The cytoplasm of this cell contains large vacuoles and very little rough endoplasmic reticulm. No nuclear or cytoplasmic inclusions typical of the pagetic osteoclast were seen in any of the osteocytes.

Conclusions

The bulk of the histologic data that we and others have collected in patients with Paget's disease points to the osteoclast as the prime mediator of bone resorption in this disease. A minor role of the osteocyte can not be excluded.

The ultrastructural features of the osteoclasts have provided a new impetus for studies concerning the etiology of the disease. The nuclear and cytoplasmic inclusions so closely resemble viral nucleocapsids that the concept of the disease as a slow virus infection must be seriously examined. Although there is no direct evidence that Paget's disease and giant cell tumor of bone share a common pathogenesis, the similarity of the inclusions in the cells of these disorders suggest that this may be a fruitful area for study. It is known that these tumors can arise in the lesions of Paget's disease.

Acknowledgments

We thank Mrs. Anne Santo and Ms. Carol Gowdy for secretarial assistance and Ms. Pat Holst for technical assistance. This study was supported in part by funds provided by USPHS grant DE 03929, General Clinical Research Centers Grant RR-43, the Armour Pharmaceutical Co., the CIBA-GEIGY Corp. and by Ms. Gracia Bremer.

REFERENCES

1. Schmorl, G., 1932. Über Ostitis deformans Paget.
   Virchows Arch. Path. Anat. 283: 694-737.

2. Belanger, L.F., Jarry, L., and Uhthoff, H.K. 1968
   Osteocytic osteolysis in Paget's disease. Rev. Canad. Biol.
   27: 37-44.

3. Bordier, P. Woodhouse, N.J.Y., Joplin, G.F. and TunChot, S.
   1972. Quantitative bone histology in Paget's disease of
   bone. J. Bone Jt. Surg. 54-B, 553-554.

4. Khairi, M.R.A., Meunier, P., Edouard, C., Courpron, P.,
   Bernard, J., Derosa, G.P. and Johnston, C.C. Jr. 1977.
   Quantitative bone histology in Paget's disease of bone:
   Influence of sodium etidronate therapy. Calc. Tiss. Res.
   (Suppl. Vol. 22), pp355-358.

5. Singer, F.R., Rude, R.K. and Mills, B.G. 1977. Studies of
   the treatment and aetiology of Paget's disease of bone.
   In: Human Calcitonin and Paget's Disease, ed. by MacIntyre,
   I., Bern, H. Huber, pp. 93-110.

6. Rubinstein, M.A., Smelin, A. and Freedman, A.L. 1953.
   Arch. Int. Med. 92: 684-696.

7. Bordier, P., Rasmussen,H. and Dorfmann, H. 1974. Effectiveness of parathyroid hormone, calcitonin and phosphate
   on bone cells in Paget's disease. Am.J. Med. 56: 850-857.

8. Rasmussen, H. and Bordier, P. 1974. The Physiological and
   Cellular Basis of Metabolic Bone Disease. Baltimore,
   Williams and Wilkins Co., pp. 292-303.

9. Mills, B.G. and Singer, F.R. 1976. Nuclear inclusions in
   Paget's disease of bone. Science 194: 201-202.

10. Rebel, A., Malkani, K. and Basle, M. 1974. Anomalies
    nuclearies des ostéoclastes de la maladie osseuse de Paget.
    Nouv. Presse Méd. 3: 1299-1301.

11. Rebel, A., Malkani, K., Basle, M. and Bregeon, C. 1974
    Particularités ultrastructurales des osteoclastes de la
    maladie de Paget. Rev. Rhum. 41: 767-771.

12. Rebel, A. Bregeon, C., Basle, M. and Malkani, K. 1975.
    Les inclusions des osteoclastes dan la maladie osseuse de
    Paget. Rev. Rhum. 42: 637-641.

13. Rebel, A., Malkani, A., Basle, M. and Bregeon, C. 1976.
    Osteoclast ultrastructure in Paget's disease. Calcif. Tiss.
    Res. 20: 187-199.

14. Baldet, P. 1975. Histopathologie de l'os pagétique. In
    La Maladie Osseuse de Paget, Paris, Galliena;

15. Welsh, R. A. and Meyer, A.T. 1970. Nuclear fragmentation and associated fibrils in giant cell tumor of bone. Lab. Invest. 22: 63-72.

16. Le Charpentier, Y., Le Charpentier, M., Forest, M., Daudet-Monsac, M., Lavenu-Vacher, M.-C., Louvel, A., Sedel, L. and Abelanet, R. 1977. Inclusions intranucleaires dans une tumeur osseuse a cellules géantes. Nouv. Presse Med. 6: 259-262.

17. Oysnagi, S., ter Meulen, V., Katz, M. and Koprowski, H. 1971. Comparison of subacute sclerosing panencephalitis and measles viruses: an electron microscope study. J. Virol. 7: 176-187.

18. Horta-Barbosa, L., Fuccillo, D.A., London, W.T., Jabbour, J.T., Zeman, W. and Sever, J.L. 1969. Isolation of measles virus from brain cell cultures of two patients with subacute sclerosing pancephalitis. Proc. Soc. Exp. Biol. Med. 132: 272-277.

19. Katz, M., Koprowski. H. and Moorhead, P. 1969. Transformation of cells cultured from human brain tissue. Exp. Cell Res. 57: 149-153.

20. Mills, B.G., Singer, F.R., Weiner, L.E. and Holst, P.A. 1977. Hormonal responses of cells cultured from pagetic bone for up to eight months. Program of the Sixth Parathyroid Conference, p.104.

21. Singer, F.R., Melvin, K.E.W. and Mills, B.G. 1976. Acute effects of calcitonin on osteoclasts in man. Clin. Endocrinol. 5: 333s-340s.

22. Duriez, J., Flautre, B. and Ghosez, J.P. 1968. Etude microscopique du tissue osseux pagétique. Presse Méd. 76: 431-434.

23. Meunier, P.J. 1977. Disturbances in morphology and dynamics of the remodelling process in pagetic bone. In Human Calcitonin and Paget's Disease, edit. by MacIntyre, I., Bern, H. Huber, pp. 78-92.

Discussion for Session V: Primary Disorders of Bone Cell
Function. Part A.

DR. MARCUS: Dr. Jowsey, I wanted to get your response to
the paper that appeared in the Journal of Nutrition earlier this
year similar to the studies which you did in varying the calcium-
to-phosphorus ratio in the diet. In rather long-term experiments, using a diet which had a calcium-to-phosphorus ratio which
was quite low, they failed to show any evidence of nutritionally-
induced bone disease whatsoever.

DR. JOWSEY: Yes. I am aware of that. It is an exception to
all the animals that have been studied, which include, mice,
rats, rabbits, tigers, parakeets, horses, donkeys, and beagles.
It is an exception to the studies that have been done, perhaps
most importantly, in man.

DR. TEITELBAUM: Dr. Jowsey, I am very attracted to the
hypothesis that osteoporosis is a disease of increased bone
resorption. But I think it would be a mistake to leave the audience with the impression that the clinical syndrome is a homogeneous phenomenon; and rather, that it is really heterogeneous.

If one looks at the bones of individuals with the crush-
fracture syndrome, one can detect subpopulations of individuals
who do not demonstrate an increase in the rate of bone resorption. So probably what we are looking at is not a homogeneous,
but a heterogeneous phenomenon.

DR. JOWSEY: I think that is true. If you noticed in that
slide where I showed the bone resorption and bone formation, we
had about three or four people with osteoporosis who fell within
the normal range. These are characteristically long-term
osteoporotics, people who have had a long history of the disease.

Clinically it is very obvious that people don't go on
resorbing bone until there is none left. There is a certain time
and a certain stage in bone loss in which you get to about one-
quarter of the initial bone mass where the bone resorption
phenomenon becomes secondarily important. Bone resorption stops,
and that amount of bone is maintained. I think this would
represent a subpopulation; you might call it a terminal stage of
the disease, where bone resorption levels drop down to within the
normal range.

The other problem, of course, is that when you are looking at patients with osteoporosis, you are looking at people who have sustained a fracture and have the clinical diagnosis of the disease. You are comparing them, usually, with age-matched people who may be developing the bone loss; in other words, have a higher bone resorption level than they may otherwise have had, but yet not have sustained a fracture. Therefore, they are not clinically osteoporotic. So there is certainly a number of people amongst our "normals" who have, perhaps, elevated bone resorption levels but have to be called controls or normal, because they haven't yet had a fracture. So there is bound to be overlap from that point of view also.

DR. TEITELBAUM: I am really talking about comparing osteo-porotics to osteoporotics; in other words, people who present with the clinical syndrome that have different types of histol-ogies in their bone biopsies.

DR. JOWSEY: I don't think at any time you could divide them into a number of very separate populations. I don't think they have a bimodal distribution. I think it is a whole spectrum, all the way from low to high. This is also true of normals; that if you take normal formation and resorption, you go all the way from a low value to a high value. So that population that you are talking about, e.g., with the low formation or normal resorption, you could also find amongst your normals and would therefore not be a distinguishing feature between normal and osteoporotic people.

DR. TEITELBAUM: Dr. Singer, how did you culture the bone? What was the technique that you used?

DR. SINGER: Under sterile conditions at surgery, we minced the bone and tried to clear away as much of the marrow as possible to get relatively a marrow-free preparation. We put this on a rat-tail collagen substrate, and watched it grow as long as possible, up to 40 or 50 days; and then passed these cells up to seven times into culture media.

DR. TEITELBAUM: Did you strip the periosteum?

DR. SINGER: This was all trabecular bone.

DR. TEITELBAUM: Were you sure you didn't have fibroblasts?

DR. SINGER: We are well aware of the interpretation of the problem; and I think that there are two aspects to this work. One is, can one identify what the inclusions are? It doesn't matter, frankly, whether those are fibroblasts or not. On the other hand, it would be very nice to have human bone cells in long-term culture.

I think we have to use the methods of Mundy and take some of these cells from the next batch that we grow and put these on a bone matrix to see if we can get more differentiated bone cells. We are not trying to say these are absolutely bone cells. We are just hopeful that they may be related.

DR. HORTON: Dr. Jowsey, Jean Aaron from Nardine's lab has been looking at what are called "micro-fractures" in trabeculations. I wonder with the loss of cortical material in the osteoporotics if you are seeing any micro-fractures in trabecular bone?

DR. JOWSEY: We haven't in the iliac crest material, but I have collected a number of samples from the vertebrae; and we certainly find microfractures there, mostly in a stage of healing, with bundles of callus around them. I have always interpreted that as you get a loss of cortex, then you get a loss of integrity of the vertical body and you get small collapses which usually aren't interpreted; i.e., they are too small to be interpreted in terms of a frank fracture. That is an observation that many people have made in vertebral body.

DR. HORTON: Dr. Singer, there are many laboratories chasing the origin of the osteoclast. In your presentation here today, you were very specific to point out that you did not see these bodies in osteocytes nor in osteoblasts. However, you failed to mention whether you have looked at peripheral blood cells, specifically mononuclear leukocytes, either circulating or derived from bone marrow, or in even various immature forms of bone marrow cells.

DR. SINGER: You bring up a very important point. That is on our list; we just haven't done it.

DR. PARFITT: I have a brief comment for each of these papers. This is a session supposedly on primary disorders of bone cell function. Dr. Jowsey evidently believes that in osteoporosis, there is no primary disorder of bone cell function; the bone cells are simply responding in an appropriate manner to whatever homeostatic insults, dietary peculiarities, impose upon them.

I would make one brief comment, however; and that is that if the bone cells do not show any impairment of function with age, they must be the only cells in the body which enjoy this privileged status.

The second comment, having to do with Dr. Singer's paper: I think the participation or supposed participation of the osteocytes in the resorptive process of Paget's disease was actually first drawn attention to by Dr. Lent Johnson several years before Dr. Belanger. But what Johnson demonstrated was that the osteocytes were only involved close to the advancing osteoclastic surface. In other words, it was an example that Dr. Baylink drew attention to, that in many situations the osteoclasts on the surface and the osteocytes immediately subjacent to the surface form a unit which together is accomplishing resorption of bone from the surface. It may not make any sense to say which comes first; that the stimuli which cause osteoclastic activity on the surface may also cause whatever changes the osteocytes are contributing to the overall process.

DR. JOWSEY: I would like to respond to the first comment Dr. Parfitt made. I think you have to be careful when you are talking about aging. It depends on when you think "old" is. The average age of our population, of our group as a whole, is 59.3 years-old, which includes the idiopathic group; and of our study patients which includes people over the age of 40, it is about 64.8 or 65. So we are looking at a population that may be different from the more commonly aged osteoporotic population of between 70 and 90, where I am sure that one might very well come up with cells that are behaving in a different manner to our younger group, who are responding mainly to the request by the serum for normal calcium levels.

DR. TALMAGE: I would like to ask Dr. Jowsey if there isn't another problem with the phosphate. You talked about the post-prandial rise in plasma phosphate. Whether the phosphate rises or falls after eating depends to a large extent on the carbohydrate content of the diet; if you have a large carbohydrate content, you are going to stimulate insulin release, and the phosphate may go down. There will be a large study, some 200 or 300 cases, coming out of Paris in the next couple of years showing that the phosphate fall after eating, or rise after eating, will depend entirely upon what was in the diet; not the phosphate, but what else was in the diet, particularly the carbohydrate. So I would like to suggest that whether or not you have carbohydrate in the diet may depend upon what time of day your parathyroid secretion may go up.

DR. JOWSEY: No. We have looked at serum phosphate levels at varying times after eating, and we do get an initial fall, which starts at about 15 minutes and it goes back to normal by about one hour, and then it goes up from there.

DR. TALMAGE: If the phosphate after eating goes down at the time calcium is coming in from the gut, you are going to have an entirely different system for calcium-phosphate to go to bone, than the rise in phosphate which only occurs much later in the fasting period where parathyroid hormone is stimulated with no calcium. It becomes a completely different picture. I think in any case study you are going to have to really know what the carbohydrate ratios are.

DR. JOWSEY: The key thing, of course, to all of the serum phosphorus and the serum calcium changes, is the ionized calcium, because that is what is stimulating parathyroid hormone. What we see with the ionized calcium is not very much change during the first hour, but then a fall between one hour and four hours in man post-prandially. In the dog it is between about one and six hours when it is back to normal. So I think that is the key thing, irrespective of the time sequence of the serum PTH. The other thing, too, is that the serum phosphorus fall immediately post-prandially is usually on the order of less than one milligram, whereas the rise is usually in the order of two milligrams.

DR. TALMAGE: But the rise is going to come during the fasting period when you also have a tendency to stimulate parathyroid hormone. So it is going to make a lot of difference in whether calcium and phosphate are going to bone or coming from bone, depending upon whether the parathyroid hormone is stimulated in the fasting period or the feeding period.

DR. JOWSEY: Yes. Well, in our control animals, we have a slight fall in the total calcium and a slight fall in PTH; but this is much greater, exaggerated greatly, in animals or people that are fed phosphate.

DR. WALLACH: Dr. Jowsey, I would ask you about the ratio of cortical to trabecular bone. Your feeling that this is as much or more a disease of cortical than trabecular bone is based obviously on the places you can biopsy most effectively, namely the rib and iliac crest. What would be your feeling about the impact of the osteoporotic condition on the femoral neck or the vertebral body, where probably the ratio of cortical to trabecular bone is quite different than 80-20, even in health? Do you still feel that cortical bone is taking the brunt here, or is it trabecular bone?

DR. JOWSEY: Iliac crest, as you mention, is a convenient place, because it is an area that you can biopsy without causing problems of fracture later. It also happens to be an area which contains cortical and trabecular bone in the same proportions as it is in the whole body, 80 to 20, which is nice.

Now the question of disease: I have been looking at it, obviously, not from the point of "disease," or pain, or symptoms, but from the point of view: is the skeleton a source of calcium for calcium homeostasis? And that is the important point, where that comes from; and it comes from the cortex.

If you are going to observe this from the point of view of a clinician who is looking at patients who come in; "Where do they have their fractures?" and the symptomatic problem, then that is certainly areas of trabecular bone, such as the vertebrae and the femoral neck. But it is not defined by the presence of trabecular bone.

For instance, one of the places that has as much trabecular bone exclusively as the vertebrae is the distal end of the tibia, which is not characteristically an area of fracture. Fractures depend more on the biomechanical properties of the bone and the relationship of that bone to stress, which is why, of course, the lumbar and thoracic vertebral areas fracture more frequently than the vertebrae higher up, and why the femoral neck fractures, as opposed to the distal femur. So I think that is a slightly different question when you are looking at calcium homeostasis and bone resorption, as opposed to areas which are symptomatic.

DR. RAISZ: Dr. Jowsey, I was fascinated by your observation that there were more osteons per unit bone in osteoporosis than in normals. There are all kinds of ways that would come about, and I would like you to expand on it. For example, do these osteons have larger empty canals or vascular canals? Is there therefore less lamellar non-osteonal bone in osteoporosis? Is there something about this that you could explain its mechanism?

DR. JOWSEY: The reason we got that data was we were looking at the relationship between osteoporosis and femoral neck fractures. There has been a suggestion, and I think it is well substantiated, that one of the problems in bone strength is lack of the intimate organization between Haversian systems and remodeling. This apparently is the cause of fractures, for instance, in osteopetrosis. So we were interested in the question, "was in fact osteoporotic bone weaker per unit volume than normal bone"; and came up with this rather surprising result that in fact it had more osteons, which therefore failed to explain the fact that it might be weaker.

Now the values that I showed you there are the amount of Haversian bone versus the amount of non-Haversian bone; so that it represents the total sum of Haversian remodeling over the years. It includes Haversian systems and the remains of Haversian systems.

DR. RAISZ: The remains of Haversian systems as well as lamellae on the surface?

DR. JOWSEY: Right. The only thing it excludes is non-Haversian lamellar bone.

DR. RAISZ: But it is cortical bone?

DR. JOWSEY: It is cortical bone. It is the cortical bone of ilium.

DR. RAISZ: Is there a possibility that the strength of bone is substantially impaired by the loss of flat lamellae on the surfaces binding that mass of osteons together?

DR. JOWSEY: No. The biomechanical studies that have been done on osteon structure and the sort of intimate relationship between the bundles of osteons that turn around would suggest it is the opposite. We didn't examine the size of the Haversian canals in those, but on the whole I would think one would expect they would be larger.

DR. HEANEY: Dr. Jowsey, as you know, there are a number of attractive features about the calcium-phosphorus ratio question in the diet, but not all the data are consistent with the interpretation which I think we might like to put on it.

As you know, Harris and I did some studies with phosphate supplementation in dogs, and we did not find the type of observation which you had cited as being found in the beagle. As a matter of fact, we found increased formation and, if anything, increased mass, rather than evidence of increased porosity or osteoporosis.

Perhaps more to the point, the data which you quoted from our study of normal perio-menopausal women fails to show any relationship at all between the calcium-phosphorus ratio of the diet and the calcium balance performance of these individuals. You and I have corresponded on this, so you know what I am talking about.

We have extended these studies now to over 250 balance studies in normal perio-menopausal women; and over a calcium-phosphorus ratio range of about 0.5 to up above 1.5, maybe to 2, we can't find any relationship whatsoever between this ratio and the balance performance; that is, the level of positive balance which an individual is able to maintain on a given diet.

DR. JOWSEY: I think my response to that would be really that you have to remember that this is one aspect of bone loss in osteoporosis, and it is obviously multifactorial in all populations, including yours; certainly, in ours.

Obviously other things like estrogen presence or absence, estrogen levels, disuse, and then a number of other things I cited here such as lactate deficiency, calcium absorption, and so on, are going to come into it and make it impossible, as I think the calcium-intake studies have not been able to show a relationship between the absence of calcium-intake and the presence or absence of osteoporosis.

But I think it remains that the preponderance of the literature, and this excludes your study with Harris in those beagles, is that if you feed phosphorus to a large number of different species and man, that you will decrease the calcium to phosphorus ratio well below one, below its normal value which is less than one, and that you will result in stimulating parathyroid hormone and losing bone.

DR. VIGNERY: Dr. Singer, did you find, in these Paget's disease biopsies, inclusions in each nucleus of each osteoclast?

DR. SINGER: No. The inclusions were maybe in roughly 20 percent; but of course we don't serial-section each cell. This is just a crude estimate.

DR. JOHNSTON: I would assume, Dr. Jowsey, that the phosphorus-intake idea would only apply to some small portion of the population, and could not be used to explain age-related changes, since the population as a whole, let's say women, start losing rapidly at 45 to 50 and it is slow at 70. This has been documented in modern man as well as ancient man.

You would not propose that there is a change in dietary habit at age 45 that would explain that, but only in a small portion, is that right, of those that have crush fractures?

DR. JOWSEY: I think first of all I would suggest that bone loss starts about age 30; the more sensitive your methods of evaluating bone mass, the earlier you find that bone loss starts.

As one gets to the ages of about most of our patients, say 70 and about, then obviously other factors such as chronic estrogen deficiency and inactivity become the overwhelming causes for the age-related bone loss. But certainly I think this is a major factor in the bone loss that you see early on.

DR. JOHNSTON: True, there may be a minimal amount of loss in the third decade, but certainly, in almost every series reported, there is an accelerated rate of loss in women in the post-menopausal age; and it would be difficult to explain that totally on the basis of switch in diet.

DR. JOWSEY: No, I don't. I can't talk about the whole of osteoporosis in 15 minutes; I could have talked about the importance of estrogens and the importance of inactivity. However, I chose to limit myself to the calcium and phosphorus implications; and I don't mean to suggest that that is the only factor by any means. In fact, that is obviously not true.

I think the estrogens certainly are very important in the acceleration of the bone loss you see post-menopausally. You only have to look at Turner's syndrome to be very convinced of that; and certainly, inactivity in the 70, maybe even the 65, 70, and 80-year-olds, is becoming a more and more important factor.

Abbrogation of Congenital Osteopetrosis by Leukocyte ·
Subpopulations.

Donald G. Walker

Department of Cell Biology and Anatomy, The Johns Hopkins
University, School of Medicine,
Baltimore, MD   21205

This progress report includes discussion of 1) past work
which revealed sources of the cells capable of restoration of
bone resorption in organisms with congenital osteopetrosis, 2)
current efforts to isolate and identify the cell type(s) with
bone resorption-restorative activity (BRRA), and 3) evidence,
pro and con, that the immune system regulates bone resorption.

1) Sources of bone resorption-restorative cells.

Restoration of bone resorption in organisms with congenital
osteopetrosis was first demonstrated through application of
parabiosis (1). Grey-lethal (gl/gl) and microphthalmic (mi/mi)
mice were symbiosed to one of their littermates. Evidence of
restoration of bone resorption was detectable in the more active
metaphyseal regions of the long bones as early as 12 days post-
operatively. Replacement of the excessive deposits of spongiosa
by marrow proceeded to completion in the parabiotic mutant while
the normal parabiont showed no adverse effects. At first it was
assumed that permanent recovery would require maintenance of the
cross-circulation. However, by severing the cross-circulation
after varying periods of parabiosis it becomes evident that the
restoration of bone resorption was permanent in mutants which
had been exposed to the normal circulation for periods as short
as ten days (2). The latter observation led directly to the
assessment of the therapeutic value of the hematopoietic tissues
in congenital osteopetrosis. Normal bone marrow and spleen were
effective in the restoration of bone resorption when administered intravenously in aliquots of 5×10^6 nucleated cells to sublethally irradiated osteopetrotic (mi and gl) littermates (3).
Thymus (4) and lymph modes were not effective in mi and gl mice
(Walker, D.G., unpublished observations). However, in osteopetrotic rats including the ia rat (5) and the op rat (6), the
normal thymus was effective in restoration of bone resorption.
The liver has also been used to restore bone resorption in newborn microphthalmic mice in the absence of radiation (7). The
number of CFU-S in the thymus and liver of very young mice and
rats may be high enough to restore bone resorption in non-
irradiated op and mi mice. Direct quantitative evidence in
support of this proposition is the object of current investigation.

In man, osteopetrosis, of the malignant (autosomal recessive gene-transmitted) type has been treated successfully by means of an intravenous infusion of HLA identical bone marrow cells. The patient, though immunologically competent, received no immunosuppressive therapy before or after transplantation (8).

2) Current efforts to isolate and identify the cell type(s) with bone resorption-restorative activity (BRRA).

a) A fifty-fold concentration of BRRA cells has been obtained through use of velocity sedimentation at unit gravity (9). The most active fractions consisted of a mixture of medium-sized, leptochromatic mononuclear cells and monocytes in a ratio of about 10 to 1. The latter fractions were effective in aliquots of 0.1×10^6 cells. In contrast, the small, pachychromatic lymphocyte-rich fractions in aliquots of 25×10^6 cells were negative for BRRA. The minimal effective dose of unfractionated normal spleen from mice of 6 to 8 weeks of age is 5×10^6 cells.

b) Immunological methods for identifying B-cells, T-cells, and macrophages are currently being applied to normal mouse spleen cell fractions prepared as described above. Initial results indicate that of the small pachychromatic cell fraction (+5-8) 75% are T-cells, 20% B-cells, 5% other (normoblast) than T or B cells. The BRRA-rich fractions contain 5-10% T and B cells, 25% monocytes and the remainder lack theta antigen, C_3- and Fc- receptors.

c) Pure fractions of B-cells, T-cells and monocytes prepared from normal mice of microphthalmic stock in aliquots of 10^6 to 10^7 cells currently are being assayed for BRRA in sublethally irradiated osteopetrotic littermates. One limitation of any attempt to assay the monocyte fraction is the possibility that the separatory method itself will induce macrophage differentiation. The macrophage is not capable of homing and is likely to be arrested in the pulmonary or hepatic capillary or sinusoidal beds.

d) CFU-S is present in the mi spleen in concentrations as high as normal littermate bone marrow (Walker, D.G., and Sensenbrenner, L., unpublished observations).

3) Evidence, pro and con, that the immune system regulates bone resorption.

Pro: 1) A lymphokine, osteoclast activating factor, stimulates bone resorption in vitro (10).

2) Production of lymphokines is deficient in the op mutant rat (11) and proliferative responses of lymphocytes to various mitogens are deficient in the mi mouse (12).

3) The thymic parenchyma may mediate the skeletal

response to bone marrow transplantation. Normal bone marrow restores bone resorption in the op rat with intact thymus but not in the thymectomized mutant (13).

Con: 1) Restoration of bone resorption in fetal mi mouse bones failed to occur in response to OAF (14).

2) Normal bone marrow and splenic transplants restore bone resorption in thymectomized mi mice (Walker, D.G., unpublished observations).

3) Bone resorption has been restored by means of normal syngeneic bone marrow transplantation to an immunologically competent, osteopetrotic infant (8).

Elucidation of the role of the immune system in osteopetrosis is engaging the interest of an increasing number of investigators. Therefore, it is reasonable to anticipate that the apparent contradictions cited above will be resolved. Until then, the most significant result of osteopetrotic research is the reversal of this congenital disease in mice, rats and man through transplantation of histocompatible, normal bone marrow.

Abbreviations

BRRA, bone resorption-restorative activity

CFU-S, colony forming unit-spleen

OAF, osteoclast activating factor

References

1. Walker, D.G. 1972. Congenital osteopetrosis in mice cured by parabiotic union with normal siblings. Endocrinology, 91, 916-20.

2. Walker, D.G. 1973. Osteopetrosis in Mice cured by temporary parabiosis. Science, 180, 875.

3. Walker, D.G. 1975. Bone resorption restored in osteopetrotic mice by transplants of normal bone marrow and spleen cells. Science, 190, 784-5.

4. Luotit, J.F. and Sansom, J.M. 1976. Osteopetrosis of microphthalmic mice - a defect of the hematopoietic stem cell? Calcif. Tiss. Res. 20, 251-9.

5. Marks, S.C., Jr. 1976. Osteopetrosis in the ia rat cured by spleen cells from a normal littermate. Am. J. Anat. 146, 331-8.

6. Milhaud, G., Labat, M.-L., Graf, B. and Thillard, M.-J. 1976. Cure of congenital osteopetrosis in the "op" rat by thymus graft. C.R. Acad. Sci. 283, 531-3.

7. Barnes, D.W.H , Loutit, J.F., and Sansom, J.M. 1975. Histocompatible cells for the resolution of osteopetrosis in microphathalmic mice. Proc. Roy. Soc. B. 188, 501-5.

8. Ballet, J.J. and Griscelli, C., Coutris, C., Milhaud, G. and Maroteaux, P., 1977. Bone Marrow transplantation in osteopetrosis. Lancet II, 1137.

9. Walker, D.G. 1977. Concentration of splenic lymphocytes with bone resorption-restorative activity (BRRA) by velocity sedimentation at unit gravity. Excepta Medica (in press).

10. Horton, J.E., Raisz, L.G., Simmons, H.A., Oppenheim, J.J. and Mergenhagen, S.E. 1972. Bone resorbing activity in supernatant fluid from cultured human peripheral blood leukocytes. Science, 1977, 793-5.

11. Milhaud, G., Labat, M.L., Parant, M., Daimais, C. and Chedid, L. 1977. Immunological defect and its correction in the osteopetrotic mutant rat. Proc. Natl. Acad. Sci. 74, 339-42.

12. Olsen, C.E., Wahl, S.M., Wahl, L.M. Sandberg, A.L. and Mergenhagen, S.E. 1977. Immunologic defects in osteopetrotic mice. Calc. Tiss. Abstr. (in press).

13. Milhaud, G., Labat, M.-L., Graf, B., and Thillard, M.-J. 1976. Endocrinologie. Guérison de l'osteopétrose congénitale du rat <<op>> par graffe de thymus. C. R. Acad. Sc. Serie D., Paris, 283, 531-3.

14. Raisz, L.G., Simmons, H.A., Gworek, S.C. and Eilon, G. 1977. Studies on congenital osteopetrosis in microphthalmic mice using organ cultures: impairment of bone resorption in response to physiologic stimulators. J. Exp. Med. 145, 857-65.

Immunological Defects in Osteopetrotic Mice.

Charles E. Olsen, Sharon M. Wahl, Larry M. Wahl, Ann L. Sandberg and Stephen E. Mergenhagen.

Laboratory of Microbiology and Immunology, National Institute of Dental Research, Bethesda, Maryland, 20014.

Mammalian osteopetrosis is an inherited defect characterized by a failure of normal bone remodelling. Four osteopetrotic mutants of mice have been identified: microphthalmic (mi), osteopetrotic (op), gray lethal (gl), and osteosclerotic (oc). The pathological defects in these mice (lack of teeth, shorter and thicker long bones and absent or minimal marrow cavities) are the result of autosomal recessive mutation. The increase in skeletal mass in the mouse mutants seems to be a result of both increased bone formation and decreased bone resorption (1).

There is evidence to suggest that the immune system is involved in bone resorption. Injection of spleen cells or bone marrow cells from normal littermates into mi mice results in normal bone resorption (2). Moreover, osteopetrosis can be induced in irradiated normal animals by injection of spleen cells from mi mice (3). Additional evidence linking the immune system with bone resorption comes from the studies of Horton et al. (4) who found a substance (osteoclast activating factor, OAF) produced by human peripheral mononuclear cells in response to PHA which stimulates bone resorption in vitro. Both lymphocytes and macrophages are required to produce this factor (5).

That a defect in the immune system may be involved in the osteopetrotic condition of the mi mice led us to investigate the functions of the lymphoid cells from these animals as well as those from op mice. Spleen cells were assayed for their ability to proliferate in response to both B cell and T cell mitogens. In both of these mouse mutants a defective proliferative response was observed.

Materials and Methods

Mice. mi mice and their phenotypically normal littermates were obtained from Dr. Donald G. Walker (Johns Hopkins University, Baltimore, Md.). The mi mice are on a C57Bl background. C57Bl, op/+, and mi/+ breeder animals were obtained from Jackson Laboratories, Bar Harbor, Maine.

Cell Collection and Culture. Spleens were minced in RPMI 1640 medium (NIH Media Unit) with scissors, filtered through gauze, and the cells pelleted by centrifugation. The

cells were suspended in ammonium chloride lysing buffer (6)
for 5 minutes to lyse red blood cells. The cells were washed
and resuspended at 3 x 10^6 cells/ml in RPMI 1640 medium supplemented with 5% fetal calf serum (GIBCO, Grand Island, N. Y.),
100 U/ml penicillin, 100 µg/ml streptomycin (Flow Laboratories,
Rockville, Md.) and 20 µg/ml gentamicin (Schering, Kenilworth,
N. J.). One ml aliquots of this spleen cell suspension were
cultured in one dram glass vials (Bellco Glass Co., Vineland,
N. J.) for 72 hrs in the presence of various mitogens. The
replicate cultures were then pulsed with 1 µCi/ml [^{3}H]-thymidine
(specific activity 6 µCi/m mole) (Schwarz/Mann, Orangeburg, New
York). Four hours later the cells were collected onto glass
fiber filters and thymidine incorporation determined by scintillation counting.

   Mitogens. The B cell mitogens used were E. coli lipopolysaccharide (LPS)(055:B5,Difco Laboratories, Detroit, Michigan)
and polyinosinic acid (Poly I, P-L Biochemicals, Inc.,
Milwaukee, Wisconsin). The T cell mitogens included concanavalin A (Con A, Calbiochem, San Diego, Calif.) and phytohemagglutinin (PHA, Burroughs-Welcome Co., Inc., Research Triangle Park,
North Carolina).

Results

   The proliferative response of spleen cells from mi mice
to B and T cell mitogens was compared with that of spleen cells
from normal C57Bl mice (Fig. 1). PHA, Con A, and LPS stimulation of mi spleen cells was significantly lower than normal
spleen cells. Because the difference could be due to a shift
in optimum concentration of mitogen rather than a depressed
proliferative response, dose response studies were carried out
utilizing spleen cells from mi mice, their phenotypically normal littermates and C57Bl mice (Fig. 2) The optimum stimulation of thymidine incorporation occurred between 0.5 and 1.0
µg/ml Con A regardless of the origin of the cells. However, the
incorporation by spleen cells from normal littermates and
C57Bl's was approximately the same and was over 4 times that by
mi spleen cells. In Fig. 3 the thymidine incorporation of the
spleen cells from the same mice in response to LPS is compared.
The incorporation by cells from littermates and C57Bl is approximately the same and at 10 µg/ml is about 7 times the incorporation by mi spleen cells. The optimal concentration of the T
cell mitogen, PHA, was the same (1 µg/ml) for the three cell
types (data not shown). The response of spleen cells from
individual mice and their littermates to the B cell mitogens
LPS and Poly I and the T cell mitogen PHA is shown in Table 1.
The response of the mi cells was always less than that of the
normal littermates, although there was variation among the
animals in each group.

   Similar studies were carried out with spleen cells from op
mice. While these mice share the osteopetrotic defect of the mi
mutant they do not have the abnormal eyes or pigment change
characteristic of the mi mice. The thymidine incorporation by
spleen cells from individual op mice and their phenotypically

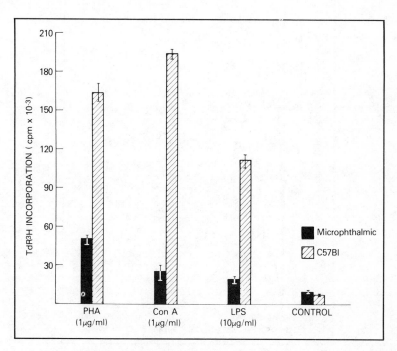

Fig.1. Spleen cells from C57Bl and mi̲ mice were stimulated with
        the indicated mitogens and the incorporation of |³H|-
        thymidine was measured. Control cells were incubated in
        the absence of mitogen. Cultures were handled as de-
        scribed in Materials and Methods. Data shown as mean
        and standard error of triplicate culture.

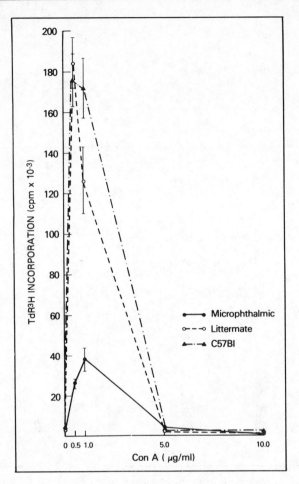

Fig.2. Spleen cells from mi mice, from their phenotypically normal littermates, and from C57Bl mice were stimulated with Con A and the incorporation of |³H|-thymidine was measured. Cultures were handled as described in Materials and Methods. Data shown as mean and standard error of triplicate cultures.

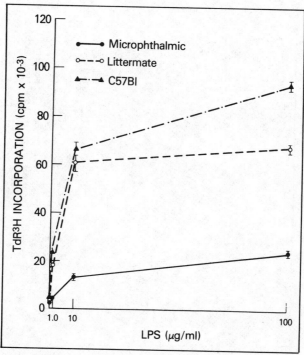

Fig.3. Spleen cells from mi mice, from their phenotypically normal littermates, and from C57Bl mice were stimulated
with LPS, and the incorporation of [³H]-thymidine was
measured. Cultures were handled as described in Materials and Methods. Data shown as mean and standard error
of triplicate cultures.

TABLE I. Proliferative Defect in Microphthalmic Mice[a]

Mouse	LPS cpm[b]	LPS E/C[c]	Poly I cpm	Poly I E/C	PHA cpm	PHA E/C	Control cpm
N1	40,167 ± 447	16.2	56,693 ± 7838	22.9	7678 ± 3512	3.1	2478 ± 163
N2	24,468 ± 3569	17.7	30,887 ± 1222	22.3	24,071 ± 933	17.4	1383 ± 58
N3	28,763 ± 335	19.8	-	-	7690 ± 226	5.3	1454 ± 42
mi1	8696 ± 807	2.6	10,578 ± 195	3.1	5230 ± 1291	1.5	3387 ± 110
mi2	3300 ± 50	0.9	-	-	4784 ± 585	1.3	3550 ± 77
mi3	7295 ± 366	2.2	-	-	3546 ± 498	1.1	3352 ± 35

a Spleen cells from 3 individual mi mice and their phenotypically normal littermates (N) were stimulated with 30 µg/ml LPS, 150 µg/ml Poly I, or 1 µg/ml PHA and the incorporation of [3H] thymidine was measured as detailed in Materials and Methods.

b Mean cpm of triplicate cultures ± standard error.

c Ratio of mean cpm of stimulated cultures (E) to mean cpm of control cultures (C).

normal littermates in response to LPS, Poly I, and PHA is shown
in Table II. Similar to the mi cells, the normal littermate's
cells always responded better than the cells from the affected
animals. The Poly I dose response of an op mouse and its normal
littermate can be seen in Table III. Increasing incorporation
of thymidine occurred up to a concentration of 150 µg/ml Poly I
at which point it plateaued. Proliferation of these stimulated
normal cells was greater than that of the op cells throughout
the entire concentration range.

Discussion

The spleen cells from both the mi and op mutant mice are defective in the proliferative response to both B and T cell
mitogens. These results are in agreement with those of Milhaud
et al. (7) who investigated the proliferative response of the
op (osteopetrotic) rat spleen cells and thymus cells.

The defects in spleen cells may be related to the lack of
bone resorption in these mutants, since the transfer of these
cells from mi mice to normal animals produces osteopetrosis (3)
and the reverse cell transfer cures the disease (2). Osteopetrotic rat mutants (ia and op) have also been cured by bone marrow
cells from normal littermates (8, 9). In the op rat the thymus
plays an important role in the cure by bone marrow cells. If
the thymus is removed prior to injection of bone marrow cells,
the mutant is not cured (10).

Other evidence for the involvement of the immune system in
bone resorption comes from studies on osteoclast activating
factor (OAF). Peripheral blood mononuclear cells stimulated with
PHA synthesize OAF which stimulates bone resorption in vitro.
The specific cell type which produces this factor is not clear,
but it is known that both macrophages and lymphocytes are needed
(5). It is of interest that Raisz et al. (11) have stimulated
spleen cells from mi mice and their littermates with PHA and
found no difference in the ability of supernatants to stimulate
in vitro resorption of normal mouse bones. The factor responsible was not characterized and could conceivably be a factor
other than OAF. However, bones from mi mice did not respond to
resorbing agents such as OAF or parathyroid hormone (11). These
findings suggest that the cure or induction of this pathological
condition is not solely attributal to a factor(s) released by
spleen cells. These studies as well as our own findings indicate
in these osteopetrotic mutants there may be a cellular defect
such as a failure of a precursor cell to differentiate or failure of the differentiated cell to perform its function in bone
resorption.

Abbreviations

Con A, concanavalin A; LPS, lipopolysaccharide; OAF, osteoclast
activating factor; PHA, phytohemagglutinin; Poly I, polyinosinic
acid.

TABLE 2. Proliferative Defect in Osteopetrotic Mice[a]

Mouse	$[^3H]$ - Thymidine Incorporation						
	LPS		Poly I		PHA		Control
	cpm[b]	E/C[c]	cpm	E/C	cpm	E/C	cpm
N1	10,118 ± 79	7.1	15,908 ± 556	11.2	35,612 ± 1631	25.1	1420 ± 169
N2	23,381 ± 994	8.2	25,349 ± 887	8.9	18,786 ± 1738	6.6	2846 ± 162
N3	18,935 ± 854	6.6	32,244 ± 1087	11.3	17,389 ± 292	6.1	2852 ± 334
op1	4701 ± 342	1.8	6865 ± 773	2.6	11,367 ± 893	4.4	2599 ± 55
op2	3452 ± 112	1.0	4203 ± 319	1.2	5,842 ± 752	1.7	3419 ± 167
op3	5917 ± 210	2.7	7209 ± 298	3.2	11,033 ± 530	5.0	2196 ± 50

[a] Spleen cells from 3 individual op mice and their phenotypically normal littermates (N) were stimulated with 30 μg/ml LPS, 150 μg/ml poly I, or 1 μg/ml PHA and the incorporation of $[^3H]$ thymidine was measured as detailed in Materials and Methods.

[b] Mean cpm of triplicate cultures ± standard error.

[c] Ratio of mean cpm of stimulated cultures (E) to mean cpm of control cultures (C).

TABLE 3.   Poly I Dose Response of Osteopetrotic
and Normal Mouse Spleen Cells[a]

Stimulant	$\left[^3_H\right]$-Thymidine Incorporation (cpm)[b]	
	Normal	Osteopetrotic
Control	1420 ± 169	2599 ± 55
Poly I		
50 µg/ml	5768 ± 443	3143 ± 98
100 µg/ml	9823 ± 887	3760 ± 372
150 µg/ml	15,908 ± 556	6865 ± 773
200 µg/ml	14,893 ± 1283	4317 ± 334
300 µg/ml	16,640 ± 1672	6210 ± 205

[a] Spleen cells from an <u>op</u> mouse and a phenotypically normal littermate were stimulated with various concentrations of poly I and the incorporation of $\left[^3_H\right]$-thymidine was measured as detailed in Materials and Methods.

[b] Mean cpm of triplicate cultures ± standard error.

References

1. Marks, S. C., Jr., and Walker D. G. 1976. Mammalian Osteo-petrosis - A Model for Studying Cellular and Humoral Factors in Bone Resorption. in "The Biochemistry and Physiology of Bone", Vol. 4. G. Bourne, ed. Academic Press, New York, 227-301.

2. Walker, D. G. 1975. Bone Resorption Restored in Osteopetro-tic Mice by Transplants of Normal Bone Marrow and Spleen Cells. Science. 190, 784-785.

3. Walker, D. G. 1975. Spleen Cells Transmit Osteopetrosis in Mice. Science 190, 785-787.

4. Horton, J. E., Raisz, L. G., Simmons, H. A., Oppenheim, J. J. and Mergenhagen, S. E. 1972. Bone Resorbing Activity in Supernatant Fluid from Cultured Human Peripheral Blood Leukocytes. Science 177, 793-794.

5. Horton, J. E., Oppenheim, J. J., Raisz, L. G. and Mergen-hagen, S. E.,1974. Macrophage Lymphocyte Synergy in the Production of Osteoclast Activating Factor (OAF). J. Immunol. 113, 1278-1287.

6. Roos, D. and Loos, J. A. 1970. Changes in the Carbohydrate Metabolism of Mitogenically Stimulated Human Peripheral Lymphocytes. Biochem. Biophys. Acta. 222, 565-582.

7. Milhaud, G. Labat, M-L, Parant, M., Damais, C. and Chedid, L. 1977. Immunological Defect and its Correction in Osteo-petrotic Mutant Rat. Proc. Natl. Acad. Sci. USA 74, 339-342.

8. Marks, S. C., Jr., 1976. Osteopetrosis in the ia Rat Cured by Spleen Cells from a Normal Littermate. Amer. J. Anat. 146, 331-338.

9. Milhaud, G., Labat, M-L, Graf, B., Juster, M., Balmain, N., Moutier, R. and Toyama, K., 1975. Kinetic, X-Ray and Histological Demonstration of the Cure of Congenital Osteopetrosis in Rats. C. R. Acad. Sci. Ser. D., 280, 2485-2488.

10. Milhaund, G., Labat, M-L., Graf, B. and Thillard, M-J. 1976. Cure of congenital osteopetrosis in the "op" rat by thymus graft. C. R. Acad. Sci. Ser D. 283, 531-533.

11. Raisz, L. G., Simmons, H. A., Gworek, S. C. and Eilon, G. 1977. Studies on Congenital Osteopetrosis in Microphthalmic Mice using Organ Cultures: Impairment of Bone Resorption in Response to Physiologic Stimulators. J. Exp. Med. 145, 857-865.

Lymphoid Cell Transplantation in Human Osteopetrosis.

Jean Jacques Ballet and Claude Griscelli

Unité d'Immunohématologie, Clinique Médicale Infantile,
Hôpital des Enfants-Malades, 149 rue de Sèvres,
75015 Paris, France

INTRODUCTION

Human osteopetrosis (1) is a congenital disease defined by a generalized increased density of bones due to a severe impairment of bone resorption (2). The progressive form (3), inherited as if determined by an autosomal and recessive gene, is often revealed in the first months of life, with severe haematological symptoms related to an absence of marrow spaces and an extramedullary hematopoiesis. Optic atrophy, frequently observed, and paralysis of other cranial nerves correlate with a narrowing of cranial foramina. Others symptoms include hydrocephalus, dental abnormalities (4) and fractures. The disease is generally fatal in the first years of life. Another form, generally autosomal and dominant, is usually discovered later, sometimes in adults, with milder manifestations (5). An association with a renal tubular defect was reported in osteopetrotic patients with a presumably dominant (6) or recessive (7) pattern. Besides blood transfusion and other symptomatic therapies, only limited improvements were obtained using calcium depleting regimes or agents, steroids or splenectomy (8, 9, 10).

We are reporting here the effects of lymphoid cell transplantation in 4 infants with severe osteopetrosis. This new approach of the disease was suggested to us by the studies performed in osteopetrotic mutants in rodents. In mutant mice (11), the decisive observation was the cure of osteopetrosis by temporary parabiosis (12). This effect was also obtained in "Op" rats (13, 14). The involvement of cellular material was demonstrated by bone marrow transplantation experiments, which induced a reversal (15, 16) as well as an induction of osteopetrosis in mice (16, 17). In "Op" rats, injections of normal syngeneic cells restored a bone resorption without immunosuppressive preparation (18), but irradiation was needed with allogeneic cells (19).

Animal osteopetrosis is genetically heterogenous (11, 20, 24). This is likely the case in human, and not only histocompatibility barriers but also the form of the disease may play a role in the response to bone marrow. However, taking also in account the risks of an immunosuppression in a situation

where mechanisms and immunological status were not entirely
defined, we decided to perform our first attempts in human
by injecting cells from related donors or fetal tissues without any immunosuppressive preparation.

PATIENTS AND METHODS.

Four infants with severe manifestations of osteopetrosis
were studied. Table I gives pertinent clinical and biological
data.

All children were born after a full-term pregnancy without
known intake of osteocondensing agents by the mother. The
general growth and development were retarded and severe early
haematological manifestations were present. Roentgenograms
revealed an increased density of the entire skeleton with an
absence of bone marrow spaces. When first studied, none of
the children had a special diet or therapy. An usual pattern
of osteopetrosis was observed on bone biopsies obtained, except
in case #1, within days following diagnosis. Immunoreactive
parathormone levels and karyotypes were normal. No abnormality
was detected on bone X rays of the parents and brothers or
sisters of the children.

Case #1. The parents, from Saudi Arabia, had a common
grandfather. No other case was recorded in the family. The
pregnancy was apparently uncomplicated. At birth, weight and
size were 2.7 kg and 47 cm. In this infant girl, the disease
was revealed at about two months. Abnormal searching eye
motions with optic atrophy were already present. Biological
data are detailed in tables and figure 1. Plasma calcium
(8.5 mg/100ml) and daily calcium urinary output (5mg) were
low. Calcium kinetic data were typical for osteopetrosis
with very low bone accretion and resorption and increased
calcium balance and intestinal absorption rate (21). Moreover, a metabolic acidosis consistent with a renal tubular
defect was detected: urinary pH was constantly over 6.5, and
plasma levels were: urea nitrogen 20 mg/ml, creatinin 0.5
mg/100 ml, Na^+ 139 mEq/l, Cl^- 117 mEq/l, K^+ 4 mEq/l, total
CO_2 12-18 mEq/l. Arterial pH was 7.2.

Case #2. A first child, a boy, from unrelated parents,
and without other case in the family. Bone X-rays of parents
were normal. At birth, a cesarean section was needed, and
for anoxic and mechanical trauma, the child (3.3 kg) was kept
for three days under artificial ventilation. For two weeks,
calcemia was at 6.8-8.0 mg/100 ml, then constantly over 8.0
mg/100 ml. X-rays revealed osteopetrotic bones in the first
days of life. At one month, of age, the anemia was stable
(7-9 g Hb/100 ml) and no transfusion was needed. No ocular
abnormality was detected. In plasma, urea, creatinin,
Na^+, Cl^- and K^+ were in normal ranges, calcium was 9-10
mg/100 ml, $PO_4 \equiv 4.4$ mg/100 ml, alkaline phosphatases =
916 mu/ml.

TABLE I

CASE	#1	#2	#3	#4	
SEX	FEMALE	MALE	FEMALE	FEMALE	
AGE (MONTHS/DAYS)	2/26	1/25	6/7	7/19	9/16
SIZE (CM)	52	60	63	64	N.A.
SPLEEN/LIVER ENLARGEMENT	+ + +	+	+ + +	+ + +	+ + +
OPTIC ATROPHY	+ +	0	+	+ +	+ +
HAEMOGLOBIN (G/100 ML)*	9.6	7.4	9.9	6.7	9.2
IMMATURE NUCLEATED CELLS IN PERIPHERAL BLOOD	+ +	+ + +	+ +	0	+
RETICULOCYTES (PER MM3)	170000	310000	312000	336000	180000
THROMBOCYTES (PER MM3)	20000	65000	35000	10000	30000

CLINICAL AND BIOLOGICAL DATA (AT THE DATES OF CELL TRANSPLANTATION)

* ALL PATIENTS, EXCEPT CASE #2, HAD RECEIVED PRIOR BLOOD TRANSFUSIONS.

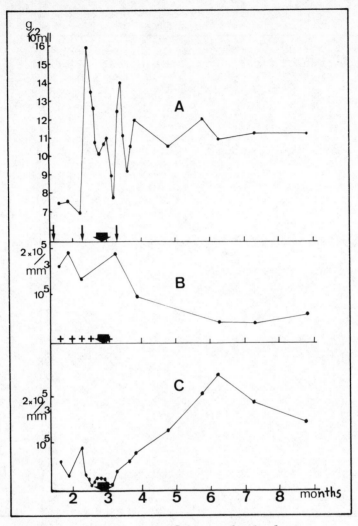

Fig. 1: Evolution of hematological
parameters in case #1

A: haemoglobin (g/100ml). Arrows indicate blood transfusions.
B: reticulocytes (per mm3) (o——o) and immature nucleated cells.
(+++) in blood.
C. platelets (per mm3).

In A, B and C, larger arrows indicate the bone marrow transplantation.

Case #3. No consanguinity or other known case in this family. X-rays of the parents and the older brother were normal. At birth, this little girl weighed 2.960 kg and her size was 49 cm. By the age (4 months) of diagnosis, she had minor infections, but clinical and haematological symptoms of osteopetrosis were present. Plasma levels were: calcium 8-8.6 mg/100 ml, PO_4 2.0-3.8 mg/100 ml and alkaline phosphatases 20 K.A. units.

Case #4. No consanguinity was found in the family. A younger brother was normal. Birth weight and size were 3.2 kg and 49 cm. At one month, after convulsions were transient hypocalcemia, X-rays revealed the disease. An anemia and optic atropy were already present. The child, a girl, was transfused twice before the age of 7 months. From the 3rd to the 6th month a discontinous (15 mg/day) prednisone therapy was given. At six months, plasma levels were: calcium 7.6-10 mg/100 ml, PO_4 3.1-3.9 mg/100 ml, alkaline phosphatases: 495-628 mU/ml.

IMMUNOLOGICAL EVALUATION

Serum immunoglobulins were measured using radial immunodiffusion techniques. Skin-tests, detection of serum haemagglutinins, E-rosetting cells, μ-bearing cells and proliferative responses to lectins and in mixed leukocyte cultures were studied as previously described (22). In cases #1 and 2, removal of large immature cells from Ficoll-Triosil populations was achieved on discontinuous bovine albumine gradients (23).

HL-A A and B types were determined on lymphocyte preparation by serological (cytotoxicity) methods.

TRANSPLANTATION PROCEDURES

In all cases, transplantations were decided after fully informed parental consent. Bone marrow cells were aspirated from donors under general anesthaesia by multiple punctures, and injected intravenously in heparinized saline. Human fetuses (12 - 14 weeks) were obtained after cesarean section in cases where no infectious or metabolic abnormality of the mother and the fetus could be detected or suspected. Fetal organs were harvested under sterile conditions, the thymus and liver fragments were chopped in sterile saline into single cell suspension, filtered, and injected (intravenously for thymocytes and intraperitoneally for liver cells).

After transplantation, (generally at days +15 and +60) the persistence of donors cells in the recipient was explored using HL-A A and B typing, and, in relevant cases, chromosomal markers (karyotype and quinacrine staining (22)). Erythrocyte groups and immunoglobulin allotypes were also verified.

RESULTS AND DISCUSSION

Results of immunological explorations and transplantation

data are summarized in tables II and III.

In case #1, the 2 year-old sister was identical for HL-A-A, B and D determinants and for all erythrocytic antigens and immunoglobulin allotypes tested. She was therefore chosen as a donor.

In the weeks following transplantation, alterations were observed and are still present 18 months later. Circulating immature nucleated cells disappeared from peripheral blood and haemoglobin levels reached 11-12 g% without any further transfusion. Three months later, the hepatosplenomegaly had disappeared and the blood picture was entirely corrected (fig. 1). X-rays revealed progressive modifications of bones (fig. 2), mainly the appearance of medullary cavities with distinct cortex and marrow space. Dense transverse metaphyseal bands became visible. The base of the cranium remained dense. Symptoms of optic atrophy persisted despite an attempt of neurosurgical decompression at 7 months of age. Plasma calcium level increased (9.0 mg% in average). Calcium kinetics (21) indicated a raised bone-accretion rate and a higher calcium balance than normal. The slowly exchangeable calcium compartment had decreased. Plasma alkaline phosphatase activity decreased (680 mU/ml). Growth and development have progressed, but size and weight are still below normal (-2 S.D.). The renal condition remained unchanged. No evidence of the survival of transplanted cells was available.

In case #2, no histocompatible related donor was available, and liver and thymus cells from a male fetus were transplanted (table III). The transplantation is still recent, and only preliminary data can be reported.

In weeks preceding transplantation, blood ranges were: erythrocytes 2.4-2.6 x 10^6/mm3, Hb 7.3-8 g/100 ml, erythroblasts and reticulocytes respectively 7.0-11.0 x 10^3/mm3 and 310-473 x 10^3/mm3, leukocytes 21-28 x 10^3/mm3 with immature cells (myeloblasts to metamyelocytes) around 3.2 x 10^3/mm3, platelets 30-65 x 10^3/mm3. No bone resorption was visible on roentgengrams. At day +30 after transplantation, erythrocyte counts reached 4 x 10^6/mm3 (with Hb = 10.5 g/100 ml), erythroblasts were 0.6 x 10^3/mm3, reticulocytes 245 x 10^3 and leukocytes around 10 x 10^3/ml. Myeloid cells disappeared (less than 0.2 x 10^3 myelocytes/mm3). Thrombocyte counts raised and remained stable at 160-180 x 10^3/mm3. The first signs of bone resorption became visible on metaphyses of long bones +30 days after transplantation. By day +60, metaphyseal resorption had progressed and disseminated resorption zones had appeared in most areas, with a slight central resorption in some long bones. By day +120 however, a generalized densification had reappeared and the number of immature cells in blood was increasing again. Plasma calcium levels were stable at 8.5-10.0 mg/100 ml. At day +30, plasma alkaline phosphatase activity fell to 576 mU/ml, and increased in the following months to 790 mU/ml. In blood, no lymphoid

TABLE II

IMMUNOLOGICAL DATA (AT THE DATE OF FIRST CELL TRANSPLANTATION)

CASE	#1	#2	#3	#4
AGE	2/26	1/25	6/7	7/19
IgG (serum, mg/100 ml)	850	320	1050	650
IgM (serum, mg/100 ml)	64	62	210	110
IgA (serum, mg/100 ml)	60	38	90	56
ALLOHEMAGGLUTININS (serum)	DETECTABLE	UNDETECTABLE		HIGH
ANTIBODY FUNCTION (serum)	-	±	+	+
LYMPHOCYTES (blood)				
- ABSOLUTE NUMBER (per mm3)	2500-5000	5000-15000	6000-8000	6000-20000
- E-ROSETTING LYMPHOCYTE * (%)	35	24	7	24
- μ-BEARING LYMPHOCYTES * (%)	N.D.	N.D.	14	8
IN VITRO PROLIFERATIVE RESPONSE OF BLOOD LYMPHOCYTES TO : **				
- LECTINS (PHYTOHAEMAGGLUTININ, POKEWEED MITOGEN, CONCANAVALIN A)	NORMAL	NORMAL	NORMAL	NORMAL
- MIXED LEUCOCYTE REACTION **	POSITIVE	POSITIVE	N.D.	POSITIVE
- SKIN TEST (PHYTOHAEMAGGLUTININ)	POSITIVE	N.D.	N.D.	N.D.

* LYMPHOCYTES SEDIMENTING ON A FICOLL HYPAQUE GRADIENT.

** LYMPHOCYTES SEDIMENTING IN LAYERS 25% TO 35% ON BOVINE SERUM ALBUMIN , RESPONSE TO LYMPHOCYTES FROM AN UNRELATED DONOR.

TABLE III

TRANSPLANTATION DATA

CASE	#1	#2	#3	#4
SEX (RECIPIENT)	FEMALE	MALE	FEMALE	FEMALE
HL-A (A, B) TYPES (RECIPIENT)	A2,W17/192,B14	A9,A1/BW25,B8	A3,-/W29,12	A3,B7/A28,B12
DONOR AND INJECTED CELLS	SISTER (BONE MARROW, I.V.)	UNRELATED FETUS (LIVER I.P., THYMUS.I.V.)	FATHER(BONE MARROW, I.V.)	1) FATHER (BONE MARROW, I.V.) (TWICE) 2) UNRELATED FETUSES (THYMUS, I.V.)
NUMBER OF INJECTED NUCLEATED CELLS (PER KG WEIGHT)	0.7×10^9	LIVER : 1.87×10^8 THYMUS : 4.5×10^5	6.3×10^9	1) 0.08 AND 1.6×10^9 2) 19×10^6

Fig. 2: Evolution of X-rays in case #1

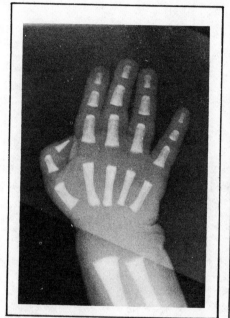 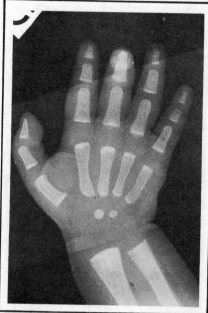

Fig. 2(a$_1$)   Fig. 2(a$_2$)

a) Ages: 2 months (a$_1$) and 9 months (a$_2$):

Fig. 2: Evolution of X-rays in case #1

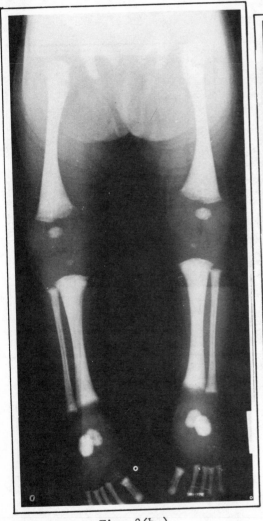

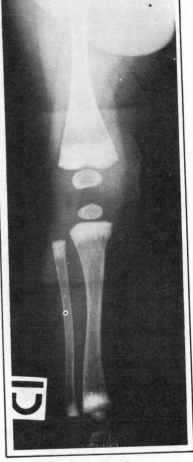

Fig. 2(b$_1$)   Fig. 2(b$_2$)

b) Ages: 2 months (b$_1$) and 9 months (b$_2$):

Fig. 2: Evolution of X-rays in case #1

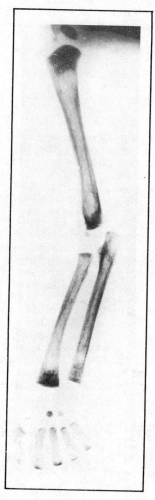

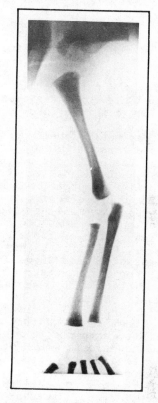

Fig. 2(c$_2$)

Fig. 2(c$_1$)

c) Ages: 2 months (c$_1$) and 10.5 months (c$_2$).

cells of donor origin have been so far detected using HL-A
typing.

In cases #3 and 4, HL-A semi-identical bone marrow cells
from the fathers were injected, and in case #4, fetal cells
from thymus. No improvement was observed in blood pictures
and bone X-rays and parameters of calcium metabolism were
not altered. No lymphoid chimerism could be detected by
HL-A and chromosome studies. Despite blood transfusions
and steroid therapy, the clinical evolution is unfavorable
after more than one year after transplantation.

More clinical and experimental data are obviously needed
to clarify the nature, the role and the fate of injected
cells, and the following questions are already raised by these
preliminary clinical results:

1. The heterogeneity of human osteopetrosis is to be
considered first. In our patients, osteopetrosis was ascer-
tained by the early osteocondensation and the lack of marrow
cavities, associated with severe hematological and, in three
cases, ocular symptons, which are distinctive of the disease.
Clinical and biological data were not compatible with other
bone diseases or manifestations, especially athyreosis or
fluor poisoning. Bone biopsies available prior to transplantation confirmed the absense of a normal bone resorption.
In case #1, the first biopsy was obtained five months after
transplantation, and showed, juxtaposed, zones with and
without resorption patterns. In all patients, symptoms
were consistent with a recessive form, and a consanguinity
was present in case #1. However, in this case, the association
with a tubulopathy may also suggest a genetically different
entity. Despite the rarity of the disease and the lack of a
known cause, attempts to a better distinction of forms in
human osteopetrosis would be supported by studies in animals.
In rat, genetically independent mutations (20, 24) are different
not only in their evolution and mechanisms (25, 26) but also
in their response to cell transplantation, and this would have
to be considered in further transplantation attempts in human.

2. In case #1, medullary spaces appeared progressively
and reached a maximal extent months after transplantation.
By reference to cell transplantation in cellular immune
deficiencies, this delay suggests a cell differentiation
process. However, the nature of transferred effector cells
remains unknown.

The demonstration, in microphthalmic mice, of an impaired
in vitro bone resorption in response to physiologic stimulators
(27) would support the hypothesis of a cell of osteoclastic
lineage. An alternative possibility could involve cells able
to activate potentially normal resorbing mechanisms. The
observation of a bone resorbing activity in lymphoid cell
cultures (28, 29, 30, 31, 32) suggests a role for resorption-
controlling lymphocytic or/and monocytic populations. (33, 34)

In both cases, the survival of syngeneic or allogeneic effector cells in patients where no cellular immune defect could be detected or suspected (absence of clinical or biological manifestations of graft versus host reactions) remains to be clarified. More data on immunological events before and after transplantation are crucially needed in order to define better transplantation criteria---namely the choice of the donor and the use of immunosuppressive preparation of recipients. In "Op" rats, which exhibit antibody responses (35), but also in vitro quantitative lymphocytic defects (36) migrations of dividing lymphoid cells to lymphoid organs were observed after syngeneic bone marrow transplantation (37), and thymic cells were also found able to restore bone resorption (38). These syngeneic situations might be compared to case #1 where HL-A compatible cells from the sister were transplanted and where bone resorption is persisting eighteen months later. However, we were unable to detect a chimerism. In allogeneic situations, a preparative irradiation was needed in rats (19). This, and our observation of a presumably transient resorption using fetal tissues in case #2 raises the question of the use of a preparative immunosuppression in incompatible or partially compatible situations (like cases #3 and #4, where no improvement was obtained with cells from a parent).

The involvement of other bone-controlling systems, hormonal (39), vascular (40) or others, needs to be more fully documented. For instance, the persistence, in case #1, of the tubulopathy and of dense metaphyseal areas in long bones seems of genetic and pathogenetic interest.

In summary, our first observations indicate that a bone resorption can be restored by lymphoid cell transplantation in human osteopetrosis. Despite the fact that all forms of the disease may not respond, and that optimal conditions are not yet entirely defined, this procedure should now be considered as early as possible in the course of a disease where no specific therapy was available.

ACKNOWLEDGEMENT.

This work was supported in part by grants INSERM ATP 27-76-59 and from DGRST, 1977.

REFERENCES.

1) Albers-Schönberg, H.1904. Roentgenbilder einer seltenen Knochenkrankunung. Münch. Mediz. Wochenschrift, 51, 365-368.

2) Fraser, D.,Kooh,S.W.,Chan,A.M.,Cherian,A.G.Congenital osteopetrosis-a failure of normal resorptive mechanisms of bone. Calcif. Tissue Res., 1968,2,52-61.

3) In Maroteaux, P.Les maladies osseuses de l'enfant (Bone diseases in childhood) 1975, Flammarion,Paris. Pages 133-138 and 155.

4)   Smith, N.H.H.Albers-Shonberg disease osteopetrosis. Report
     of a case and review of the literature. Oral Surg.,
     1966,22,699-710.

5)   Hasenhuttl K. , Orange, N.J.Osteopetrosis. Review of the
     literature and comparative studies of a case with a twenty
     four year follow-up. J.Bone Jt. Surg. 1962,44A,359-363

6)   Guibaud,P.,Larbre,F.,Freycon,M.T.,Genoud, J.Osteopetrose
     et acidose renale tubulaire.Deux cas de cette association
     dans une fratrie.Arch.Franc.Péd.,1972,269-286.

7)   Vainsel,M.,Fondu,P.,Cadranel,S.,Rocmans,C.,Gepts,W.
     Osteopetrosis associated with proximal and distal tubular
     acidosis.Acta Paed.Scand. 1972,61,429-434.

8)   Dent,C.E.,Smellie,J.M.,Watson,L.Studies in osteopetrosis.
     Arch.Dis.Childh.,1965,40,7-15.

9)   Yu,J.S.,Oates, R.K.Walsh,K.H.Stuckey,S.J.Osteopetrosis.
     Arch.Dis.Childh. 1971, 46, 257-263.

10) Moe P.J.,Sklaeveland A.Therapeutic studies in osteopetrosis.
     Acta Paed.Scand.1969,58,593-600.

11) Murphy,H.M.A Review of inherited osteopetrosis in mouse.
     Man and other mammals also considered.Clin.Orthopaed.Rel.
     Res.1969,45,97-103.

12) Walker,D.G.Osteopetrosis cured by temporary parabiosis.
     Science,1973,180,875.

13) Moutier,R.,Lamendin,H.,Berenholc,S.Ostéopétrose par mutation
     spontanée chez le rat (Osteopetrosis by spontaneous mutation
     in the rat) Expér. Animale, 1973, 6, 87-101.

14) Toyama, K.,Moutier,R.,Lamendin,H.Resorption osseuse après
     parabiose chez le rat "Op"(ostéopétrose) (Bone resorption
     after parabiosis in "Op"(osteopetrosis) rat).C.R.Acad.Sci.
     Paris,1974 D,278,115-117.

15) Walker,D.G.Bone resorption restored in osteopetrotic mice
     by transplants of normal bone marrow and spleen.Science,
     1975,784-785.

16) Walker,D.G.Control of bone resorption by hematopoietic
     tissue. The induction and reversal of congenital osteo-
     petrosis in mice through use of bone marrow and splenic
     transplants. J.Exp.Med.,1975,142,651-663.

17) Walker,D.G. Spleen cells transmit osteopetrosis in mice.
     Science,1975,190,785-787.

18) Milhaud,G.,Labat,M.L.,Graf,B.,Juster,M.,Balmain,N.,
     Moutier,R.,Toyama,K. Démonstration cinétique, radio-
     graphique et histologique de la guérison de l'ostéopétrose

congénitale du rat. C.R.Acad.Sci. Paris, 1975. D,280, 2485-2488. (Kinetic, radiographic and histologic demonstration of the curing of congenital osteopetrosis in rats.)

19) Moutier,R.,Toyama,K.,Lamendin,H.,Guérison de l'ostéopétrose par injection de moelle allogénéique chez le rat "Op"3.C.R. Acad.Sci.Paris,1977. D,284,1697-1699.

20) Moutier,R.,Toyama,K.,Cotton,W.R.,Gaines,J.F.Three recessive genes for congenital osteopetrosis in the Norway rat.J.Hered., 1976,67,189-190.

21) Ballet,J.J.,Griscelli,C.,Courtris,G.,Milhaud,G.,Maroteaux, P. Bone marrow transplantation in osteopetrosis. Lancet, 1977, in press.

2) Griscelli, C.,Durandy, A.,Ballet, J.J.,Prieur A.M.,Hors J. T- and B- cell chimerism in two patients with severe combined immunodeficiency (SCID) after transplantation.1977, Transpl. Proc., 9(1),171-175.

3) Ballet,J.J.,Agrapart,M.,Durandy,A.,Griscelli,C.Daguillard, F.,Separation of precursor T-Cells and Ig-secreting B cells from the large lymphocytic cells of human tonsil. Cell.Imm.,1977,33,291-296.

4) Moutier,R.,Toyama,K.,Charrier,M.F. Genetic study of osteopetrosis in the Norway rat.J.Hered.,1974,65,373-375.

5) Leonard,E.P.,Cotton,W.R. Morphological and histochemical observations on the lack of osteoclasts in the "tl" strain of rats. Proc.Soc.Exp.Biol.Med.,1974,147,596-598.

6) Marks,S.C.,Jr. Pathogenesis of osteopetrosis in the ia rat. Reduced bone resorption due to reduced osteoclastic function. AM.J.Anat.,1973,138,165-189.

7) Raisz,L.G.,Simmons,H.A.,Gworek,S.C.,Eilon,G. Studies on congenital osteopetrosis in microphtalmic mice using organ cultures: impairment of bone resorption in response to physiologic stimulators. 1977, J.Exp. Med., 145, 857-865.

8) Horton, J.E.,Raisz,L.G.,Simmons,H.A.,Oppenheim,J.J., Mergenhagen, S.E. Bone resorbing activity in supernatant fluid from cultured human peripheral blood leukocytes, 1972.Science,177,793-795.

9) Marks,S.C.,Jr.,A discrepancy between measurements of bone resorption in vivo and in vitro in newborn osteopetrotic rats. 1974, Am.J.Anat., 141, 329-339.

10) Raisz,L.G.,Luben,R.A.,Mundy,G.R.,Dietrich,J.W.,Horton, J.E.,Trmmel,C.L. Effect of osteoclst activating factor from human leukocytes on bone metabolism. J.Clin.Inv., 1975,56,408-413.

31) Luben,R.A.,Mundy,G.R.,Trummel,C.L.,Raisz,L.G.Partial purification of osteoclast activating factor from phythohaemagglutinin -stimulated human leukocytes.J.Clin. Invest.,1974,53,1473-1480.

32) Mundy,G.R.,Luben,R.A.,Raisz,L.G.,Oppenheim,J.J.,Buell, D.N. Bone -resorbing activity in supernatants from lymphoid cell lines.New Eng.J.Med.,1974,290,867-871.

33) Horton,J.E.,Oppenheim J.J.,Raisz,L.G.,Mergenhagen,S.E. Macrophage -lymphocyte synergy in the production of osteoclast activating factor (OAF)J.Imm.,1974,113, 1278-1287.

34) Chen,P.,Trummel,C.,Horton,J.,Baker,J.J.,Oppenheim,J.J. Production of osteoclast activating factor by normal human peripheral blood rosetting and non-rosetting lymphocytes.Eur.J.Imm.,1976,6,732-736.

35) Aschkenasy,A.,Quelques données sur les réactions immunitaires humarales chez des rats atteints d'ostéopétrose. C.R.Soc.Biol.,Paris,1974,168,417-421. (Data on humoral immunological reactions in rats with osteopetrosis).

36) Milhaud,G.,Labat,M.L.,Parant,M.,Damais,C.,Chedid,L. Immunological defect and its correction in the osteopetrotic mutant rat.proc.Natl.Acad.Sci.USA,1977,339-342.

37) Milhaud,G.,Labat,M.L.,Viegas-Péquignot,E.,Dutrillaux,B., Moutier,R.,Toyama,K. Migrations cellulaires au cours de la guérison provoquée de l'osteopetrose du rat Op et thymus. (Cellular migrations during the curing of osteopetrosis of Op rat and thymus). C.R.Acad.Sci.Paris,1975 D, 281,1929-1932.

38) Milhaud,G.,Labat,M.L.,Graf,B.,Thillard,M.J.Guérison de l'ostéopétrose congénitale du rat "Op" par greffe de thymus.C.R.Acad.Sci.Paris,1977,D 283,531-533.

39) Brown,C.E.,Dent,P.B.Pathogenesis of osteopetrosis: a comparison of human and animal spectra.Pediat.Res.,1971,5, 181-191.

40) Brem,H.,Folkman,J.Inhibition of tumor angiogenesis mediated by cartilage. J.Exp.Med.,1975,141,427-438.

ACKNOWLEDGEMENTS

We wish to thank Drs. Maroteaux, Blondet and Saudubray, Dr. Nezelof for bone biopsy studies and Drs. Coutris and Milhaud for calcium kinetics studies, and Miss Agrapart for her help in immunological explorations.

Discussion for Session V: Primary Disorders of Bone Cell
Function.   Part B.

DR. KAHN: Dr. Olsen, did you mention during the course of
your presentation that these op or osteopetrotic animals have
reduced or increased rates of bone formation?

DR. OLSEN: It is increased rates of bone formation. All of
the mouse mutants seem to have increased rates of bone formation,
whereas some of the osteopetrotic rat mutants have decreased
rates of bone formation. Dr. Walker has published on the bone
synthesis studies.

DR. PECK: Dr. Olsen, could you tell us whether you have
done any receptor studies with lectins in your lymphocyte
preparations, or whether you have any idea about the mechanism
for the increases in responsivity?

DR. OLSEN: No, we haven't.

DR. PECK: The cyclic AMP generation, calcium uptake, and so
forth?

DR. OLSEN: Not in these mutants; not yet.

DR. DUNCAN: I would like to ask a question and pass a
comment. Did either Dr. Walker or Dr. Olsen identify the morphology of cells which might rest now on the endosteal surface,
presumably the source or site of the mineral removal? Was there
any relationship to the cells we have already discussed yester-
day and today?

DR. WALKER: You mean in vivo, after transplantation?

DR. DUNCAN: Correct.

DR. WALKER: No, there wasn't a thorough study of this. It
was studied in routine histologic preparations and, to a very
limited extent, with the electron microscope; but this hasn't
been evaluated thoroughly enough to give a definitive answer.

DR. DUNCAN: The question arises whether there is any osteoclastic activity; is there an increased number of osteoclasts on
the endosteal surface which is, after all, where the disease is?

DR. WALKER: That is a hard thing to evaluate; to quantitate osteoclast population in a very rapidly-changed situation is difficult.

DR. DUNCAN: Obviously, the situation occurring is that you have removed the excessive bone and it has arrived at a point of correction, much as the osteoporosis in the adult individual, where bone removal occurs and then ceases. So for this reason, I think there is no necessity to invoke immunological systems, but rather some local phenomenon which controls the continuation of this population of corrector cells.

DR. WALKER: I didn't mention this, but these untreated osteopetrotic mutants have osteoclasts; and the animals with the induced disease have abundant osteoclasts in the lesions. They are different in qualitative study, in the electron microscopic study, in that the mutant osteoclasts are deficient in ruffled borders and in other ways, but they are usually applied to the bone matrix, or calcified cartilage matrix. In the case of those osteoclasts observed in the mutants that have recovered, they are normal in having all the features of the active osteoclasts, including ruffled borders.

DR. RAISZ: I just want to comment on the OAF studies in this discussion. We did not work up OAF from mutant mice; so it is quite possible that it was not typical. It is clear that the osteoclasts of the mutant mice did not respond to good OAF, nor did they respond to any of the six or seven resorbers which we published. And I can just fill in the negative data which we will now never publish, that all the other resorbers that have come down the pike since then, 823187, mellitin, whatever; all of those failed to work that we have tested so far in the system.

I think the cells are cytologically typical osteoclasts, as Dr. Walker just alluded to, which are sitting there with all of the morphologic features of osteoclasts except for ruffled borders and the ability to resorb bone. This, to me, is the central issue. I guess I don't understand where in the derivation of cells, from mononuclear cells in the spleen or anywhere else, such an aberrancy could be developed or overcome.

DR. MINKIN: We too have been working on immuno-function in osteopetrotic animals; and we chose to look at the ability of spleen cells from microphthalmic mice and phenotypically normal litter-mates to respond in a plaque-forming assay in vitro to thymus-independent or thymus-dependent antigens.

I have a couple of slides which will demonstrate that in three separate experiments the mutant animals had a significantly decreased PFC response to either thymus-independent or thymus-dependent antigens. (Slide.) Now, in an attempt to begin to understand this phenomenon, we decided that one thing to look for would be a defective monocyte or macrophage or adherent-cell helper function; and so we conducted an experiment where we co-cultured these cells in the presence of serial dilutions of peritoneal-exudate cells from phenotypically normal litter-mates.

The next slide shows that as we added peritoneal cells, instead of augmenting the response, we diminished the response.

I now have a question for Dr. Walker. You made the statement that the cellular defect is a defective osteoclast precursor. I would like to know what you choose as evidence for that, because that statement may be premature.

DR. WALKER: That is as you put it. I said the findings are consistent with that hypothesis. Of course, that means a derivative of the hematopoetic stem cell; I don't mean all derivatives, but the line that leads to the osteoclasts; probably, the macrophage line. I think it is reasonable that they may have a common stem cell. It is a profitable place to look; but that is not the only place.

DR. HORTON: I wonder whether in Dr. Olsen's and Dr. Wahl's laboratories, where they are looking at the immunocompetence of these animals and also at collagenase production by other macrophages, whether in fact you people have begun to look at peritoneal-exudate monocytes and macrophages from these microphthalmic mice, and found other changed parameters in relation to cell functions.

DR. OLSEN: One of the big problems is getting enough macrophages to do the collagenase assay from these mice, because they are so small.

We have looked at prostaglandin production by these peritoneal-exudate macrophages. At this point I would say that in older microphthalmic mice, our data are fairly clear that there is no difference between the microphthalmic macrophages and normal macrophages in prostaglandin production in response to endotoxin. However, with younger animals, the results are not as clear. In the cells from animals one to two months old, there seems to be a slight decrease in prostaglandin production in response to endotoxin. Since we believe that the prostaglandins play an important role in collagenase production, this is a possible connection.

DR. HORTON: Since some lymphoid cells have receptors for PTH, have you looked for this?

DR. OLSEN: No, we have not.

DR. KAHN: A question to the whole panel: I wonder if you gentlemen would care to tackle the apparent difference between the kind of system that Dr. Olsen and his group are looking at, where there appears to be immunological defects in this series of mutant mice, and perhaps the circumstance that Dr. Ballet described in the human condition, where they did not find any evidence for such defects; and perhaps tie that, in turn, to what I gather is the absence of evidence for skeletal defects in thymectomized or other kinds of athymic experimental animals like the "nude" mouse.

DR. WALKER: Of course, one "out" is that these different mutants involve a different gene in each case, and they might represent, in a sense, different diseases.

DR. KRANE: I was very much interested in Dr. Ballet's presentation. We have seen recently one case where we also could pick up no defect in T-cell or B-cell function, including the child normally rejected a skin graft; and was transplanted with fetal thymus. We couldn't get a match, and we don't know yet what happened. Dr. Dayer studied the macrophages that he isolated from peripheral blood, which produced normal amounts of our collagenase-activating principal, and looked like normal peripheral blood monocytes.

For the record, at the Vancouver parathyroid meeting, Dr. Milhaud presented a case. Was this case one of the ones that you are reporting?

DR. BALLET: Yes. This case was my first case.

DR. KRANE: Your first case? For the record, Dr. Milhaud claimed there were no studies on that case. The immunological functions, then, of the studies that you reported, were entirely normal?

DR. BALLET: Entirely normal, with the restriction of the technical difficulties involved; and I would insist on that. I don't know rats very well; but I think that the proliferative responses may be different, not only the response of the cells, but also the technical system used, for instance, the number of cells, and the population one has. I noticed in those experiments that the spontaneous incorporation was high in the microphthalmic mice. This could show that, in fact, one has a different population, and I wonder if it is not difficult to compare, in these conditions, results only with the time of thymidine incorporation.

DR. HEERSCHE: Do I understand the speakers correctly that this syndrome also demonstrates an increased bone formation? If that is so, what is the evidence?

DR. WALKER: The evidence is from an in vivo study which assayed the bone at nine hours after the administration of tritiated proline for tritiated hydroxyproline and tritiated proline in the mutants as compared with the normal litter-mates. In the mice, the levels of the tritiated hydroxyproline and proline were about 50 percent higher than normal. This was in young animals that were usually two to three weeks of age; and it is an effect that, if studied at older ages, disappears by six weeks to two months.

But it is not observed in the ia rat during their period of osteopetrosis. It is not observed in the osteopetrotic rabbit; in fact, it is just the opposite.

DR. HEERSCHE: So it may be caused then by resorption in the

controls; or is that --

DR. WALKER: I am sorry. There is no question that there is a deficiency in resorption in all the mutants; but in the mouse mutants, it is aggravated by increased osteogenic activity; but this is not entirely acceptable data yet.

DR. RAISZ: The bone formation data in vitro, using cal-varia, show a slightly greater rate of proline incorporation under conditions where we have attempted to flood out pool size; so I think there may be a slightly greater number of osteoblasts in those tissues.

The other point, however, which is quite clear, is that those bones show marked inhibition of osteoblastic activity in response to PTH and OAF preparations. Now, I don't know what it is in OAF preparations that inhibits bone formation, but it is there. So the receptors for PTH in those osteoblastic, separate, different cell lines are present.

DR. HOLTROP: Right now, in the lab, we are looking at an osteopetrotic patient, using light microscopy. It looks like there are a lot of osteoid seams. We haven't done the right staining yet; but under electron microscopy, it is very clear that there is a lot of unmineralized collagen fibers. It is demineralized material, but I can recognize very well the previously mineralized matrix and never-mineralized matrix because of the collagen banding. This appears where it has been mineralized. And there I see a lot of, unusually, much more than normal, unmineralized collagen. That is one case, and I haven't looked at enough.

DR. WALKER: In the literature, although I am prepared to quantify this, there is frequent reference to the complication in the osteopetrotic patients of rickets, or ricketic changes.

In the osteopetrotic mouse mutants, again, a similar observation is usually made in the young animals. There is a great increase in the amount of osteoid in the long bones, in the spongy bone.

DR. HORTON: Dr. Ballet, I would like to come back to the baseline data on tritiated thymidine incorporation in your studies. When you presented the material, I was under the assumption that when you eradicated the nucleated cells your baseline control returned to a more normal level. Now, I know you didn't say that. I would like to clarify whether in fact once the nucleated cells were removed, did those mononuclear cell populations now devoid of the nucleated population have a more normal baseline, as we know it, for in vitro lymphocyte trans-formation? Or were they, indeed, still increased?

DR. BALLET: If one takes the Ficoll-Triosil population from osteopetrotic patients with immature cells in the blood, we have generally very high spontaneous incorporation; more than 100,000 cpm per million cells. We used BSA gradients to separate

ymphoid cells, for we knew that the larger nucleated cells sedi-
ent in the upper layers. Taking the small lymphocytes in the
ower layers, we had the usual background we have with one
illion cells per ml of lymphocytes; that is about 1,000 cpm per
illion cells at the third day. The mitogenic index in this
ase, for all the lectins we studied, were in the ranges for a
ormal population. It ran something like 50 to 100 times for
HA, and so on. That is what I meant.

DR. HORTON: That is the way I understood it. Thank you.
'he other question: what percentage of the circulating cells
rere indeed nucleated?

DR. BALLET: Not including reticulocytes, we had in all
atients between 5 and 20 percent of cells being immature and
iucleated, expressed, of course, by comparing them to the total
white cell number. It is the same thing for all patients.

DR. PECK: Dr. Walker, can you give us any information about
the lifespan of the osteoclast in the osteopetrotic model? Is
there a turnover of osteoclasts at all? And the second question
is, what is the earliest time after the injection of normal cells
that you can see the appearance of a brush border?

DR. WALKER: These two questions are related in so far as I
can answer them. It is a little crude, but when you administer
normal bone marrow transplant or a splenic transplant to a
mutant, there is a lag time of about 12 days before you see
evidence of recovery in the areas that are most responsive, which
is the metaphyseal line adjacent to the most active growth
plates; the proximal tibia and the distal femur are good
examples. Correspondingly, when you induce the disease by
administering spleen cells from an osteopetrotic mutant to a
lethally-irradiated normal litter-mate, there is a lag time of
about 12 days before you see evidence of failure, again along
those metaphyseal lines, and it is manifested by the number of
calcified cartilage trabeculae crossing this line; I mean the
concentration. So I think this might represent an upper limit of
the lifespan of the osteoclasts, because of the resolution of the
method, histologic, as well as they are prepared as you would for
electronmicroscopy.

DR. HIRSCH: Dr. Ballet, I think your number one case is a
very impressive one, because it did look like you had a positive
response. If you fail to get one in a future case, it may
indicate that you have a more difficult job than the other people
here who work with standard mutants; and it may be that you have
a different etiology for different osteopetrotic conditions. You
may fail in another case, which wouldn't take anything away from
your Case Number One. I wonder if you would comment on this,
i.e., different etiologies for the osteopetrosis in humans?

DR. BALLET: Do you mean on the immunological status of
these patients?

DR. HIRSCH: It is like the difference between the mutant

mice and the op rat. You may find that a spleen cell might cure
one kind of human osteopetrosis and a bone transplant might cure
another.

DR. BALLET: In humans we have a choice between some sort of
donors, and we have a choice between some cells; but not all
cells can be used. For instance, spleen cells couldn't be used.
We have the choice between cells from bone marrow, from peripheral bloods, maybe, with a cell sorter; and we have the choice
between fetal tissues. These fetal tissues may be liver or
thymus, and I think that is all. I think our main difficulty now
is to know if we should or not use immunosuppression in cases
where we are not able to find a compatible donor; because in this
first case I think we were very lucky to have a sort of syngeneic
situation. As a model, I would take the op rat, which is quite
syngeneic, and which has now 13 or maybe 14 generations of
inbreeding.

DR. KAHN: I wonder if anyone on the panel has either done
or considered looking at the change that might occur in the
immunological status of some of these mutant animals which undergo spontaneous remission. I think the ia rat is among them, and
I don't know about the mouse lines, but it might be an interesting situation to look at.

DR. SCHNEIDER: The problem with the ia is that it doesn't,
at least with regard to the T-cell system, have any immunological
defect that I can find. Rather than using mitogens, I have
looked at some contact sensitivity and delayed hypersensitivity
reactions in the ia's, and they are normal. And this is both
before remission and after.

DR. HORTON: Dr. Doty presented an abstract whereby he
showed that in one of these mutants, he was able to spontaneously
have a remission by taking the suckling animals away from the
mother for 24 hours. Since it is known that in such mother's
milk there are cells, would you speculate as to whether there is
a transference into the suckling animals which is either humeral
or cellular which maintains this defect; and that the remission
that you see by taking the animals away from the mother has, in
fact, abrogated this transference of something from the mother.

DR. DOTY: The effects that we got, as far as overnight
fasting, were the same as we got for putting the animals on a
calcium-free diet, or by giving parathyroid hormone. So we have
kind of lumped all of these things together. That may not be the
right way to do it, and in fact, you may have a good suggestion.
I am not sure, but it seems to me back in the early days of this
work, when Dr. Irving was doing some of these studies, he
actually took some of these animals and put them with normal
mothers and they did not spontaneously undergo remission. I am
not sure of that information, or whether it is actually in the
literature.

SESSION VI

SUMMARY

Current Status - Future Directions

Dr. J.L. Matthews

Baylor University Medical Center,
Dallas, Texas 75226

First, the members of the organizing committee are to be congratulated for bringing together a group representing diverse specialties to focus on local factors controlling bone resorption. The importance of local factors have been recognized for some time. McLean and Urist's book BONE[1] includes a statement on growth and regulatory phenomena of resorption and formation with the perceptive sentence, "Some of the factors, at least, are local." Years later, Heaney elaborated on this at a conference on the Biology of Hard Tissue sponsored by the New York Academy of Science and NASA[2]. At that conference, many of the questions facing us today were posed. At that time, they did not have the benefit of many of the elegant approaches reported here, but the necessity for further study of the cells, their origins, modulating factors, inductors, inhibitors, precursors, and fate and the influence of other local factors was clearly evidenced.

Bone researchers have long recognized that there are numerous substances that influence bone metabolism. This long list includes PTH, CT, Vitamins D and A, cortisone, estradiol, etc. We recognize, however, that although we speak in general terms of these agents exerting catabolic or anabolic bone tissue effects (or cell effects), that regions of a given bone respond to an agent while other regions are less affected or even respond in an opposite manner! Thus, one has to speak in terms of bone envelopes, and to contrast effects at the periosteum with those at the endosteum, the metaphysis from the diaphysis, one side of a trabecula from the other, select osteon resorption, etc., i.e., local effects. Thus, the factors influencing the localization of effects and the responsiveness of select cell populations defined by both type and location and biochemical activity must be an integral part of delineating factors involved in resorption.

Appropriately, this conference opened with a consideration of the features of the cells involved in the resorption scenario and was further developed with discussions on bone cell origins, and the influence of many factors, both humoral and matrix related that modulate bone cells, macrophages, and other phagocytes.

In 1853, Tomes and DeMorean described osteoclasts in resorption tunnels of compact bone[3]. A succession of studies on these cells by Hancox[4], Gaillard[5] and others have established this multi-nucleated cell as the workhorse in bone matrix resorption. As described at this workshop, the osteoclast has a functional, highly motile brush border, a glycoprotein and actin-like rich peripheral area, and an abundance of mitochondria and intracellular vacuoles. From recent studies we learn that this is able to respond within minutes to stimuli, the reaction being characterized by both morphological changes and biochemical responses. The membrane of the ruffled border of active cells is translocated to infoldings and membrane lamellae on the non-resorbing surface of the cell; i.e., it is polarized with respect to its action on matrices and its polarization is coupled to its state of activation! Investigators have clearly established the presence of microfilaments in these cells that account for both motility and translocation events and have used morphometric technics to quantify its time course of response. The factors that activate this cell, or its precursors continue to grow as observations from both in vitro and in vivo systems yield new data on factors that serve as primary or secondary activators. Cortisone, PTH, and Vitamin D influence were early recognized, but we must now add the more potent Vitamin D metabolites, OAF, functional fragments of PTH, a class of prostaglandins, lymphokines, extracts of fungi and anaerobic microorganisms, plasma albumen factors, tumor factors, possible viral influence, and some relationship to the events of complement activation, cell mediated immunity, cAMP, the presence of immune complexes, collagenase activation, clotting factor activation, pharmacologic agents such as melittin, phorbol, colchicine, heparin. Other hormones are being investigated for select bone cell effects, especially estradiol and insulin, and lymphocyte macrophage interactions are now coupled to synovial cell and bone cell activation or inhibition. Thus, bone cell modulation at the local level is a multifactorial complex and it is likely that other effectors will be found. It remains to be determined how the domains of each of these factors are defined and how their interactions are expressed in resorption activation. It seems attractive at this point, to encourage work which will delineate what specific resorptive cell receptors are present on the involved cells such that determination of primary or secondary activation could be learned. The specific localization of 1-25 binding to osteoclast nuclei, for example, would indicate a primary effect as would the presence of specific cell surface agonist and antagonist action of some of the peptide moieties.

Interestingly, much less is known about inhibitory factors, the diphosphonates, glucocorticoids and calcitonin being notable exceptions. More work should be directed towards assessing the possible role of resorption inhibition factors as the obvious select localization of resorption fronts cannot be totally understood on the basis of systemic changes or circulating levels of related substances. The discussion on AIF and cell-collagen binding substances which compete with collagenase binding sites presented at this meeting give exciting new possibilities for correlating local resorption with inhibition.

Other local inhibitory factors may also be directly related

to the determination of site. What influences do the matrix
constituents exert? In the past two decades, localized resorption was explained on the basis that "osteoclasts can sense the
presence of dead bone" and will seek to remove it so that it can
be replaced by structure more suitable for its organ support
function. No one agent has been identified that leaves a fracture site, or dead Haversian system, or a trabeculum with a
micro-fracture that serves this physiological "activator" function. Dead cell products have been suggested to have modified
matrices that hypothetically have been made "tasty" to osteoclasts as a consequence of partial degradation or modified
synthesis. The present concepts of functional metabolic units,
and the coupling of resorption to compensatory formation (ARF)
must be included in our quest for control factors. Whether
"aged" matrices or cells elaborate different substances or
whether "aging" is simply a matter of changes in concentration of
normal constituents that are rate limiting is still not clear.
The general condition of osteopenia alone does not necessarily
reflect excessive resorption. Possibly, other factors such as
trauma play a significant role in determining where micro- and
macro-fractures occur in the elderly and in post-menopausal
osteoporosis. Few, if any, studies have adequately studied the
three-dimensional architecture of normal and osteopenic bones to
determine whether the biomechanical signals are being properly
processed in these bones.

Among the many provocative discussions presented here are
the growing number of cell lines used in culture, recognition of
additional hormones that appear to help modulate bone cells.
Insulin and some steroid metabolites are specifically cited.
Additionally, the use of genetic strains of osteopetrotic
animals also point to new avenues of research to be explored.

From all of the papers presented, I have used a scheme
suggested by Dr. Montgomery of Southwestern Medical College to
bring this symposium to a focus (Figure 1). If one approaches
the question of local bone control as a jig-saw puzzle, one
starts with the established facts and readily perceived corner
pieces, and fills in the puzzle as additional bits begin to
"fit". The key pieces are the primary bone cells but, as clearly
reported in this conference, consideration has to be extended to
mononucleated cells, precursor cells, lymphoid organs, and interactions with other systems involved in inflammation, neoplasm
influence, the immune system, the endocrine system, and a host of
kinins related to chemotaxis, permeability, lysis, enzyme
activation, suppression, motility factors, agonist and antagonist
interactions, as well as other factors such as stress, deforma-
tion, bioelectric phenomenon, pH, depolarization, cell-cell
interaction, and ion concentrations. From the puzzle, you can
see that many pieces are beginning to fit, but unlike a good
puzzle, when we have put all the available pieces together, no
clear picture emerges. Likely, pieces are missing, perhaps the
existent pieces are placed in the wrong relationship. We may
still be looking at a mosaic piece of a still larger puzzle.

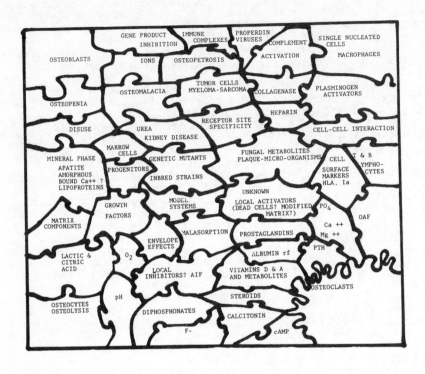

In summary, it is clear that multiple systems, organs.
tissues, cells, subcellular components and matrix and fluid
constituents are integrally involved in modulating bone. Our
future direction must thus encourage more interdisciplinary
research; we must look further for better in vivo and in vitro
models that better reflect the whole and to address ourselves to
the question of specificity of action, and raison d'etre for
select localization of these phenomena. The model systems
developed must move in the direction of studying cell systems
that show polarity, and select cell-matrix relationships. We,
ultimately, wish to move from the pathology states of osteopenia,
osteomalacia, and osteoporosis discussed in this conference to a
healthy whole skeleton in individuals of all ages.

References

1. McLean, F. C., Urist, M. R. (1961): Bone: An Introduction to the Physiology of Skeletal Tissue. Second Ed., University of Chicago Press.

2. Heaney, R. P. (1966). Local (Nonhormonal) Factors Controlling Bone Reconstruction in: Biology of Hard Tissue, National Aeronautics and Space Administration, Washington, D. C., Pp. 83-133.

3. Tomes, J., DeMorgan, C. (1853): Observations on the Structure and Development of Bone. Phil. Trans. Roy. Soc., London, 143: 109-139.

4. Hancox, N. M. (1972): The Osteoclast, in The Biochemistry and Physiology of Bone. G. Bourne, Ed., Academic Press, New York, Pp. 45-67.

5. Gaillard, P. J. (1957): Parathyroid Gland and Bone in vivo. Schweiz Med. Wochenschr. 14: 447-450.

PRELIMINARY SESSION

SELECTED ABSTRACTS
IN POSTER MODE

Treatment of Senile Osteoporosis. R. Agrawal, S. Wallach, R. Peabody, M. Tessier and S. Cohn. (Albany VA Hospital and Albany Medical College, Albany, N.Y. 12208 and Brookhaven National Laboratory, Upton, N. Y. 11973).
Spontaneous osteoporosis is not uncommon in male veterans. The efficacy of synthetic salmon calcitonin (SCT), a potent inhibitor of bone resorption, in the treatment of such osteoporotics was studied using the objective parameters of total body calcium (TBCa) and bone mineral content (BMC) at six month invervals. Male veterans, 50 years or older, with diffuse demineralization and collapse of one or more vertebrae were included in the study. TBCa was measured in vivo neutron activation analysis utilizing the Brookhaven whole body counter. BMC of the radial shaft was measured by photon beam absorptiometry using the Norland-Cameron densitometer. Thirty-one patients were randomly divided into three groups: (1) a control group receiving multivitamins, (2) a calcium supplemented group receiving 1 g Ca and multivitamins, and (3) a calcitonin group receiving 100 MRC units SCT daily plus calcium and multivitamins. There were no siginificant changes in TBCa among the three groups during the first year of observation. In contrast the SCT treated group showed significant increases in TBCa (+4% to +6%) at 18 and 24 months whereas no changes were present in the other two groups. Increases in TBCa were not reflected by BMC measurements. These data indicate that TBCa can be used as an objective parameter of bone mass during treatment of osteoporosis and suggest that salmon calcitonin may increase skeletal mass in male osteoporotics after prolonged treatment.

Failure of Prostaglandins E to induce local bone resorption in vivo
R. Baron, J.R. Nefussi, A. Duflot-Vignery, J.J. Lasfargues, F. Cohen and E. Puzas. (U. of Paris 5, Dental Faculty, 92120-Montrouge, France and Yale U. School of Med., Dept. of Pathology, 310 Cedar St, New Haven, Ct 06510, USA).
Prostaglandins E1 and E2 have been shown to induce CA45 release from bone in culture and to be as potent as parathyroid hormone (Klein and Raisz, Endocrinology, 86: 1436-40, 1970). Bone resorption in vitro occurs with inflamed gingival fragments and is inhibited by indomethacin, suggesting Prostaglandins involvement (Goldhaber et al., JADA, 87: 1027-33, 1973). An in vivo study suggests that Prostaglandins E1 are able to induce local bone resorption (Goodson et al., J. Dent. Res., 53: 670-677, 1973). However, the results of this study are not convincing as far as no osteoclasts were observed and no quantitative data were recorded.

The present study was undertaken in order to check the ability of PGE1 and 2 to induce in vivo local bone resorption in the rat, using a wide range of concentrations (10-4 to 10-1M), different areas (calvaria, vertebrae, alveolar bone), different vehicles (Phosphate buffer, glycerol), different time lags between injection and sacrifice (1 to 7 days) and single or repetitive injections. PGE2-15-methylated and Arachidonic acid were also tested. The technics used involved undecalcified thin sections and fluorescent labelings. Bone resorption was not observed in

any of these experiments. Osteoclasts were rarely present along
the bone surfaces, despite the presence of large inflammatory
areas. On the other hand, bone formation seems to be stimulated
by the injection trauma and may be influenced by the Prostaglandins. The results of constant perfusions and cultures will
be presented.

Diphosphonates as an inhibitor of hydroxyapatite formation by
phospholipids. A. L. Boskey , M.R. Goldberg, A.S. Posner
(Hospital For Special Surgery, Cornell University Medical
College, New York, N. Y. 10021).
Many workers have shown that diphosphonates prevent the dissolution of synthetic and biological apatites. This is a report
on the effect of the diphosphonate, disodium ethane 1-hydroxy-1,
1-diphosphonate (EHDP), on the formation of Ca-phospholipid-PO$_4$
complexes and their ability to nucleate hydroxyapatite (HA).
The complexes which can be extracted from all mineralized
tissues can be formed in vitro by the combination of acid phospholipids (Phosphatidyl serine, PS, and phosphatidyl inositol,
PI) with Ca and inorganic PO$_4$. It is believed that the source
of phospholipids (PLs) in vivo are the membranes of cells and
extracellular matrix vesicles of calcifying tissues. The effect
of EHDP on the kinetics of HA formation was studied in the
presence of the following substrates: complexes isolated from a
variety of tissues; purified PS and PI; HA seed crystals. In
each reaction chemical analysis of the solution and x-ray
diffraction of crystalline phases were determined as a function
of time. When 2×10^{-5} moles of EHDP were present per mg. of
substrate, there was a complete blockage of HA formation and/or
HA growth by any of the substrates. Furthermore, this EHDP
concentration in addition to increasing the amount of PL dispersed in solution prevented in vitro formation of the complex
by the acidic PLs. Thus, EHDP which inhibits hard tissue
resorption, also interferes with the formation of and nucleating
properties of Ca-PL-PO$_4$ complexes. Supported by NIH Grants
DE-04141, DE-00002 and AM-18412.

Immune Complex Induced Immunopathologic Bone Resorption in vivo.
J. Clagett, M. Torabinejad, L. Engel. (U.W., Seattle, WA 98195).
Resorption of bone is an important pathologic feature of many
long-term inflammatory disease states, such as rheumatoid
arthritis, bacterial arthritis, Reiter's syndrome, and
periodontitis. Specific etiologic agents have not been identified but the inflammatory cell infiltrate, which is a
consistent feature of these diseases, is believed to be responsible for the connective tissue alterations and bone loss. It
has been suggested that one likely phlogogenic agent important
in the pathogenesis of these diseases is an antigen-antibody or
immune complex (IC) that is deposited from the circulation or is
formed at the affected site. Although in vitro models for bone
resorption exist, no adequate animal model has yet been developed for studying immunopathologically induced bone destruction.
We report methods for an in vivo model to study bone destruction,
and present evidence that immune complexes may cause bony lesions

via induction of an inflammatory response. A central role for
prostaglandin is predicted by these studies since the bone
destruction is inhibited by administration of indomethacin.
Several lines of evidence support these conclusions: 2) simulated
immune complexes (heat aggregated human IgG) induced a connective
tissue and bone loss to a greater extent and more quickly than
did monomeric human IgG; b) neutrophils and macrophages composed
the inflammatory infiltrates associated with osteoclastic bone
resorption; c) however, bone loss may be a separate event from
soft-tissue destruction because inhibition of prostaglandin
synthetase by indomethacin did not prevent the accumulation of
inflammatory cells at the periapex or the loss of connective
tissue elements but did block bone loss.

Effect of lipopolysaccharides on bone cell calcium and cyclic AMP.
R. Dziak, E. Hausmann, Y. Chang (S.U.N.Y. at Buffalo, School of
Dentistry, Buffalo, N.Y. 14226).
The effect of lipopolysaccharides on bone cell calcium and cyclic
AMP were studied to understand their mechanism of action on bone.
Bone cells were isolated by collagenase digestion of 19-21 day-
old fetal rat calvaria. Calcium uptake was studied with ^{45}Ca.
Cyclic AMP was measured by radioimmunoassay. Lipopolysaccharide
(LPS-S) prepared from S-form of S. minnesota and purified
lipid A obtained from Luderitz and Galanos were used. Incubation
of bone cells at 37°C with either LPS-S or lipid A (0.01-10.0
µg/ml) for 5-60 min. produced no effect on cyclic AMP levels
whereas PGE$_2$ produced 30-fold increases. At 37°C, 1.0 µg/ml
LPS-S decreased calcium uptake 30-60% below control values with
no effect on lactate production. The decrease in calcium was
evident 3-5 min. after the simultaneous addition of LPS-S and
^{45}Ca but was not observed at later times (30-60 min.) when
the cells were in isotopic equilibrium. A 4°C, LPS-S
(1.0 µg/ml) produced 100-900% increases in calcium uptake
1-30 min. after its simultaneous addition with ^{45}Ca. Incubation
with 1.0 µg/ml lipid A produced effects similar to LPS-S
at 37°C and 4°C. We have previously shown that calcium uptake
at 37°C represents primarily uptake by an active intracellular
pool whereas at 4°C calcium taken up from the medium represents
binding by the cell membrane. LPS-S and lipid A appear to
increase calcium binding by the cell membrane with a subsequent
decrease in the rate of uptake by an intracellular pool. This
effect does not seem to be mediated by cyclic AMP. This project
was supported by Grants Nos. DE01932 and DE04637 awarded by the
NIDR, DHEW.

Cellular Basis of Bone Erosion in Rheumatoid Arthritis
H. Duncan, C. Mathews, M. Parfitt (Henry Ford Hospital, Detroit,
MI 48202).
Erosion of periarticular bone in rheumatoid arthritis is a well
known radiographic phenomenon. We have studied this in 20
surgically excised joints using undemineralized sections 5-10
µm thick stained by the Goldner or Villenueva methods, examined
with fluorescence and polarized microscopy. There is a local
response extending approximately 100 µm from the rheumatoid
inflammatory tissue, consisting of both new woven bone formation,
and increased resorption of both the pre-existing lamellar bone

and the new woven bone, by a complex three component process:
1) There is an increase in the number of osteoclasts producing
classic Howship's lacunae. 2) There is periosteocytic demineralization often with coalescense of adjacent zones; preservation of
periosteocytic matrix is demonstrated by red staining with the
Goldner method. This phenomenon can be distinguished from the
enlarged osteocytes and lacunae normally found in woven bone.
In contrast to other reports, we do not find so called osteocytic
osteolysis to be a major component of either normal or abnormal
bone resorption. 3) Many of the surfaces apparently undergoing
resorption show Howship's lacunae containing only mononuclear
cells which are identical to those present within the rheumatoid
inflammatory tissue. We postulate that the initial demineralization occurs in response to a humoral agent released by the
inflammatory tissue and that exposed collagen is rendered susceptible to collagenase and other proteolytic enzymes secreted
by cells which are not normally able to resorb bone. There are
many similarities between the processes we have observed and
those found by Galasko in relation to osseous metastases.

Prostaglandins and cyclic AMP in human gingiva with periodontal
disease. T.M.A. ElAttar and H.S. Lin. (U. of Missouri School of
Dentistry, Kansas City, Missouri 64108).
Previous studies in our laboratory (ElAttar, Prostaglandins,
1976, 11(2): 331-341) have shown that PGE_2 levels in human
gingiva with periodontal disease are twenty-fold greater than
that present in healthy gingiva. We have also shown that
estradiol could enhance significantly the in vitro synthesis of
PGE_2 (I) in gingival tissue homogenate. Since PGs could act
as major mediators of the inflammatory response as well as
potent stimulators of bone resorption with a controlling
mechanism supplied by cAMP (II), the present investigation was
designed to study simultaneously: (1) The levels of (I) and (II)
in gingiva of patients with periodontal disease and which have
been evaluated histologically, (2) the effect of (I) on the
synthesis of (II) in gingiva in vitro. By using ^{3}H-cAMP
protein binding assay, it was found that the mean concentrations
of (II) in 20 gingival samples with no inflammatory cells and
43 gingival samples with various aggregations of inflammatory
cells were 340 and 552 pmol/gm wet tissue weight respectively.
The corresponding values of (I) were 40 and 171 pmol/gm tissue
weight. The addition of exogenous PGE2, PGE_1, $PGF_{2\alpha}$ or
estradiol to four different samples of gingival slices in Tris
buffer solution (pH 7.4) and incubation for 40 min. at 37°C
caused a 38-110% increase in the concentration of cAMP in
gingiva. The data indicate that tissue inflammatory response to
(I) could be mediated by (II). Supported by NIH Grant DE
04276-01A1.

Diphenylhydantoin (DPH) Effects on Hormonal Mediation of
Resorption in Cultured Fetal Rat Bone. T. J. Hahn, S.L.
Teitelbaum and A.J. Kahn. (Washington University School of
Medicine, St. Louis, Mo.).
The mechanism of DPH inhibition of PTH (1-34) - induced ^{45}Ca
release was examined in fetal rat forelimb rudiments maintained
in 5-day culture. DPH over a concentration range of 25-200
µg/ml significantly inhibited PTH (50 ng/ml) induced resorption.
Additionaly DPH had a synergistic interaction with the inhibitory effects of HCT; DPH (200 µg/ml) inhibited PTH (50 ng/ml) -
induced resorption by $27.8 \pm 1.5\%$, while PTH (50 ng/ml) +
HCT (5 ng/ml) - mediated resorption was inhibited by $52.4 \pm$
2.8% ($p<0.001$) in the presence of DPH. To examine effects on
cAMP generation, rudiments were preincubated for 24 hours with
or without DHP, and cAMP content determined by radioimmunoassay
after a 7 minute incubation with hormone. The following results
were obtained: control 0.70 ± 0.04 pM/4 rudiments, PTH - 3.13
± 0.15 ($p<0.001$ vs control); PTH + DPH - 1.98 ± 0.17 ($p<0.001$
vs PTH): PTH + HCT - 3.59 ± 0.14 ($p<0.05$ vs PTH): PTH + HCT +
DPH 2.29 ± 0.20 ($p<0.001$ vs PTH + HCT). Thus while DPH
markedly augmented HCT inhibition of PTH resorption, DPH and HCT
were not additive with regard to effects on cAMP generation.
Additionally, calcium ionophore A23187 - induced resorption was
completely abolished and A23187 - induced increases in bone cAMP
content were suppressed by DPH (200 µg/ml). It was concluded
that (i) DPH may inhibit PTH - induced resorption via suppression
of cAMP generation (ii) DPH and HCT have different modes of
action and (iii) the effect of DPH may be at the level of trans-
membrane transport of calcium ion.

The mechanism of osteoclastic bone resorption: a new hypothesis.
J.N.M.Heersche. (MRC Group in Periodontal Physiology, University
of Toronto, Toronto, Ontario, Canada, M5S 1A8).
The possibiltity that, during the osteoclastic dissociation of
bone matrix, demineralized collagen fibers are phagocytosed and
digested by mononuclear cells adjacent to the osteoclast has
never been considered. The present communication offers evidence
to support this possibility. Firstly, we conclude from our finding that parathyroid hormone (PTH)-induced resorption of
non-mineralized osteoid is not inhibited by calcitonin while
PTH-stimulated resorption of mineralized bone collagen is inhibited that degradation of mineralized and non-mineralized bone
matrix are regulated by separate mechanisms. That different
cell types might be involved in these two processes is suggested
by the finding of Wong and Cohn (Nature, 252, 713, 1974), that
cells could be isolated from bone responding either to PTH
exclusively or to both PTH and calcitonin. Further support can
be derived from a recent observation of Garant (J. Periodontal
47, 380, 1976), who found fibroblast-like cells containing
phagocytosed collagen immediately adjacent to osteoclasts in
the periodontal ligament, and from recent work of Sakamoto
(Proc. 6th Parathyroid Conference, in press, 1978) showing

collagenase to be present in resorbing bone in all cell types with the exception of the osteoclast. We believe that these findings are compatible with the hypothesis that one cell type, presumably the osteoclast, responds to both PTH and calcitonin and is responsible for demineralization whereas resorption of non-mineralized and demineralized organic bone matrix is accomplished by a second cell type, responsive to PTH but not to calcitonin. We are currently attempting to obtain further evidence in support of this theory.

Development of an assay for osteoclast activating factor in biological fluids. Richard A. Luben. (Program in Biomedical Sciences, University of California, Riverside, Ca 92521). Osteoclast Activating Factor (OAF) is a lymphokine which stimulates bone resorption. Attempts to evaluate the role of OAF in human disease have been limited by the absence of specific assays for it in samples such as serum or tissue. For this study, we used the electrophoretic properties and biological characteristics of OAF to develop an unequivocal assay of OAF in biological samples. Serum, culture medium and tissue homogenates were concentrated and dialyzed into appropriate buffers, then separated on polyacrylamide slab gels using discontinuous buffer systems. To some samples were added aliquots of purified OAF, or of parathyroid hormone, 1, 25 dihydroxyvitamin D_3, prostaglandin E_2 or bacterial endotoxin. After electrophoresis the gels were cut into segments, eluted, and assayed at multiple dilutions for either bone resorption or the ability to increase cyclic AMP in isolated bone cells. Each assay was carried out in the presence or absence of $10^{-8}M$ dexamethasone, an inhibitor of OAF activity. Samples with biological activity which a) migrated in the same position as authentic purified OAF, and b) was dexamethasone-inhibitable, were classified as containing OAF. None of the other bone resorbing agents tested was identical to OAF in either of these criteria. OAF was quantitated in the samples by parallel-line bioassay using authentic OAF (subjected to identical procedures) as a standard. The results of assays on human normal and diseased samples will be presented. (Supported by NIH-DE04766 and American Cancer Society #BC-263).

Mononuclear Phagocytes & bone remodeling: bone mediated macrophage chemotaxis. C. Minkin. (Univ. of Southen California, School of Dentistry - Dept. of Biochemistry, Los Angeles, CA 90007).
An increasing amount of evidence implicates cells of the mononuclear phagocyte series as participants in the process of bone remodeling and resorption. Since the macrophage accumulates in areas of inflammation & tissue repair in response to chemotatic gradients, it would be reasonable to examine this as a possible mechanism for attracting this cell type to areas of active bone remodeling and resorption. A series of experiments are in progress in an attempt to answer specific questions relating to bone mediated macrophage chemotaxis. Peritoneal macrophages, elicited by injection of Brewers thioglycollate medium, were tested for chemotactic response using lucite blind well chambers. Bone homogenate, of newborn mouse calvaria were found to possess

significant chemotactic activity. Several factors present in the
homogenate could account for this activity. For example collagen
and collagenous peptides have been found to be chemotatic for
human peripheral monocytes. Preliminary experiments indicate that
collagen subunits ($\alpha 1$ 1 chains) are not chemotatic for peritoneal mononuclear phagocytes. Several other factors which are
potentially responsible for bone mediated macrophage chemotaxis
are currently under investigation. Supported by: Program Project
Research Grant #DE02848 and Training Grant #DE07006.

Isolation of osteoclast activating factor from human cancer
ascites fluid. R. B. Nimberg, A. Badger, D. Humphries, W. Lloyd,
K. Schmid and H. Wells. (Boston U. School of Medicine and
Graduate Dentistry, Boston, MA 02118).
Osteoclast activating factor (OAF), a protein first identified
in 1972, has been shown to induce the resorption of bone explants
in organ culture. OAF has been isolated in crude form from
activated human peripheral lymphocyte cultures, but has not yet
been purified. The purpose of this study was to determine
whether OAF could be isolated from sources other than small aliquots of human blood. Ascites fluid from a patient with colon
carcinoma and from 10 patients with a variety of cancers were
employed as starting materials. Fractionation was achieved by
gel filtration, affinity chromatography and by ion exchange
chromatography on DEAE-cellulose. At a dose of 20 µg/ml, the
active fraction isolated from DEAE-cellulose produced an
increase in ^{45}Ca release from newborn mouse calvaria in organ
culture equivalent to that produced by 2U/ml of parathyroid
hormone. The active fraction, whose components possessed a
molecular weight of about 60,000 daltons, did not contain PTH,
PGE_2 or vitamin D metabolites. All of the bone resorptive
activity was lost after incubation with pronase. To compare
cancer ascites OAF with that produced by human leukocyte
cultures, the supernatants of phytohemmaglutinin stimulated
normal human peripheral lymphocytes were also fractionated as
described above. The results demonstrated that ascites OAF
and lymphocyte OAF chromatographed similarly on gel filtration,
affinity and ion exchange chromatography.

Calcitonin Treatment in Hereditary Bone Dysplasia: A Morphologic Study of Bone and Cartilage. E.A. Nunez (Columbia
University, Collage of P&S, New York, N.Y. 10032) and M.
Horwith, L. Krook, J.P. Whalen (Cornell University Medical
College, New York, N.Y. 10021).
The morphologic response of bone and cartilage of two siblings
with familial bone dysplasia with hyperphosphatasemia to 12
months of calcitonin treatment has been studied radiographically,
histologically and ultrastructurally. Before treatment bone was
characterized radiographically by the absence of a normal cortex
and medullary cavity and histologically by an intense osteocytic
osteolysis. During the course of calcitonin therapy, there was
a progressive development of a normal cortex and inhibition of
osteocytic osteolysis. At the ultrastructural level, mitochondria of all three bone cell types (osteocytes, osteoclasts and
osteoblasts) contained dense intramitochondrial crystalline

bodies. Moreover, osteocytes exhibited poor organellar development. During calcitonin treatment, mitochondria of osteocytes
and osteoclasts, but not those of osteoblasts, lost the intramitochondrial crystalline bodies. In addition, osteocytes underwent a proliferation of organellar development. Chondrocytes,
before hormone administration, contained normal mitochondria but
minimal glycogen. During the course of calcitonin treatment,
chondrocytes started to exhibit large deposits of glycogen.

Role of mononuclear cells in cultured fetal long bones: B. Rifkin,
R. Baker, M. Somerman, S. Pointon, W. Au, and A. Newman. (U.
of Rochester, Rochester, N. Y. 14642).
The fetal rat long bone organ culture system has been utilized
extensively to identify agents which stimulate or inhibit bone
resorption. In this system, much attention has been focused on
the structure and function of osteoclasts, while other cell types
have received little notice. The purpose of the present study
was to determine whether cells other than osteoclasts have a role
in removal of calcified matrix. Nineteen-day fetal rat radii and
ulnae were cultured in a chemically defined medium (BGJ). Stimulation of bone resorption was induced by appropriate doses of
PGE_2, PTH, and 1,25-DHCC. At various time periods, cultured
bones were fixed by standard techniques and processed for
electron microscopy. Mononuclear cells, containing mineral
deposits and collagen fibrils within cytoplasmic vacuoles or
multivesicular bodies, were found near regions of abundant
osteoid. Macrophages with numerous lipid droplets, as well as
vacuoles with cellular debris, were identified throughout the
cultured bones. Occasionally, macrophages were seen closely
apposed to bone surfaces. In some instances, the bone surface
near such cells appeared disrupted. This study suggests that
in organ culture the partially calcified matrix of osteoid is
removed and degraded by active mononuclear cell phagocytosis
and intracellular digestion. The nature of these mononuclear
cells remains uncertain. Macrophages located diffusely throughout cultured bone appear to be largely engaged in phagocytosis
and digestion of cellular debris, but may also have a role in the
resorption of fetal bone. Supported by USPHS Grant No. DE04443-
02.

Quantitative bone remodeling changes during experimental periodontal disease in the golden hamster. J.L. Saffar, G. Makris,
and R. Baron. (U. of Paris 5, Dental Faculty, 92120-Montrouge
France, & Yale U. School of Medicine, Dept of Pathology, New
Haven, CT 06510, USA).
In a previous study (Saffar and Baron, J. of Periodont. Res.,
1977, in press) we reported variations in the number of osteoclasts along the periosteal, endosteal and alveolar wall surfaces
after experimental periodontal disease in the golden hamster.
This study reports the effects of Keyes 2000 diet induced periodontal disease on the bone remodeling sequence. The results
indicate that: 1) the extension of resorption surfaces with
osteoclasts increases along the endosteum (p 0.01) but remains
unmodified along the alveolar wall, 2) the extension of the
Howship's lacunae with no osteoclasts (reversal phase) increases

along both the endosteum (p<0.001) and the alveolar wall (p<0.01), 3) the extension of the osteoid seams decreases along both the endosteum (p<0.01) and the alveolar wall (p<0.02), 4) the extent of the resting areas seems to remain unmodified along both surfaces.

The classically reported increase in resorption is consequently not the only feature of bone reactions during experimental periodontal disease. The present study shows that the different steps of the remodeling sequence are also modified, namely an increase in lacunae with no osteoclasts and a marked decrease in the extension of bone formation occur.

A further study on these reactions using double fluorescent labelings to assess bone formation, and a comparison with human biopsies, will also be presented and discussed.

Immunocytochemical studies of collagenase localization in normal mouse tissues with special reference to cartilage and bone. M. Sakamoto, S. Sakamoto, P.Goldhaber and M.J. Glimcher. (Harvard Sch. of Dent. Med. & Harvard Med. Sch., Boston, MA 02115).

A specific collagenase has been isolated from mouse bone. The enzyme has been purified by heparin-Sepharose affinity chromatography. Antiserum to this mouse bone collagenase (MBC) has been produced and the antibody has been purified by an immunoadsorbent method using MBC-Sepharose. The localization of tissue collagenase has been studied in normal tissue of adult mouse and undecalcified calvaria and tibiae of 2-6 day old mouse by an indirect immunofluorescent antibody technique. Various organs and soft tissues revealed specific fluorescence extracellularly on collagen bundles, on reticular fibers and on basement membranes. The cytoplasm of fibrolasts, endothelial cells and other mesenchymal cells revealed specific fluorescence to a lesser extent. Collagenase was present extracellularly on collagen . fibers of periosteum and perichondrium, at the osteoid surface, in Howship's lacunae, and in the walls of the lacunae of osteocytes. Collagenase was also present to a lesser extent intracellularly in the cytoplasm of osteoblasts, osteocytes, osteoclasts and cartilage cells. It is not certain whether the immunofluorescence associated with Howship's lacunae and with osteoclasts is any greater than that associated with other structures and cells. (Supported by NIH grants DE 02849, AM 15671 and 1K04 DE00048-01).

Chick bone latent collagenase: A reversible enzyme-inhibitor complex. S. Sakamoto, M. Sakamoto, A. Matsumoto, P. Goldhaber and M.J. Glimcher. (Harvard Sch. of Dent. Med.& Harvard Med. Sch., Boston, MA 02115).

Collagenase isolated from tissues only after treatment with trypsin or NaSCN have been termed latent enzymes. No collagenase activity is detected in the culture media of 14 d embryo chick bone, however, if the culture medium is treated with trypsin or NaSCN, considerable collagenase activity can be demonstrated: 2.35 units/ml and 3.25 units/ml respectively. The molecular weights of latent and active forms of chick bone collagenases as determined by molecular sieving on Sephadex G-200 are 54,000 and 43,000 daltons respectively. Latent collagenase was activated instantaneously by mixing with NaI. The subsequent gel-filtration of the mixture of latent collagenase and NaI revealed activated collagenase. When the mixture was dialyzed against a buffer no activity could be demonstrated, but subsequent treatment of such samples with trypsin revealed activity. The results indicate that latent collagenase is activated by NaI, but re-inhibited during dialysis. Therefore, the activation of latent collagenase with NaI is dissociation of enzyme and inhibitor. These results are evidence in favor of latent collagenase from the cultre medium of embryonic chick bones being an enzyme-inhibitor complex. (Supported by NIH grants DE 02849, AM 15671 and 1K04 DE 00048-01 and by New England Peabody Home for Crippled Children).

Uptake of ^{45}Ca by hard tissue cells. F. Sayegh, K. Porter, and G. Sun. (U. of Mo. K.C., School of Dentistry and Sinclair Research Farm, U. Mo. Col.).

The cellular role in mineralization of hard tissues has not yet been established. This report of a study of ^{45}Ca uptake by the alveolus osteoblast and tooth germ cells is an attempt to elucidate the cell role in mineralization process at the subcellular level. Two hundred tooth germs and the adjacent alveolar bone were obtained from mice, ages 19 and 20 days in utero and 1-7 days old. The mice were injected by (Ip) with ^{45}CaCl$_2$ in isotonic saline at 5 and 10 μc/gm body wt. At 5, 15, and 30 min. after injection, the animals were killed, tooth germs were dissected out and were incubated in a 1% trypsin for 30 min. at 37°C. Bone samples were also taken but were not trypsinized. The enamel organ was separated from the dental papillae by trypsinization. Specimens were fixed for EM, light microscopy and autoradiography and scintillation counting. EM studies were also made on each pellet which resulted from cell fractions and centrifugation. Scintillation counting showed that ^{45}Ca was incorporated within the various tooth germ cells and the osteoblasts of the alveolar bone. Uptake was seen at 5 min., but the optimal uptake was at 15 min. after injection in all fractions. The subcellular distribution revealed that the ^{45}Ca activity was within the microsomal fraction and the mitochondrial pellets. EM studies revealed both the orthodox and condensed forms of mitochondria.

Activation of osteoclasts in the "incisor absent" (ia) rat. B.H. Scholfield[1], L.S. Levin[1], and S.B. Doty[2]. ([1]Johns Hopkins University School of Medicine, Baltimore, Md. 21205. [2]National Institute of Dental Research, Bethesda, Md. 20014).

Osteoclasts in the young "incisor absent" (ia) rat are known to be deficient in bone resorbing ability. Using electron microscopy and histochemistry we have previously shown (B.H.

Schofield, L. Stefan Levin, and S.B. Doty, Calcif. Tiss. Res.
14: 153-160, 1974) that these cells contain large numbers of
lysosomes with hydrolytic activity but these osteoclasts do not
form ruffled borders and do not resorb significant amounts of
mineralized bone matrix.
The "IA" osteoclasts can be activated to resorb bone by an in
vivo administration of parathyroid hormone, by placing animals
on calcium free diet, or by fasting animals overnight. The
activation sequence consists of: (1) the rapid appearance of
large cytoplasmic vacuoles, (2) the formation of ruffled borders
which consist of numerous membrane infoldings, (3) the fusion
of lysosomal membranes with cytoplasmic vacuoles and infoldings
of the ruffled border, and (4) the extracellular release of
lysosomal enzymes onto the bone surface being resorbed.

Contact-mediated bone resorption by human monocytes in vitro.
S.L. Teitelbaum, C.C. Stewart, and A.J. Kahn. (Washington University Schools of Medicine and Dental Medicine, St. Louis, MO.
63110).
Normal human monocytes were cultured with devitalized fragments
of adult human and rat bone. Time lapse microcinematography
revealed selective adhesion of these cells to the mineralized
substrate. Matrix resorption was demonstrated morphologically
by alterations in the profiles of these particles as well as
by a net release of radioisotopically labeled calcium. Furthermore, intracellular accumulation of skeletal matrix occurred.
The cultured monocytes assumed osteoclast-like features. These
include multinucleation, and formation of a "clear-zone" at the
point of attachment to the substrate. Polarization of acid
phosphatase containing organelles towards the skeletal matrix
occurred and the enzyme was present extracellularly on the bone
surface.
It is concluded that cultured monocytes adhere to bone and are
capable of its resorption, a phenomenon mediated at least in part
through cell-matrix contact.

Disappearing Bone Disease. Two Cases of Localized Osteolysis.
I. Zanzi and H. L. Atkins. (Medical Research Center, Brookhaven
National Laboratory, Upton, N.Y. 11973).
Disappearing Bone Disease is a rare clinical condition of undet-
ermined etiology and physiopathology and with no known method of
treatment. Two cases are reported of Caucasian women, 45 and 51
years old, respectively. The younger patient had a 3 year
history of pain in the pelvis with multiple fractures of rib and
pelvis. Laboratory studies and x-ray films reported progressive
osteolysis of segments of pubic bones, substantiated by histological diagnosis. The second case had an established diagnosis
of multiple sclerosis of long duration. The patient gradually
developed osteolytic lesions during a period of three years,
first in the pubic area and then in a sacral wing. She also
incurred some fractures of the ribs. There was no laboratory
evidence of a diffuse or metabolic bone abnormality. The
mechanism of these dramatic localized resorptive lesions of bone
remains speculative.

REGISTRANTS

Avioli, Dr. Louis V.
Washington University
School of Medicine
St. Louis, MO 63110

Baker, Dr. Bill R.
University of Texas
Health Science Center
San Antonio, TX 78201

Baker, Dr. Richard L.
University of Rochester
School of Medicine
Rochester, NY 14627

Ballet, Dr. Jean Jacques
Hospital des Enfants Malades
149 Rue de Sevres
Paris   75015, France

Barnett, Dr. Michael L.
SUNY at Buffalo
School of Dentistry
Buffalo, NY 14214

Baron, Dr. Roland
Yale University
School of Medicine,
New Haven, CT 06510

Battistone, Dr. Gino C.
U.S. Army
Institute of Dental Research
Washington, D.C. 20012

Bergmann, Dr. Pierre
University of Connecticut
Health Center
Farmington, CT 06032

Binderman, Dr. Itshak
12226 Greenleaf Avenue
Potomac, MD 20854

Bockman, Dr. Richard S.
Sloan-Kettering Institute
1275 York Avenue
New York, NY 10021

Boskey, Dr. Adele L.
Hospital for Special Surgery
535 East 70th Street
New York, NY 10021

Branham, Dr. Gerald B.
Navy Medical Research Institute
National Naval Medical Center
Bethesda, MD 20014

Bringhurst, Dr. F. Richard
Endocrine Unit
Massachusetts General Hospital
Boston, MA 02115

Bynum, Dr. Gaither
GRC/NIA
Baltimore City Hospital
Baltimore, MD 21205

Casciani, Dr. Frank S.
National Institute of Dental
    Research
National Institutes of Health
Bethesda, MD 20014

Canterbury, Dr. Janet M.
University of Miami,
School of Medicine,
Miami, FL 33152

Chase, Dr. Donald C.
1924 Accoa Highway
Knoxville, TN 37919

Chen, Dr. Priscilla
4510 Main Street
Buffalo, NY 14226

Clagett, Dr. James
University of Washington
Schools of Medicine and
    Dentistry
Seattle, WA 98195

Cohn, Dr. David V.
University of Kansas
V.A. Hospital
Kansas City, KS 64128

Coleman, Dr. Richard A.
404 Hillview Drive #301
Linthicum, MD 21090

Cooper, Dr. Cary W.
University of North Carolina
Chapel Hill, NC 27514

Corio, Dr. Russell
15 Bentana Way
Rockville, MD 20850

D'Amato, Dr. Robert A.
The Proctor and Gamble Company
Miami Valley Laboratories
Cincinnati, OH 45247

Davis, Dr. William F.
Division of Research Grants
National Institutes of Health
Bethesda, MD 20014

Dayer, Dr. Jean-Michel
Massachusetts General Hospital
Boston, MA 02114

Deftos, Dr. Leonard J.
University of California
San Diego, CA 92161

De Leon, Dr. Lino Diaz
National Institute of Dental
    Research
National Institutes of Health
Bethesda, MD 20014

Douglass, Dr. Carl D.
Division of Research Grants
National Institutes of Health
Bethesda, MD 20014

Duncan, Dr. Howard
Henry Ford Hospital
Detroit, Michigan 48202

Durie, Dr. B.G.M.
The University of Arizona
Health Science Center
Tucson, AZ 85724

Dziak, Dr. Rosemary
SUNY at Buffalo
Buffalo, NY 14221

Dziewiatrowski, Dr. Dominic
School of Dentistry
University of Michigan
Ann Arbor, MI 48109

Eilon, Dr. Gabriel
University of Connecticut
Health Center
Farmington, CT 06032

El Attar, Dr. T.M.A.
University of Kansas
Kansas City, KS 66205

Ellison, Dr. Dolon A.
SUNY at Buffalo
Buffalo, NY 14214

Eman, Dr. Nabil
Golar House 410
Rochester, NY 14620

Fica, Dr. Juan
263 Camp
Bristol, CT 06010

Figueroa, Dr. Alvaro
4506 Jones Bridge Road
Bethesda, MD 20014

Flora, Dr. L.
P.O. Box 39175
M.V.L.
Cincinnati, OH 45247

Forrest, Dr. William R.
801 Braeburn Drive
Oxon Hill, MD 20022

Frame, Dr. B.
2799 W. Grand Boulevard
Detroit, MI 48202

Frazier, Dr. Paul D.
National Institute of Dental
    Research
National Institutes of Health
Bethesda, MD 20014

Frederick, Ms. Joan D.
NIAMD
National Institutes of Health
Bethesda, MD 20014

Fuentes, Dr. Elia I.
8202-2C Kramer Ct.
Glen Burnie, MD 21061

Garant, Dr. Philias
SUNY at Stony Brook
Dental School
Stony Brook, NY 11794

Gaston, Dr. Gerald W.
New Jersey Dental School
Newark, NJ 07094

Gay, Dr. Carol
508 Life Science Building
University Park, PA 16802

Gibson, Dr. William A.
Louisiana State University
Medical Center
New Orleans, LA 70119

Goldhaber, Dr. Paul
Dean, Harvard School of
    Dental Medicine
Boston, MA 02115

Goldring, Dr. Steven
Massachusetts General Hospital
Boston, MA 02114

Gomes, Dr. Blasco C.
SUNY at Stony Brook
School of Dental Medicine
Stony Brook, NY 11794

Gross, Dr. Arthur
USAIDR, WRAMC
Washington, DC 20012

Grubb, Dr. Stephen
University of North Carolina
School of Medicine
Chapel Hill, NC 27514

Gworek, Ms. Susan C.
University of Connecticut
Medical School
Farmington, CT 06032

Harris, Dr. Suzanne S.
IDR, UAB
Birmingham, AL 35294

Hausmann, Dr. Ernest
SUNY at Buffalo
School of Dentistry
Buffalo, NY 14226

Hawley, Dr. Charles
USAIDR, WRAMC
Washington, D.C. 20012

Heaney, Dr. Robert P.
Creighton University
Omaha, NE 68178

Heath, Dr. Hunter III
Mayo Clinic
Rochester, MN 55901

Hedglin, Dr. W.L.
Miami Valley Laboratories
Proctor and Gamble Company
Cincinnati, OH 45247

Hicks, Dr. M. Lamar
National Naval Research Cntr.
Dental Institute
Bethesda, MD 20014

Hirsch, Dr. Philip F.
University of North Carolina
Dental Research Center
Chapel Hill, NC 27514

Hoffeld, Dr. J. Terrell
Nat. Inst. of Dental Research
National Institutes of Health
Bethesda, MD 20014

Holtrop, Dr. Marijke E.
Childrens Hospital
Boston, MA 02108

Horton, Dr. John E.
Harvard School of Dental
    Medicine
Boston, MA 02115

Horwith, Dr. Mel
New York Hospital
New York, NY 10021

Isaacson, Dr. Robert J.
620 Greystone
Orinda, CA 94563

Jain, Dr. R.
8 Winding Brook Drive
Guilderland, NY 12084

Johnson, Dr. Lent C.
Armed Forces Institute of
    Pathology
Washington, DC 20306

Johnston, Dr. C.C., Jr.
Indiana University
School of Medicine
Indianapolis, IN 46202

Jowsey, Dr. Jenifer
Mayo Clinic
Rochester, MN 55901

Kahn, Dr. Arnold J.
Washington University
School of Dental Medicine
St.Louis, MO 63110

Kahn, Dr. Deborah
512 Deming Place
Chicago, IL 60614

Kakehashi, Dr. Samuel
National Institute of Dental
    Research
National Institutes of Health
Bethesda, MD 20014

Kenny, Dr. Alexander E.
Texas Tech University
School of Medicine
Lubbock, TX 79409

Kim, Dr. Jin
NIAID
National Institutes of Health
Bethesda, MD 20014

King, Dr. William R.
3968 Sharonview Drive
Cincinnati, OH 45241

Kinnard, Dr. Matthew
National Institute of Dental
    Research
National Institutes of Health
Bethesda, MD 20014

Klein, Dr. LeRoy
2065 Adelbert Road
Cleveland, OH 44106

Kleinman, Dr. Hynda K.
National Institute of Dental
    Research
National Institutes of Health
Bethesda, MD 20014

Kopp, Major William M.
U.S. Air Force Hospital
Seymour Johnson Air Force Base,
    NC 27530

Kowalski, Ms. Mary Ann
University of Connecticut
School of Medicine
Farmington, CT 06032

Krane, Dr. Stephen M.
Massachusetts General Hospital
    and Harvard Medical School
Boston, MA 02114

Kream, Dr. Barbara E.
University of Connecticut
School of Medicine
Farmington, CT 06032

Kuettner, Dr. K.E.
Department of Biochemistry and
    Orthopedic Surgery
Presbyterian-St.Luke's Hospital
    and Rush Medical College
Chicago, IL 60612

Levin, Dr. Stefan
113 West Monument Street
BAltimore, MD 20906

Lewis, Dr. David M.
3030 Hewitt Street
Silver Spring, MD 20906

Lifschitz, Dr. Mervyn L.
78 Blessing Road
Slingerlands, NY 12159

Luben, Dr. Richard A.
University of California
Riverside, CA 92521

Mahaffey, Dr. Jane
Massachusetts General Hospital
Boston, MA 02114

Marcus, Dr. Robert
Veterans Administration Hospital
Sepulveda, CA 91343

Marx, Dr. Stephen J.
NIAMD
National Institutes of Health
Bethesda, MD 20014

Mathews, Ms. Catharina H.E.
3623 Merritt Lake Drive
Metamora, MI 48455

Matsumoto, Dr. A.
188 Longwood Avenue
Boston, MA 02115

Matthews, Dr. J.L.
Baylor University Medical Center
Dallas, TX 75226

McArthur, Dr. William
University of Pennsylvania
Philadelphia, PA 19106

McCabe Dr. Mead M.
12901 S.W. 63rd Ct.
Miami, FL 33156

McDonald, Dr. Daniel
1142 Sherwood Avenue
Baltimore, MD 21239

Mechanic, Dr. Gerald
University of North Carolina
Dental Research Center
Chapel Hill, NC 27514

Mellonig, Dr. James T.
Naval Medical Research Institute
Bethesda, MD 20014

Miller, Dr. Scott T.
2693 Glenmare Street
Salt Lake City, UT 84106

Mills, Dr. Barbara G.
University of Southern California
Los Angeles, CA 90007

Minkin, Dr. Cedric
1885 Peterson
South Pasadena, CA 91030

Mundy, Dr. Gregory R.
University of Connecticut
Health Center
Farmington, CT 06032

Munson, Dr. Paul L.
University of North Carolina
School of Medicine
Chapel Hill, NC 27514

Nardell, Dr. Birgit E.
University of Maryland
School of Dentistry
Baltimore, MD 21201

Nefussi, Dr. J. Raphael
Dental Faculty of Paris V
Paris, France 92120

Neiders, Dr. Mirdza E.
SUNY at Buffalo
School of Dentistry
Buffalo, NY 14214

Newbrey, Dr. Jerry
Washington State University
Pullman, WA 99163

Newcombe, Dr. David S.
1115 Bellemore Road
Baltimore, MD 21210

Nimberg, Dr. R.B.
80 E. Concord Street
Boston, MA 02118

Nisengard, Dr. Russell
SUNY at Buffalo
School of Dentistry
Buffalo, NY 14214

Norimatsu, Dr. Hiromichi
University of North Carolina
School of Medicine
Chapel Hill, NC 27514

Nunez, Dr. Eladio A.
149-41 Cherry Avenue
Flushing, NY 11355

Nylen, Dr. Marie U.
National Institute of Dental
    Research
National Institutes of Health
Bethesda, MD 20014

Olsen, Dr. Charles E.
National Institute of Dental
    Research
National Institutes of Health
Bethesda, MD 20014

Parakkal, Dr. Paul F.
National Institute of Dental
    Research
National Institutes of Health
Bethesda, MD 20014

Peck, Dr. William A.
Washington University
School of Medicine
St. Louis, MO 63178

Posek, Dr. Robert J.
8740 Tuscany Avenue
Playa Del Rey, CA 90291

Puzas, Dr. J. Edward
Yale University
School of Medicine
New Haven, CT 06510

Ragsdale, Dr. Bruce D.
Armed Forces Institute of
    Pathology
Washington, DC 20306

Raisz, Dr. Lawrence G.
University of Connecticut
Health Center
Farmington, CT 06032

Ram, Dr. Agrawal
1381 Philomena Drive
Schenectady, NY 12309

Reddi, Dr. A.H.
National Institute of Dental
    Research
National INstitutes of Health
Bethesda, MD 20014

Reich, Dr. E.
111 East 88th Street
New York, NY 10028

Rifkin, Dr. Barry
601 Elmwood Avenue
Rochester, NY 14642

Rizzo, Dr. Anthony A.
9801 Parkwood Drive
Bethesda, MD 20014

Robinovitch, Dr. Murray R.
University of Washington
School of Medicine
Seattle, WA 98195

Rowe, Dr. Dorothy J.
University of Iowa
College of Dentistry
Iowa City, IA 52242

Saffer, Dr. Jean Louis
Dental Faculty
Montrouge, France 92120

Sakamoto, Dr. Seizaburo
188 Longwood Avenue
Boston, MA 02115

Sammon, Dr. P.J.
University of Kentucky
College of Dentistry
Lexington, KY 40503

Sandberg, Dr. A.L.
National Institute of Dental
    Research
National Institutes of Health
Bethesda, MD 20014

Sayegh, Dr. F.
650 East 25th Street
Kansas City, MO 64108

Schechter, Dr. Geraldine P.
Veterans Administration
    Hospital
Washington, DC 20042

Schneider, Dr. Gary B.
University of Massachusetts
Medical School
Worcester, MA 01605

Schofield, Dr. Brian
Johns Hopkins University
School of Medicine
Baltimore, MD 21205

Schraer, Dr. Harald
Pennsylvania State University
University Park, PA 16802

Schwartz, Dr. Ruth
Cornell University
Medical College
Ithaca, NY 14850

Scott, Dr. David B.
National Institute of Dental
  Research
National Institutes of Health
Bethesda, MD 20014

Shapiro, Dr. Irving M.
University of Pennsylvania
School of Medicine
Philadelphia, PA 19174

Shapiro, Dr. Jay R.
4028 Glenrose Street
Kensington, MD 20795

Sherwood, Dr. Louis M.
Michael Reese Hospital and
  Medical Center
Chicago, IL 60616

Shigeto, Dr. Abe
25-F Congressional Lane
Rockville, MD 20852

Singer, Dr. Frederick R.
Clinical Research Center
University of Southern
  California
Los Angeles, CA 90033

Slatolpolsky, Dr. Eduardo
Washington University
School of Medicine
St. Louis, MO 63124

Smallridge, Dr. Robert C.
7815 Overhill Road
Bethesda, MD 20014

Somerman, Dr. Martha
1899 South Avenue
Rochester, NY 14620

Sonis, Dr. Stephen
Harvard University
Medical School
Boston MA 02115

Steinmann, Dr. Beat U.
National Institute of Dental
  Research
National Institutes of Health
Bethesda, MD 20014

Stern, Dr. Paula H.
Northwestern University
Medical School
Chicago, IL 60611

Sweet, Dr. Donald
Armed Forces Institute of
  Pathology
Washington, D.C. 20306

Talmage, Dr. Roy
University of North Carolina
School of Medicine
Chapel Hill, NC 27514

Tarpley, Dr. Thomas M., Jr.
Division of Research Grants
National Institutes of Health
Bethesda, MD 20014

Tashjian, Dr. Armin H.
Harvard SChool of Dental Medi-
  cine and Harvard Medical
  School
Boston, MA 02114

Terry, Dr. Roger
1200 North State Street
Los Angeles, CA 90033

Thompson, Dr. Trink
University of Rochester
School of Medicine
Rochester, NY 14627

Trummel, Dr. Clarence L.
University of Connecticut
Health Center
Farmington, CT 06032

Turner, Dr. Russell T.
American Lake Hospital
Tacoma Washington

Vander Wiel, Dr. Carol
University of North Carolina
School of Medicine
Chapel Hill, NC 27514

Vassalli, Dr. Jean-Dominique
Rockefeller University
New York, NY 10021

Vignery, Dr. Agnes M.C.
Yale University
School of Medicine
New Haven, CT 06510

Wahl, Dr. Larry M.
National Institute of Dental
    Research
National Institutes of Health
Bethesda, MD 20014

Walker, Dr. Donald G.
The Johns Hopkins University
School of Medicine
Baltimore, MD 21205

Wallach, Dr. Stanley
RD 2
Petersburg, NY 12138

Walser, Dr. Paul F.
2040 Tanglewood Road
Iowa City, IA 52240

Weatherred, Dr. Jackie G.
Medical College of Georgia
Augusta, GA 30902

Wells, Dr. Herbert
Boston University
Boston, MA 02118

Werb, Dr. Z.
University of California
School of Medicine
San Francisco, CA 94122

Whedon, Dr. G. Donald
National Institute of Arthritis,
    Metabolism, and Digestive
    Diseases
National Institutes of Health
Bethesda, MD 20014

Wigley, Dr. F.M.
34 Dowling Circle
Baltimore, MD 21234

Williams, Dr. Betsy L.
University of Washington
Seattle, WA 98195

Wong, Dr. Glenda
Veterans Administration
    Hospital
Kansas City, KS 64128

Wray, Dr. H. Linton
Walter Reed Army Medical
    Center
Washington, DC 20012

Wuthier, Dr. Roy E.
University of South Carolina
Columbia, SC 29208

Yaari, Dr. Abraham
University of Pennsylvania
School of Medicine
Philadelphia, PA 19104

Zanzi, Dr. Italo
Brookhaven National Laboratory
Upton, NY 11973

Zorsky, Dr. Paul
University of Connecticut
Health Center
Farmington, CT 06032